PSYCHOTHERAPY OF ABUSED AND NEGLECTED CHILDREN

Psychotherapy of Abused and Neglected Children

Second Edition

JOHN W. PEARCE
TERRY D. PEZZOT-PEARCE

THE GUILFORD PRESS
New York London

A Division of Guilford Publications, Inc.
72 Spring Street, New York, NY 10012
www.guilford.com

Printed in the United States of America

This book is printed on acid-free paper.

Last digit is print number: 8 7 6 5 4 3 2 1

Library of Congress Cataloging-in-Publication Data

Pearce, John W.
Psychotherapy of abused and neglected children / by John W. Pearce, Terry D. Pezzot-Pearce. — 2nd ed.
p. ; cm.
Includes bibliographical references and index.
ISBN-10: 1-59385-213-4 ISBN-13: 978-1-59385-213-9 (hardcover : alk. paper)
1. Abused children—Rehabilitation. 2. Child psychotherapy.
I. Pezzot-Pearce, Terry D. II. Title.
[DNLM: 1. Child Abuse—psychology. 2. Child Abuse—rehabilitation.
3. Child. 4. Infant. 5. Psychotherapy. WS 350.2 P359p 2006]
RJ507.A29P43 2006
618.92′8582230651—dc22

2006008759

About the Authors

John W. Pearce, PhD, is a staff psychologist in the Child Abuse Service at Alberta Children's Hospital, Calgary, Alberta, Canada. He also serves as the Coordinator of Consultation Services for the local Calgary child welfare authority, and is an Adjunct Associate Professor in the Clinical Psychology Program at the University of Calgary. With his wife, Terry D. Pezzot-Pearce, he coauthored *Parenting Assessments in Child Welfare Cases: A Practical Guide* (University of Toronto Press, 2004).

Terry D. Pezzot-Pearce, PhD, is a therapist and evaluator who sees children and parents from the child welfare system among other clinical cases. She is a Practice Advisor for the Psychologists Association of Alberta and serves as a consultant to various programs and professionals regarding parenting assessments and other clinical and professional issues. Dr. Pezzot-Pearce utilizes an interdisciplinary collaborative law approach in some cases and is actively involved in the Round Table in Family Law in Alberta.

Preface

The principal goal of this second edition is the same as the first edition's goal: to provide a comprehensive description of strategies to assess and treat children who have suffered various types of abuse and neglect. There have been exciting and important developments in research examining the effects of maltreatment on children and what we can do to help them. In the first edition we reported that there were few empirical investigations of the efficacy of interventions commonly employed with maltreated children. Clinicians had some ideas of what might work, but evidence backing up such claims was slim. There has been a radical change: Empirically supported therapies (ESTs) have received enormous attention from clinical scientists (and have generated considerable controversy). Identification of ESTs initially focused on adult psychotherapy, but there is now evidence for the efficacy of certain treatments for children, including those who have been maltreated. Given the importance and prominence of the EST literature, we review what we know about what works with abused and neglected youngsters.

Some readers may dread that this book is a manual that rigidly dictates what to do in a prescribed number of sessions, without taking into account the daily demands of clinical practice with maltreated children, who often present with myriad comorbid diagnoses and who live in impoverished environments with caregivers with their own complex problems. While the EST literature can teach us much, another goal of this book is to describe how ESTs can, and must, be modified to meet the unique demands of our young clients and their families. Our model of clinical practice is empirically informed, not empirically dictated.

A further decade of treating many children and reviewing the recent literature has deepened our belief in the importance of the therapeutic relationship for outcome, especially from the perspective of attachment theory. The second edition offers practical recommendations for the strategic use of the relationship between the clinician and child as a principal way of promoting change. A major criticism of the EST movement has been its apparent neglect of the therapeutic relationship. We emphasize that the application of ESTs and a focus on the therapeutic relationship are not antithetical; in fact, considerable evidence supports the notion of "empirically supported relationships" (Norcross, 2002; Shirk & Karver, 2003).

Like the first edition, the second emphasizes ecological, comprehensive assessments grounded in the basic tenets of developmental psychopathology. Evaluations not only must identify the clinically problematic behaviors of children according to a formal nosological system (i.e., the diagnosis), but should describe the "pathogenic processes" or mechanisms that contribute to and maintain pathological behaviors (Shirk & Russell, 1996). An understanding of pathogenic processes guides treatment planning and the choice of effective interventions, in conjunction with our knowledge of the EST research and literature. As most clinicians realize, development of a treatment plan for a child based *solely* on evidence that a randomized control study demonstrated efficacy of certain interventions with children with the same diagnosis may not optimize outcome. For example, children's developmental characteristics are often powerful moderators of their response to particular interventions (Grave & Blissett, 2004). Developmentally delayed children with little capacity to identify and articulate thoughts and cognitive processes may not do well in cognitive-behavioral therapy, despite the research that demonstrates its efficacy for children with certain disorders. Initiating cognitive-behavioral therapy for such children may even prove to be detrimental, because they may experience a real sense of failure and frustration, thereby exacerbating their difficulties.

The second edition also includes recent developments in the assessment of children's abuse-related attributions and appraisals and strategies to modify them. We have included more information about the assessment of attachment disorders, and highlight the prominent role of internal working models and interpersonal schemas as significant pathogenic processes and targets of intervention. The last decade has witnessed more clinical and research attention directed to sexual behavior problems and posttraumatic stress disorders of maltreated school-age children, and this edition offers an expanded discussion of relevant assessment and intervention strategies.

Our discussion focuses exclusively on individual therapy. We do not dismiss the utility of other psychotherapeutic approaches, especially group therapy for victimized youngsters and family therapy. Space limitations, as well as our own relative lack of expertise with these other interventions, preclude a description of these modalities. We describe family interventions designed to complement and support individual child psychotherapy, but we spend no time discussing interventions designed to help abusive or neglectful caregivers develop healthier parenting practices.

The book is intended for clinicians who work with preadolescent school-age children, although a few of the case examples incorporate material from sessions with young adolescents. Given this focus, we have deleted our previous discussions of parent-based interventions for infants and toddlers, such as infant–parent psychotherapy.

Acknowledgments

In 2005 The Guilford Press invited us to prepare a second edition of *Psychotherapy of Abused and Neglected Children*. We were delighted with the invitation but apprehensive about recommitting to a process that can be both exhilarating and arduous. We overcame our worries and accepted Guilford's invitation, and have spent the last 15 months reading, critically analyzing, and reformulating our ideas and preparing the manuscript.

Although writing the second edition was easier than the first, it would have been impossible to do without the encouragement, support, and advice of many individuals. Jim Nageotte and the staff at Guilford were unfailing in their support, sage advice, and guidance. They adeptly guided the book from its inception to its final version. We are indebted to our colleagues and students who have stimulated our thinking and have proved to be exemplary models of clinical practice. The good will and encouragement of close friends—Doug and Diane Lindblom, Pat Petrie, Don Schwartz, Karen Walsh, Jane Matheson, David Westelmajer, and Elva Jolly—never flagged. We have saved our final thanks for our family. Bob and Victoria Pezzot, Susan and John Kennedy, and Claire Pearce have always supported us, and this project was no exception. Finally, we wish to thank our children, Clarissa, Tim, and Kathleen. They graciously tolerated a household turned topsy-turvy while the book was being written and again showed us what is really important in our lives.

Contents

PSYCHOTHERAPY OF ABUSED AND NEGLECTED CHILDREN

CHAPTER ONE

Child Maltreatment and Developmental Outcome

INTRODUCTION TO THE SECOND EDITION

Despite considerable attention to child maltreatment since the publication of this book's first edition in 1997, thousands of children continue to be abused and neglected every year. Child maltreatment remains a serious legal, medical, and psychosocial problem with often grave consequences for its victims and society. A survey in Washington State assessed the mental health status of children ages 3–18 years who were recipients of protective services. Seventy-two percent were statistically indistinguishable from children in the state's most intensive mental health treatment programs (Trupin, Tarico, Low, Jemelka, & McClellan, 1993). More recent research suggests that, sadly, a significant proportion of maltreated youngsters do not receive appropriate intervention. Swenson, Brown, and Sheidow (2003) reported that services are not offered to the majority of physically abused youngsters who show clinical elevations on caregiver ratings of behavior problems. Besides the human costs associated with child maltreatment, vast financial resources are spent on professional treatment and social service programs.

This first chapter summarizes what is currently known about the impact of maltreatment on children's development, revised in accordance with the latest research. It would have been easier to write a book without reviewing this vast body of research. A book dealing exclusively with therapeutic strategies and techniques would probably be easier to read, too. Some readers may find the literature review dry and academic and begin to question its relevance for their daily clinical practice. Clinicians are often searching for creative and useful interventions, especially when confronted with children and families whose progress in therapy seems almost imperceptible and whose pain is all too apparent. Although we focus on practical interventions, we strongly believe that restricting the book's scope to technique alone would do our clients a real disservice. We refine our clinical skills and acumen by understanding and appreciating maltreatment's effects and the mechanisms and processes responsible for developmental sequelae. An awareness of the diverse array of outcomes of maltreatment alerts us to the need for comprehensive assessments that evaluate many domains of functioning. Literature, theory, and research guide clinical decision making, facilitate the selection and development of specific interventions, and eventually lead, we hope, to more rigorous evaluations of treatment techniques. Being a skilled clinician and being a good scholar should be synonymous.

THE IMPACT OF MALTREATMENT: A THEORETICAL OVERVIEW

In this section we examine the impact of maltreatment on the child's journey from infancy to early adolescence within the context of the model proposed by developmental psychopathology. Developmental psychopathology's basic tenets, especially the transactional model espoused by Cicchetti (Cicchetti, 2004; Cicchetti & Rizley, 1981) and elaborated by others (Sroufe, Carlson, Levy, & Egeland, 1999), offer researchers and clinicians a useful way to understand the heterogeneous effects of maltreatment. One hallmark of this approach is the attempt to integrate knowledge from different disciplines: clinical and experimental psychology and psychiatry, sociology, and the biological sciences, including genetics and the neurosciences. Developmental psychopathologists maintain that attempts to understand human development from the perspective of just one discipline do injustice to its complexity. Likewise, exclusive focus on one factor or variable to explain human behavior (e.g., attributing abusive behavior solely to a parent's own history of maltreatment) is simplistic and can result in an inaccurate picture. Considering development across a broad range of functioning and behavioral organization is an approach well suited to the study of child maltreatment's diverse effects.

According to Cicchetti and Rogosch (1994), developmental psychopathology "adopts an organizational view, conceptualizing development as a series of qualitative reorganizations among and within biologic and behavioral systems as growth of the individual proceeds" (p. 760). These various systems and processes include the biological, behavioral, and psychological, as well as broader systems such as the environment, society, and culture. They are in dynamic transaction (i.e., interaction) with one another throughout a person's lifespan. This concept of the primacy of interrelations among various systems for human development is antithetical to the notion of a direct, linear (i.e., main-effects) relationship between maltreatment and specific developmental sequelae first used to explain causes of child abuse. Theorists and clinicians had regarded one factor, a parental history of victimization, as the causative variable of abusive behavior (Steele & Pollock, 1968). There is now general agreement that abusive or neglectful parenting is determined by the interaction of many different variables. Belsky's (1980, 1993) ecological model of child maltreatment is typical of such an approach. He proposes that child maltreatment is more likely to occur when there is a confluence of factors at four different levels: the psychological characteristics of the parents, the family setting and its dynamics, the immediate social network of the family members, and the current state of society as it pertains to maltreatment (Figure 1.1).

Similarly, child maltreatment can be regarded as one of many variables that may contribute to specific developmental outcomes. Clinicians and researchers must remain cognizant of the complexity of the association between maltreatment and outcome; indeed, this is one of the guiding principles of this book. Given the influence of multiple variables, there are multiple pathways to adaptive and maladaptive developmental outcomes (Sroufe et al., 1999). Likewise, interventions may have to be directed at a

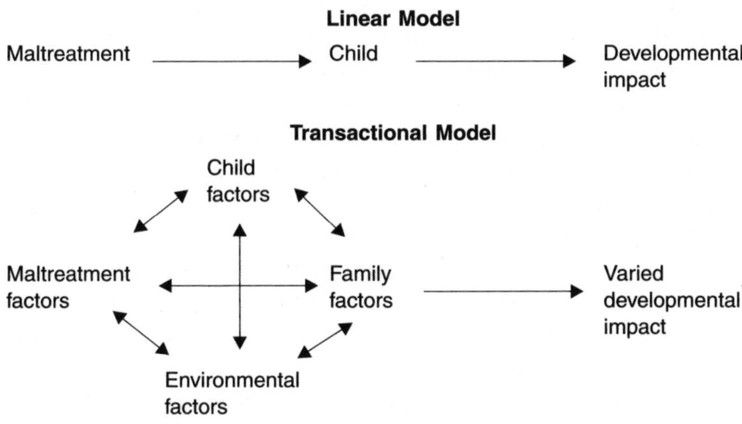

FIGURE 1.1. Linear/transactional models.

number of different targets or variables. A history of maltreatment, although a significant risk factor for many serious emotional, behavioral, and interpersonal problems, does not necessarily condemn individuals to such fates. Sroufe and colleagues' (1999) comment that "cause is probabilistic not deterministic" (p. 3) is similar to Cicchetti's (2004) notion that maltreatment has a number of possible outcomes (multifinality). In other words, a history of child maltreatment does not necessarily result in significant psychopathology.

The proposition that not every child succumbs to dire circumstances, including maltreatment, is well supported in the literature and central to the concept of resilience. According to Bonanno (2004), resilience "pertains to the ability of adults in otherwise normal circumstances who are exposed to an isolated and potentially highly disruptive event, such as the death of a close relation or a violent or life-threatening situation, to maintain relatively stable, healthy levels of psychological and physical functioning" (p. 20). Citing the adult literature, Bonnano contends that the vast majority of adults exposed to such events do not exhibit chronic symptoms. Likewise, studies of resilient children have shown that one-third of children in a sample who experienced perinatal stress, poverty, parental psychopathology, and family disruption developed into competent and well-adjusted young adults (Werner, 1989). Rutter (1985) estimated that one-half of children exposed to severe stress and adversity do not develop symptoms of psychopathology. Similarly, there are maltreated children who do not show evidence of major dysfunction. For example, estimates of the rates of asymptomatic sexually abused children in four studies range from 21 to 49% (Caffaro-Rouget, Lang, & van Santen, 1989 [49%]; Conte & Schuerman, 1987 [21%]; Mannarino & Cohen, 1986 [31%]; Tong, Gates, & McDowell, 1987 [36%]).

However, the research indicates that some asymptomatic children will subsequently develop problems. This is why we prefer the term "resilience" to "invulnerability." As Rutter (1993) points out, "invulnerability" seems to imply an absolute resistance to damage. Although abatement of symptoms has been shown in at least seven longitudinal studies of sexually abused children, with one-half to two-thirds of all children becoming less symptomatic (for a review, see Kendall-Tackett, Williams, & Finkelhor, 1993), studies have demonstrated that a sizable proportion (10–24%) of children get worse (Bentovim, van Elberg, & Boston, 1988 [10%]; Gomes-Schwartz, Horowitz, Cardarelli, & Sauzier, 1990 [24%]; Hewitt & Friedrich, 1991 [18%]; Runyan, Everson, Edelsohn, Hunter, & Coulter, 1988, [14%]). Some children whose condition subsequently deteriorated were asymptomatic at the time of the initial assessment (Gomes-Schwartz et al., 1990).

How do we explain the diversity of outcome associated with child maltreatment? We turn again to developmental psychopathology. A central focus in the study of resilience and developmental psychopathology has been the attempt to identify moderator variables. Baron and Kenny (1986) define a moderator variable as a qualitative or quantitative variable that "affects the direction and/or strength of the relation between an independent or predictor variable and a dependent or criterion variable" (p. 1174). Cicchetti and Rizley (1981) and Cicchetti and Rogosch (1994) classify moderator variables into two broad categories: "potentiating factors" increase the probability of negative developmental outcomes, and "compensatory factors" decrease the risk of negative outcome. Within each of these broad classifications, Cicchetti and Olsen (1990) distinguish between "transient" factors, which are temporary and fluctuating influences, and "trait" factors, which represent more enduring conditions or characteristics. We can also classify moderator variables into four broad domains: (1) maltreatment factors, (2) individual child factors, (3) family factors, and (4) environmental factors (Malinosky-Rummell & Hansen, 1993).

We provide here a brief overview of these variables, a number of which we discuss in much more depth in subsequent chapters. Some of these have been found to moderate the impact of maltreatment. Although the relevance of some variables for maltreated children's developmental outcomes has received empirical support, others have not yet been investigated empirically. We should also avoid thinking of these variables in categorical ways. As Rutter (1993) points out, the same variable may be a risk factor in one situation and a protective factor in another. Table 1.1 supplements our narrative description.

Maltreatment Factors

Kendall-Tackett and colleagues (1993) reviewed the influence of characteristics of maltreatment on the outcomes of sexually abused children as documented in 25 studies. The following factors are associated with more symptoms: high frequency of sexual contact; longer duration; use of force; oral, anal, or vaginal penetration; and a close relationship between child and perpetrator. Factors such as frequency, duration, and the relationship between the child and the perpetrator have not been sufficiently explored in the literature pertaining to physically abused children, although severity of abuse, frequency of child protective services reports, and the interaction between frequency and severity were significant predictors of outcome in youngsters subjected to different types of maltreatment, including physical abuse and neglect (Manly, Cicchetti, & Barnett, 1994).

Individual Factors

The developmental level of children influences the impact of maltreatment in a variety of ways. Their interpretation and understanding of the mal-

TABLE 1.1. Known or Suspected Moderator Variables for Developmental Outcome of Maltreated Children

1. Maltreatment factors
   - Frequency
   - Duration
   - Relationship between child and perpetrator
   - Penetration (in child sexual abuse)/severity of the maltreatment
   - Use of force
   - Occurrence of other forms of maltreatment/frequency of child protective services reports
2. Individual factors
   - Child's age and stage of development
   - Gender of the child
   - Temperament
   - Medical, biological, or physical conditions
   - Premaltreatment adjustment (e.g., intelligence and cognitive skills, self-esteem)
   - Child's appraisals and attributions regarding the maltreatment
3. Family factors
   - Family's support of the child postmaltreatment
     - Acknowledgment of the maltreatment
     - Belief in the child
     - Emotional support
     - Ability to protect the child from further maltreatment
     - Securing appropriate services (e.g., medical examination, therapy)
     - Provision of adequate parenting postmaltreatment
   - Family functioning and parenting premaltreatment
     - Attachment between child and parents, including accurate perception of the child's needs and capacity to respond to them
     - Adequacy and health of marital relationship (e.g., communication, support, spousal abuse, discord, problem solving)
     - Individual functioning of parents (e.g., psychiatric illness, substance abuse, depression)
     - Poverty; stability of residence, income; social network and supports
     - Single parent
     - Discipline/parenting effectiveness and appropriateness
4. Environmental factors
   - Cultural–societal toleration of maltreatment/community's reaction to the child and family
   - Cultural and religious factors
   - Supportive social relationships for child and family
   - Provision of appropriate services for child and family (including continuing protection of the child)
   - Criminal justice involvement

treatment play a significant role in subsequent adjustment: maltreatment may have different meanings and significance for children at different developmental stages. Some very young children may not even recognize that they have been abused (e.g., sexual abuse), but become cognizant of the significance of what happened to them only as they become older and more aware of the social prohibitions and sanctions attached to this behavior (Finkelhor, 1995).

A child's cognitive development may affect his or her responses to abuse or neglect in other ways. Children's thinking becomes "decentered" as they enter the concrete operational stage of thought. They recognize that other people may have both positive and negative traits, and they may harbor simultaneously positive and negative feelings toward others (Harter, 1977). The attainment of this developmental stage contributes to feelings of ambivalence toward a perpetrator, leading to even greater confusion and conflicted feelings.

Developmental level also affects the symptom pattern evidenced by maltreated children. For example, sexually maltreated adolescents may be more likely to engage in running away, substance abuse, or suicidal behavior when distressed, because these behaviors are within their repertoires. Younger children are much less likely to show these patterns and more likely to display behavior more common to their age group (e.g., disruptive behavior or sexualized behavior).

Clinicians often fail to consider the child's medical status and temperament as moderator variables when evaluating the developmental impact of maltreatment. For example, a 5-year-old with a difficult temperament may react differently to abuse or neglect than a same-age child with a placid, regular temperament. The former might become distressed, not only by the maltreatment but also by subsequent changes in family routine or structure, such as placement in foster care. In general, an easy temperament serves as a compensatory factor (Grizenko & Pawliuk, 1994). Besides eliciting more positive responses from their caregivers and being better equipped to cope with changing environmental circumstances, children with easy temperaments appear to have higher intelligence and more advanced problem-solving skills, cognitive/integrative abilities, social skills, and coping strategies (Mantzicopoulos & Morrison, 1994; Werner, 1993).

Medical, biological, or physical conditions (e.g., sensory deficits, such as blindness or hearing impairments, fetal alcohol spectrum disorders [FAS-D]) may mediate a child's adjustment to maltreatment. A number of children whom we have assessed and treated have had primary attention deficit disorders that significantly affected their social, behavioral, and academic functioning. Other diagnoses like FAS-D are associated with conditions (e.g., irritability and difficulties in behavioral regulation, failure to consider the consequences of one's actions, social/communicative difficulties, disrupted school experience, mental health diagnoses) (Streissguth, 1997) that in turn may moderate a child's response to maltreatment. For example, preexisting problems in behavioral and emotional self-regulation may seriously compromise a child's ability to cope adaptively with the anger elicited by physical abuse. Of course, some problems may result from the maltreatment and in turn influence the child's subsequent adaptation to the trauma. In a fascinating series of early papers, Lewis and her colleagues (Lewis, 1992; Lewis, Lovely, Yeager, & Delia Femina, 1989; Lewis et al., 1988, 1991) reported that a constellation of neurological–neuropsychiatric vulnerabilities and a violent, abusive upbringing were closely associated with physical aggression. Lewis et al. (1989) described elements of a transactional model to account for this association. For example, family violence serves as a model of aggressive behavior and elicits intense feelings of rage. As well, it may result in those very neurological vulnerabilities that make it difficult for children to resist these aggressive models and control their anger. Lewis and colleagues (1989) also suggested that neuropsychiatrically impaired children, by virtue of their impulsivity, irritability, and hyperactivity, may be at higher risk for being abused. Chapter 2 reviews the more recent research on the neurobiological mechanisms of impact.

Clinicians must also evaluate children's precrisis adjustment and general level of functioning. For example, above-average IQ and positive experiences at school may serve as compensatory factors (Rutter, 1993). Success in these areas generates and strengthens feelings of self-esteem and self-efficacy that attenuate the impact of adverse events. Masten, Best, and Garmezy (1990) and Werner (1993) broaden these areas to include athletic, mechanical, and artistic pursuits as well as academic ones. Consequently, a child with such areas of strength may withstand more strongly the negative impact of being abused or neglected.

Family Factors

As we shall discuss in detail, sensitive care increases children's chances of establishing a secure attachment with parents, which in turn is a significant compensatory factor for those who are subsequently maltreated. A child whose relationships are characterized by basic trust may not be as seriously compromised by abuse, especially if it is time limited and committed by someone without a particularly close relationship to the child. Such children may regard the maltreatment as unfortunate incidents that speak more to the untrustworthiness or even dangerousness of a specific offender than evidence of the ubiquitous badness of people. Consequently, their subsequent relationships may not be deleteriously affected, although they may display some localized effects such as anxiety-related symptoms. Furthermore, a secure attachment organization increases chances that they will approach their caregivers for help and support because they expect them to respond in a sensitive and helpful manner. Parental support may attenuate their distress and increase the probability of a good outcome. We discuss the importance of attributions, internal working models, and interpersonal schemas in subsequent chapters.

Other aspects of parenting and family support can also moderate the impact of maltreatment. Indeed, support from the family seems critical for children's adjustment to almost any kind of trauma. There may be many mechanisms that account for this association. Via the phenomenon of "social referencing," young children take their cues from their caretakers regarding how to respond to situations of potential or actual threat (Lewandowski & Baranoski, 1994). Parents can transmit their own anxiety about the trauma or maltreatment, thus escalating children's apprehension and distress. Maltreated children whose parents disbelieve their accounts or blame them for the abuse may feel even greater stigmatization, which contributes to a poorer outcome (Finkelhor & Browne, 1985). As well, children's adjustment is significantly dependent on the actual parenting they receive, especially when they display behavioral or emotional problems associated with maltreatment. Parents who cannot apply firm and consistent limits to their children's behavior and who cannot maintain a regular and consistent routine for their offspring may inadvertently contribute to their children's behavior problems. Deterioration in parenting may reflect a situational reaction to the child's disclosure or a chronic and long-standing pattern of parenting difficulties that predated the maltreatment. Many variables affect parenting, including the parents' own victimization history, psychiatric illness, and broader factors such as poverty and social isolation. Chapter 3 discusses the assessment of these family factors, especially the reactions of nonoffending parents and caregivers. Chapter 6 describes some interventions designed to increase the support parents or caregivers can offer to their victimized children.

Environmental Factors

Mental health professionals have tended to ignore environmental variables, despite their importance for a child's and the family's adjustment. Broad social factors such as poverty pose significant risk to developmental outcome in general (Duncan, Brooks-Gunn, & Klebanov, 1994; Lipman, Offord, & Boyle, 1994). Cultural and religious factors often have a significant impact on children's and families' response to maltreatment, as well as having important implications for how we conduct subsequent assessments and interventions. Other factors, such as the community's negative reaction to children's disclosure of maltreatment (e.g., peers and neighbors), exacerbate their sense of stigmatization. A criminal justice system that is unresponsive and insensitive to the idiosyncratic needs of child witnesses may compound feelings of powerlessness and stigmatization. For example, Kendall-Tackett and colleagues (1993) reviewed studies pertaining to sexually abused children's court involvement. Children's adjustment deteriorated when cases were not resolved quickly or when children were compelled to testify on multiple occasions. Children who were frightened of the accused also fared poorly. Although these variables functioned as potentiating factors, the same variable (i.e., testifying in court) can be a compensatory factor under somewhat different circumstances. For example, Runyan and colleagues (1988) reported that children who testified in juvenile court proceedings recovered more quickly when cases were resolved with a conviction or a plea bargain.

We should not discount the influence of other social relationships as a compensatory, albeit indirect, factor for maltreated children. Egeland, Jacobvitz, and Sroufe (1988) demonstrated that high-risk mothers pose less risk to their children if they have been able to form a supportive relationship with another adult, such as a spouse, or if they had participated in psychotherapy.

Stage-Salient Developmental Issues

The concept of stage-salient developmental issues also contributes to our understanding of maltreatment's diverse impacts. At each developmental stage, the individual confronts specific developmental tasks that are central to that age (Cicchetti & Rogosch, 1994). Upon emergence, each remains critical to the child's continual adaptation, although decreasing in salience relative to newly emerging tasks. In optimal development, the child successfully negotiates the progression of stage-salient issues and moves through a course of increasing competence and adaptation. In other words, later competencies build on earlier competencies.

This notion of maltreatment's impact on children's progression through different developmental stages is consistent with one of the two major types of effects arising from child victimization proposed by Finkelhor (1995). *Developmental effects* "refer to deeper and generalized types of impact, more specific to children, that result when a victimization experience and its related trauma interfere with developmental tasks or dysfunctionally distort their course" (Finkelhor, 1995, p. 184). Possibly affected areas include attachment, behavioral and emotional self-regulation, development of the self, cognitive and academic functioning, and peer relations. These developmental outcomes in turn may significantly affect the attainment of future developmental tasks (Finklehor, 1995). In contrast, *localized effects* are "those specific to the trauma experience but without major developmental ramifications . . . these symptoms can be called localized not only in the sense that they are short-term, which they often are (Kendall-Tackett et al., 1993), but also in the sense that they primarily affect behavior associated with the victimization experience and similar classes of experience" (Finkelhor, 1995, p. 184). Although localized effects can be pervasive and persistent, they do not interfere to a great extent with development. Among localized effects, Finkelhor includes nightmares and fears of being in the environment where victimization occurred. Developmental and localized effects are not mutually exclusive; maltreatment may produce a mixture of both types of effects.

We now turn to a description of the potential effects of maltreatment on child development.

ATTACHMENT

An Overview of Attachment Theory

The establishment of a secure attachment with a primary caregiver is the stage-salient task children confront between the ages of 6 and 12 months (Sroufe, 1979; Sroufe & Rutter, 1984). The attachment system refers to the organization of a diverse set of behaviors in the infant that maintains proximity to the caregiver when the child is distressed, in danger, or hurt. Attachment is not an issue for the first year of life alone. Once an attachment develops, it undergoes transformations and reintegrations with subsequent developmental accomplishments; it has importance for human development throughout the lifespan. We begin this section with a review of attachment theory's basic concepts and seminal research with infants and very young children, and then examine attachment in the school-age population. As we shall demonstrate, abuse and neglect often have a profound impact on the child's ability to form secure attachments to others, and that attachment insecurity is a significant risk factor for the development of psychopathology.

There are two individuals who dominated the early formative years of attachment theory and who were responsible for its core concepts: John Bowlby, a British child psychiatrist and psychoanalyst, and Mary Ainsworth, a Canadian-born psychologist who relocated to the United States, taught at several American universities, and trained many of the leading thinkers and researchers in the area. To understand the revolutionary nature of Bowlby's thinking and how it represented a radical departure from the traditional psychoanalytic model, a little history is in order (see Brisch [2002] and Karen [1994] for cogent reviews). In 1944, Bowlby published a paper describing his experiences with young thieves at the London Child Guidance Clinic. The paper, entitled "Forty-Four Juvenile Thieves: Their Characters and Home Life," was his attempt to demonstrate the influence of children's environments, especially experiences of loss and separation, on the genesis of problematic behavior. This represented a profound change in thinking, as the psychoanalytic world at this time was dominated by the concept that children's fantasies, such as the Oedipus complex, were the primary forces responsible for personality formation and psychopathology. Actual experiences were relegated to a minor role.

In 1949 the World Health Organization asked Bowlby to prepare a report on the condition of children left homeless and orphaned by World War II. This stimulated his interest in attachment and a quest to develop a theory to explain the nature of the child's ties to the mother, which is reflected in the title of his 1958 article (Bowlby, 1958) wherein he maintained that attachment between a mother and child is biologically based. Drawing upon some concepts of ethology (the study of animal behavior), Bowlby (1973, 1980, 1982, 1988a, 1988b) and colleagues (Ainsworth, 1989; Ainsworth & Bowlby, 1991) proposed that attachment behavior keeps the infant close to one or a few principal caregivers through complementary caregiver and infant behavior. The infant is equipped at birth with species-characteristic behaviors (e.g., crying) that elicit certain behaviors in the caregiver, and these behaviors emerge when the child is stressed. The child is an active partner and not merely a passive recipient of the parent's ministrations. This is a central point: The attachment system is activated when the child is stressed. This includes situations in which the child is hurt, in pain, or separated from the caregiver. Harmonious play between a child and parent may be an important component of their relationship but does not reflect the attachment system. Caregiving behavior (e.g., feeding the child, protecting the child from harm) that sensitively and appropriately meets the child's needs helps ensure infant survival and that of the species, thereby conferring evolutionary value upon the attachment system. The caregiver's behavior generates a feeling of security in the child. At first, the infant's behaviors are not directed at a specific individual. Gradually, the child begins to discriminate among people and establishes an attachment to one or a few select individuals. Activation of the attachment system also suppresses exploration in the child. A distressed, frightened youngster with a secure attachment will seek proximity to his or her primary attachment figure rather than exploring the environment.

Mary Ainsworth began a series of observational field studies of infants and their mothers in Uganda and Baltimore. This work constituted the basis of Ainsworth's strange situation paradigm, a strategy designed to assess the security of mother–infant attachment (Ainsworth, Blehar, Waters, & Wall, 1978). In this 20-minute videotaped procedure, the infant is exposed to a series of increasingly stressful events that culminate in being left alone. Remember, the attachment system is activated when the child is under stress; the strange situation's separation episodes stress the child and activate the system. The infant's reactions to separations, and especially to reunions, are believed to measure the degree to which the infant's perceptions and expectations of the mother provide feelings of security and trust.

Ainsworth and colleagues (1978) found that infants with a *secure attachment* (type B) greeted their mothers positively after being separated, actively sought proximity or interaction, and readily accepted comfort if distressed. They directed little, if any, negative behavior toward their mothers in the reunion and calmed down after several minutes. These mothers were responsive, accessible, and sensitive to their children's needs. Infants who manifested an *avoidant attachment* (type A) showed little stress when separated and, upon reunion, avoided their mothers by turning and looking away and ignoring them. These infants showed little preference for their mothers over a stranger and evidenced little affective interchange in the preseparation episodes. The mothers ignored or rejected their children's needs, avoided physical contact, and were intrusive in interactions with their infants. These interactions were also characterized by instances of covert hostility and rejection. Infants who demonstrated an *ambivalent–resistant attachment* (type C) exhibited a high level of distress upon separation. Upon reunion, they showed angry resistance and appeared ambivalent. They actively sought proximity but angrily pushed away from their mothers. Unlike avoidant children, these youngsters appear to have learned to overexaggerate the attachment system to maximize the chances that caregivers will respond to them. These mothers responded inconsistently and interacted in a very passive, withdrawn manner.

Main and Weston (1982) describe these three attachment patterns as coherent, organized strategies for achieving "felt security" and regulating distress. According to Main (1990) and Cassidy and Mohr (2001), infants achieve their goal of attaining proximity to attachment figures by developing a strategy tailored to the specifics of the caregiving relationship. Parents of securely attached infants react promptly to their infants' arousal, thereby reducing their distress and allowing them to attend to and explore the environment. As most parents know, it is very difficult for a baby screaming with hunger or fright to settle down and interact with others or explore the environment. The securely attached child readily seeks comfort in the strange situation because of an expectation that the attachment figure will respond sensitively and appropriately. Moreover, the child can freely explore the environment because of the expectation that the attachment figure is readily available if the child becomes distraught or anxious during these explorations.

The avoidantly attached child expects the parent to rebuff, reject, or become angry and hostile if he or she makes demands in stressful situations. Consequently, the child begins to avoid closeness or intimacy with the attachment figure (Crittenden, 1992a; Main, 1981). For these children, closeness, intimacy, and the expression of negative affects are fraught with danger. Others have learned that parents ignore their distress rather than reacting angrily or punitively. Parental neglect of the child who needs soothing or comfort leads to continued intense, emotional arousal, an exceedingly disorganizing effect. To cope, the child excludes feelings and thoughts that would normally arouse the attachment system and begins to suppress or falsify the expression of affects typically used to signal for appropriate parental response (Cassidy & Kobak, 1988; Crittenden, 1992b; Main, 1990). According to Cassidy and Mohr (2001), "insecure/avoidant babies have learned to suppress the expression of attachment behavior (i.e., learned to deactivate the attachment system) in order to maintain protective access to caregivers who are uncomfortable with closeness" (p. 277). The child dismisses the importance of the attachment relationship and the associated feelings and thoughts. This strategy also protects the child from further trauma if the parents have reacted in punitive, angry, or even abusive ways when the child was distressed. Although this strategy provides relief from intense, emotional arousal, ultimately it may lead to problems in perceiving, interpreting, and displaying feelings. It may preclude children from forming close interpersonal relationships that fulfill affectional needs. Instead, it encourages expectations that relationships are a source of danger and rejection. Main and Goldwyn (1984) also suggest that children with an avoidant attachment may idealize caregivers. They portray the rejecting, hostile parent as a wonderful caregiver, thereby attenuating troublesome feelings of anger, sadness, and anxiety associated with an accurate perception of the relationship.

The child with an ambivalent–resistant attachment attempts to provoke the attachment figure to meet his or her needs via angry and aggressive behavior. Unlike avoidant children, these youngsters learn to overexpress their feelings and needs to increase the chances that their inconsistent caregiver will respond to their distress or alarm. They become "hypervigilant and responsive to signals of maternal unavailability and also . . . intensify their signals" (Crittenden, 1992b, p. 581). Furthermore, with uncertainty about whether the mother will be available, responsive, or helpful, the child becomes dependent and clingy and manifests the kind of anger just described. The child's ability to explore the environment is restricted by this preoccupation with parental unavailability.

This description of these attachment patterns as organized strategies reflects one of Bowlby's (1969, 1973, 1980, 1982; Sroufe & Fleeson, 1986) most important theoretical concepts of attachment theory. The child's *internal working model* of attachment (mental representations of the self and the parent) is inferred from the infant's responses and behavior in the structured separation and reunion episodes of the strange situation. Infants with a secure attachment organization who freely seek comfort, proximity, and contact in the reunion episode and then gradually explore the environment or return to play are inferred to have an expectation that parents can meet their needs for reassurance, comfort, and protection. Infants with an avoidant attachment organization actively avoid and ignore the parent in the reunion because of an expectation that their proximity-seeking advances will be rejected or ignored. Their mental representation of the relationship seems to be characterized by danger, rejection, or neglect. Infants with an ambivalent–resistant attachment expect that their parents cannot meet their needs consistently. This expectation is evidenced by their angry yet clingy and dependent behavior in the reunion episode, which seems designed to evoke an appropriate response from their parents.

Main and Solomon (1986, 1990) reviewed more than 200 videotapes of infants who had not been previously classified or did not fit the criteria of these three patterns. They identified criteria for an additional insecure pattern, *disorganized–disoriented attachment* (type D). When confronted with the mother's return, these infants displayed an array of diverse and contradictory behavior patterns: strong initial proximity seeking followed by strong avoidance; approaching but with head averted; undirected, misdirected, incomplete, and interrupted movements or expressions; odd movements and postures, asymmetrical movements, and mistimed movements; freezing, stilling, and slowed "underwater" movements and expressions; and expressions of fear and distress, dazed or disoriented facial expressions, and apprehension (Cassidy & Mohr, 2001).

Disorganized–disoriented behaviors do not represent a fourth organized strategy for maintaining access to an attachment figure (Main & Solomon, 1990). Rather, these behaviors make sense only if interpreted as reflecting fear and confusion about the caregiver and irresolvable (i.e., unorganized) conflict concerning whether or how to maintain access to the attachment figure in times of stress (Goldberg, 1991; Main & Solomon, 1990). Main and Hesse (1990) and Lyons-Ruth, Repacholi, McLeod, and Silva (1991) suggest that this pattern reflects a relationship in which the child suddenly experiences a previously positive and caring parent as threatening. Negative interactions with the caregiver activate the attachment system and motivate the child to turn to the caregiver as a source of comfort. However, the child is in a real bind; the attachment figure is both the source of the stress and the figure who might alleviate it, which in turn is reflected in the approach–avoidance behavior so characteristic of children with a disorganized attachment classification (e.g., approaching the mother by walking backward). This represents a breakdown of organized, coherent attachment strategies or "the breakdown of an otherwise consistent and organized strategy of emotion regulation" (van IJzendoorn, Schuengel, & Bakermans-Kranenburg, 1999, p. 226).

If pervasive enough, this conflict impedes the infant's organization of a consistent attachment-oriented strategy. However, Main and Solomon (1990) propose that this conflict and disorganization might occur in the context of a strategy that was otherwise secure. Likewise, disorganization might exist in relation to the two other coherent strategies, avoidant and ambivalent. Consequently, Main and Solomon advise investigators to code the best-fitting classification according to the infant's underlying attachment strategy. Such best-fitting classifications are usually described as "forced" classifications. Lyons-Ruth and colleagues (1991) reviewed the disorganized forms of secure and insecure attachment behavior and their correlates. Disorganized behavior in infants with serious social risks (e.g., infants from low-income backgrounds or who have been maltreated) has been predominantly the forced–insecure and, especially, forced–avoidant types. Disorganized behavior in infants from low-risk, middle-class backgrounds has been predominantly of the forced–secure type.

Attachment Organizations of School-Age Children

As researchers began to consider the attachment organizations of school-age youngsters, they were confronted with several dilemmas: What constitutes attachment in older children and how can it be measured? An underlying assumption of the strange situation is that separations from the mother alarm the child, thereby activating the attachment system, as reflected in the child's behaviors that increase proximity to or maintain contact with a particular attachment figure. Although this works well for infants and young children, separations lose their power to induce alarm and distress by the time children begin attending elementary school. Most early school-age children have had considerable experience in separating from their parents, and they know their parents will return; they do not need the actual physical proximity that infants and toddlers require. Furthermore, school-age children's greater cognitive and linguistic abilities allow them to express attachment organization, including internal working models of attachment, through words or play behavior (representational level) (Solomon & George, 1999). One evaluation strategy developed to evaluate school-age children's attachment organization at the representational level involves presenting children with a story stem, using small dolls. The experimenter describes what has happened, such as the parents departing for a trip, and then asks the children to depict what happens next, using the dolls. The representational models of older children have direct analogues to qualitative differences in infant–parent interaction. For example, Solomon and George (1999) reported that secure kindergarten children freely express separation anxiety in the doll play, but also confidence that these fears and anxieties will be resolved. This symbolic play is similar to their open and direct expression of emotions and attachment behavior in actual separations and reunions with their mothers. Chapter 4 describes representational measures of attachment and the variations in response exhibited by maltreated school-age children.

Attachment Organizations of Maltreated Children

The type of attachment depends on the quality of care the infant has received (Sroufe, 1988). Following Ainsworth's original investigations (Ainsworth et al., 1978), studies confirmed that mothers of secure infants were rated as more sensitive, responsive, accessible, and cooperative during the infants' first year than mothers of insecure infants (e.g., Belsky, Rovine, & Taylor, 1984). Results of early studies of the attachment patterns of maltreated children consistently showed that physically abused and neglected children are less likely to develop secure attachments, with 70–100% of maltreated infants exhibiting insecure attachment organizations (e.g., Cicchetti, 1989; Crittenden, 1988). The disorganized–disoriented category also has been found to characterize maltreated infants. Approximately 80% of maltreated infants were classified as disorganized–disoriented, as compared with less than 20% of a nonmaltreated comparison group (Carlson, Barnett, Braunwald, & Cicchetti, 1989).

Investigations of the attachment classifications of preschoolers (2–5 years of age) have shown that maltreated children continue to exhibit insecure attachments. Cicchetti and Barnett (1991) examined maltreated preschoolers' attachment relationships with their mothers at one or more of three ages: 30 months, 36 months, and 48 months. They evaluated children who were physically abused, neglected, emotionally maltreated, and a fourth group judged to have experienced multiple types of maltreatment. There were few statistically significant relations between the types of maltreatment and specific classifications of insecure attachment. However, a significantly greater proportion of maltreated youngsters were insecurely attached than nonmaltreated children in each age group. Moreover, a small number of maltreated children with secure attachments at 30 months were likely to be classified as insecure at later assessments.

More recent studies have demonstrated the association between maltreatment and insecure attachments, especially disorganized attachments. van IJzendoorn and colleagues (1999) conducted a meta-analysis of nearly 80 studies on disorganized attachment. They reported that the percentage of disorganized infant attachment in "normal," middle-class, nonclinical groups in North America was 15%, which was identical to the percentage of older children. The percentage of children with disorganized attachment was significantly higher in low socioeconomic samples (25%) than in middle-class samples and markedly elevated in children of maltreating parents: 48% of these children were found to be disorganized, a rate three times higher than that found in nonclinical middle-class samples.

Maltreatment's importance as an antecedent of disorganized attachment is no surprise. Maltreating parents frighten their children through abusive actions, in turn activating the attachment system. But as we have seen, the parent is also the source of comfort, and the resulting "incompatible behaviors of proximity seeking and flight lead to a breakdown of organized attachment behavior" (van IJzendoorn et al. 1999, p. 227). van IJzendoorn and colleagues (1999) also point out that maltreatment is not the only antecedent to disorganized attachment. Parents may become frightened themselves when they remember a loss of an important attachment figure, and this unexpected display of parental fear frightens the child. Lyons-Ruth has identified a number of very specific caregiver behaviors associated with disorganized infant attachment, such as maternal disorientation (e.g., a "haunted" or frightened voice, disoriented facial expressions), which frighten the child (Bronfman, Parsons, & Lyons-Ruth, n.d). Owen and Cox (1997) speculate that children who witness serious marital discord, such as domestic violence, become frightened and are therefore more prone to developing a disorganized attachment.

Other types of maltreatment such as neglect are associated with insecure attachment organizations. Several research teams have investigated the impact of severe deprivation on the attachment organization of Eastern European children raised in large institutions and orphanages and then adopted in Canada and the United Kingdom. MacLean (2003) and Zeanah and colleagues (2003) have prepared excellent reviews of this work, which we briefly summarize here. A Canadian team conducted a longitudinal study of babies from Romanian orphanages adopted by Canadian families (Chisholm, 1998). They reported that 67% of children had either secure or typical insecure attachment patterns identical to those displayed by 95% of Canadian-born and early-adopted youngsters. Most children were still able to form an attachment with their adoptive parents, but one-third of the orphanage sample had established an atypical insecure attachment pattern, as compared with 7% of Canadian-born and 4% of early-adopted children.

O'Connor, Rutter, and the English and Romanian Adoptees Study Team (O'Connor, Bredenkamp, Rutter, and the English and Romanian Adoptees Study Team, 1999; O'Connor, Marvin, Rutter, Olrick, Britner, and the English and Romanian Adoptees Team, 2003; O'Connor, Rutter, and the English and Romanian Adoptees Study Team, 2000) found that duration of deprivation was associated with the number of signs of attachment disturbance at 6 years; these signs included an indiscriminate style of relating, which was also reported by Chisholm (1998). However, approximately 70% of children exposed to severe deprivation did not exhibit marked or severe attachment disorder behaviors. According to O'Connor and colleagues (2000), "grossly pathogenic care is not a sufficient condition for attachment disorder behavior to result" (p. 710). This is consistent with the transactional model's emphasis on the interaction of an array of variables rather than the simple, linear effects model that characterized early theorizing regarding maltreatment's outcome.

Attachment and Child Development

At this point, readers may be wondering why we have spent considerable effort reviewing the basic concepts of attachment theory and the relevant research. We contend that attachment theory is not merely a construct confined to the academic lab or classroom. An extensive body of research demonstrates a significant association between attachment organization and children's functioning across a number of domains. Attachment insecurity, especially disorganized attachment, represents a potent risk factor for the development of psychopathology in children. Clinicians who assess and treat these youngsters need to be solidly grounded in this literature to understand, as comprehensively as possible, the impact of their young clients' attachments, the mechanisms underlying these effects, and the implications for clinical practice.

What follows is a brief summary of the literature describing the association between attachment organization and developmental outcome: to do it justice would be way beyond the scope of this book, although we do highlight the sequelae of disorganized attachments. We refer the reader to several sources for more detailed information (Cassidy & Mohr, 2001; Greenberg, 1999; Thompson, 1999; van IJzendoorn et al., 1999) and in the next chapter discuss the mechanisms through which attachment organization influences developmental outcome. The following summary is based on the reviews prepared by Greenberg (1999) and Thompson (1999).

- Children classified as securely attached to a caregiver during infancy later approach problem-solving tasks more positively and with greater persistence than insecurely attached children.
- Securely attached children are more likely to be more empathic, compliant, and generally competent in relationships with peers. Children with insecure attachment organizations have trouble relat-

ing to other people because their behavior is often distant or overdependent.

- The Minnesota Longitudinal Study demonstrated that, as compared with children who were insecurely attached to their mothers at 12 months, those with secure attachments at that age were more resilient, cooperative, happier, and more likely to be leaders at 3 and 6 years of age.
- Among children from low-income families, those who had been insecurely attached during infancy were, at ages 10–11 and 14–15 years, more dependent, less socially competent, and had lower self-esteem that those who had been securely attached.
- Mothers' prenatal attachment classification is a significant predictor of their infants' attachment.

Recent evidence suggests that the link between disorganized attachment and disturbed child functioning is significant (see Cassidy & Mohr, 2001, Lyons-Ruth & Jacobvitz, 1999, and van IJzendoorn et al., 1999, for comprehensive reviews). In their meta-analysis, van IJzendoorn and colleagues (1999) reported that disorganized attachment was associated with more externalizing behavior problems as assessed by parents, teachers, or observers. Furthermore, the association appeared stable, from infancy into the school-age period and even beyond. Similarly, disorganized children are more likely to exhibit social skill deficits. In adolescence they are at higher risk for exhibiting overall behavior problems, internalizing difficulties, and dissociative symptoms.

Although the association between insecure attachment, especially the disorganized classification, and the emergence of childhood psychopathology is well established, there are two important points to remember. First, this association is far from perfect. Lyons-Ruth, Easterbrooks, and Cibelli (1997) reported that only 25% of disorganized infants in a high-risk sample were rated as engaging in significant externalizing behavior at age 7. Moreover, other factors mediated this relationship. Children's mild cognitive delays combined with disorganization at 18 months increased the risk for externalizing behaviors. Maternal depression also interacted with children's disorganized attachment and was associated with higher rates of externalizing behaviors. Greenberg and colleagues examined attachments of children referred to a clinic for oppositional–defiant disorder (ODD) (reviewed in Greenberg, 1999). Approximately 80% of clinic children demonstrated insecure attachments as compared with 30% of the comparison children. The clinic children also showed a disproportionately higher rate of the disorganized–controlling classification. However, 15–20% of the clinic sample had secure attachments, leading Greenberg (1999) to suggest,

"Attachment may be a component of only some pathways leading to ODD" (p. 479). We strongly agree with Greenberg's assertion that attachment insecurity represents a nonspecific risk factor that increases the likelihood of future problems in combination with other factors, a notion consistent with the transactional model.

Second, given this perspective on attachment, we should not equate insecure attachment organization with psychopathology. Sroufe and colleagues (1999) expressed this concept in the following passage:

> In this perspective, early attachment variations generally are not viewed as pathology or even as directly causing pathology. Rather, varying patterns of attachment represent "initiating conditions" in systems terms. In this regard, they do play a dynamic role in pathological development because of the way in which environmental engagement is framed by established tendencies and expectations. (pp. 10–11)

However, there is another way of considering attachment's influence on development. Rather than regarding attachment organization as a risk factor for the emergence of psychopathology, we may consider atypical attachment patterns themselves as disorders (Greenberg, 1999). Probably the clearest example of this approach is reactive attachment disorder (RAD), a DSM-IV diagnosis (American Psychiatric Association, 1994). RAD's essential feature is markedly disturbed and developmentally inappropriate social relatedness that is associated with grossly pathological care. In the inhibited type, the youngster shows a pattern of excessively inhibited, hypervigilant, or highly ambivalent responses. Children with the disinhibited type exhibit indiscriminate sociability or a lack of selectivity in the choice of attachment figures. Zeanah and colleagues (2004) interviewed clinicians treating 94 maltreated toddlers in foster care regarding signs of RAD. Both types could be reliably diagnosed, and 17% of the sample were diagnosed with both types. To determine the effects of being reared in socially depriving caregiving environments, Zeanah and his colleagues investigated attachment disturbance in toddlers living in a large institution in Bucharest, Romania (Smyke, Dumitrescu, & Zeanah, 2002; Zeanah, Smyke, & Dumitrescu, 2002). Children residing in the large institution exhibited more signs of disordered attachment than youngsters living in the same institution in a unit designed to reduce the number of adults caring for each child, or than toddlers living at home. Children in the first group showed both the inhibited and disinhibited types. We discuss RAD in more depth in Chapter 4.

Our review demonstrates the contribution of attachment to child development, the risk maltreatment poses to the formation of a secure attachment, and, in some cases, its association with particular disorders (e.g., RAD). Despite the significance of insecure attachments and attachment-disordered behavior, maltreated children present with a number of other significant problems that deserve our clinical attention.

EXTERNALIZING BEHAVIOR PROBLEMS

Physical Aggression and Antisocial Behavior

An important component of adaptive functioning in childhood and later life is the ability to regulate both emotions and behaviors. The successful negotiation of this stage-salient task in toddlerhood and early childhood increases chances of competency in later developmentally salient tasks (Shields, Cicchetti, & Ryan, 1994). For example, a child who has previously learned to regulate and modulate feelings may have a greater chance of making and keeping friends. The child is more likely to cope adaptively with classroom demands where students are expected to exert some self-control by sitting quietly and inhibiting the urge to yell out or hit someone. Maltreated children show numerous difficulties in their emotional and behavioral self-regulation, including externalizing behaviors, such as physical aggression directed toward others, and antisocial behavior.

The first edition's review of the earlier research revealed that maltreatment is a significant risk factor for the development of childhood physical aggression (see reviews by Cicchetti & Rogosch, 1994; Wolfe & Wolfe, 1988, for summaries of this work). Researchers had identified both physical and verbal abuse as antecedents of physical aggression in preschool and school-age children (e.g., Cicchetti, Lynch, Shonk, & Manley, 1992; Vissing, Straus, Gelles, & Harrop, 1991).

More recent literature reinforces these conclusions. Six- to 8-year-old physically abused children exhibited significantly more aggression as measured by caregiver reports on the Child Behavior Checklist (CBCL) than those not physically victimized (Johnson et al., 2002). Jaffee, Caspi, Moffitt, and Taylor (2004) reported that physical abuse prospectively predicted antisocial outcome in young school-age children and that physical maltreatment was followed by the emergence of new antisocial behaviors. Other studies have demonstrated that childhood physical abuse increases an individual's risk of engaging in violent, antisocial behavior in adolescence and adulthood (Lansford et al., 2002; Widom & Maxfield, 2001).

There are, of course, moderator variables that influence the association between physical abuse and aggressive and antisocial behavior. Earlier studies examined the impact of various aspects of maltreatment, such as its frequency, severity, and chronicity. Manly and colleagues (1994) showed that severity of the maltreatment, frequency of child protective services reports, and the interaction between severity and frequency of maltreatment were significant predictors of functioning, including aggression. Other studies have confirmed this link between chronicity of physical abuse and aggressive behaviors (Bolger & Patterson, 2001; Ethier, Lemelin, & Lacharité, 2004). Jaffee and colleagues (2004) reported a dose–response association between physical maltreatment and children's antisocial behavior; at age 7, youngsters who definitely had been maltreated had more antisocial behavior problems than children who possibly had been maltreated.

Research has identified other moderator variables. Although maltreatment posed a risk for outcome in adolescence, the risk was even greater for children who experienced a greater number of caretaker transitions. The total number of caretaker changes significantly predicted delinquent behavior, alcohol use, drug use, status offenses, and high school dropout (Herrenkohl, Herrenkohl, & Egolf, 2003). Newton, Litrownick, and Landsverk (2000) also demonstrated that for foster children who did not evidence any externalizing behaviors at the initial assessment, number of foster home changes was a consistent predictor of externalizing, internalizing, and total behavior problems on the CBCL at a second assessment 18 months later. Moreover, for those children initially exhibiting some behavior problems, externalizing behaviors were significant predictors of subsequent placement changes. Foster parents may be less tolerant of aggressive or antisocial behavior in their homes and respond by requesting the children's removal. Interpreting the removal as yet another rejection may exacerbate children's feelings of anger and erode trust or confidence in relationships, thereby potentiating the likelihood of more acting-out and externalizing behaviors. These studies reinforce the need for clinicians to attend to a diverse array of moderator variables and appreciate the complexity of these interactions when attempting to understand children's responses to maltreatment.

This complexity becomes even more apparent when we consider recent research on the significance of the interplay between maltreatment and genetic vulnerabilities for antisocial behavior. Jaffee and colleagues (2005) reported that the experience of maltreatment was associated with a 2% increase in the probability of a conduct disorder diagnosis among children at low genetic risk for conduct disorder, but an increase of 24% among children at high genetic risk. Although this seems to be compelling evidence for the role of genetic variables in maltreated children's outcome, Jaffee and colleagues caution us to avoid making assumptions that genetic vulnerabilities code directly for aggression or conduct problems. Consistent with developmental psychopathology's transactional model, Jaffee and colleagues state, "This study and others . . . suggest that genes may not influence behavior disorders directly, but, in some complex disorders, genes may act to influence people's susceptibility or resistance to stressful environmental experiences" (p. 79).

The last decade has seen many more investigations of the effects of witnessing violence on child outcome. This has been an important development, given the problem's high incidence rate. Finkelhor, Ormrod, Turner, and Hamby (2005) reported that 1 in 3 children 2–17 years of age (357 per 1,000) had been a witness to violence or experienced another form of indirect violence. This included youngsters who witnessed domestic violence (35/1,000), physical abuse of a sibling (11/1,000), and an assault with a weapon (138/1,000) and without a weapon (209/1,000).

Although these findings are alarming, the sequelae are just as concerning. Kitzmann, Gaylord, Holt, and Kenny (2003) conducted a meta-analytic examination of 118 studies of the psychosocial outcomes of children exposed to interparental (domestic) violence and reported that such exposure is significantly associated with externalizing problems; children exposed to domestic violence and who were physically abused did not show worse outcomes that those exposed only to domestic violence, "suggesting that violence anywhere in the family may be sufficient to disrupt child development" (Kitzmann et al., 2003, p. 346).

Despite mixed evidence on gender effects, Yates, Dodds, Sroufe, and Egeland (2003) confirmed the contribution of domestic violence to externalizing problems for boys but not girls, who exhibited more internalizing difficulties. They also showed that developmental status at the time of exposure to violence moderates impact. Behavior problems in boys in middle childhood were related to contemporaneous exposure, whereas behavior problems for both boys and girls at 16 years were significantly associated with exposure to domestic violence during their preschool years. While demonstrating that exposure to domestic violence predicted preschoolers' behavior problems, Lieberman, Van Horn, and Ozer (2005) presented evidence of the important role of their mothers' psychological responses as moderator variables. Children whose mothers evidenced higher levels of life stress had more behavior problems, but this association was moderated by mothers' individual functioning, particularly the presence of posttraumatic stress disorder (PTSD) and the quality of the parent–child relationship. These findings offer further support for the ecological–transactional model.

Earlier studies found evidence of behavioral dysregulation in sexually abused children (Dubowitz, Black, Harrington, & Verschoore, 1993; Tufts' New England Medical Center, 1984). However, Kendall-Tackett and colleagues (1993) demonstrated the importance of including appropriate comparison groups in order to draw valid conclusions. Of the 11 studies in which the frequency of aggression and antisocial behavior problems of sexually abused children was compared with that of nonsexually abused, nonclinical children, 10 studies showed that sexually abused children were significantly more aggressive or antisocial. However, the comparison between sexually abused children and other clinical but nonabused children showed a different pattern. Of the 7 studies in which this design was used, 6 demonstrated that sexually abused children were less aggressive and antisocial than nonabused, clinical children. The other study revealed no differences.

Sexualized Behaviors and Sexual Behavior Problems

Although sexually abused children do not exhibit more physical aggression than clinical controls, they are at significant risk for exhibiting sexual behaviors in general and for developing sexual behavior problems (SBPs). Kendall-Tackett and colleagues' (1993) review demonstrated that sexually abused children showed significantly more sexual behavior than did the clinical comparison groups (six of eight studies). Sexual behavior was only one of two symptoms sexually abused children showed more consistently than nonabused clinical children; the other was PTSD. However, sexual behavior is still not shown by a majority of sexually abused children. Kendall-Tackett and colleagues calculated the percentage of victims manifesting inappropriate sexualized behavior in 13 studies as 28%.

Friedrich and his colleagues (Friedrich, Grambsch, Broughton, Kuiper, & Beilke, 1991; Friedrich et al., 1992) developed a rating scale for parents, the Child Sexual Behavior Inventory (CSBI), to assess children's specific sexual behaviors. A more recent study by Friedrich and colleagues (2001) confirmed earlier results: Sexually abused children exhibited a greater frequency of sexual behaviors than either normative or psychiatric outpatient samples. However, the psychiatric sample also exhibited more sexual behaviors relative to the normative sample, and Friedrich and colleagues suggested, "Sexual behavior was not unique to sexually abused children and may be present in other non-sexually abused samples, particularly boundary problems and heightened sexual knowledge" (p. 46). Variables such as penetration (oral, vaginal, or anal), the presence of medical evidence, abuse perpetrated by a family member or by more than one perpetrator, and abuse of greater frequency and longer duration were related to higher frequency of sexual behaviors (Friedrich et al., 2001).

Although we discuss assessment and intervention strategies for SBPs in subsequent chapters, we want to provide a brief description of what is meant by the term "sexual behavior problem" before we discuss the impact of maltreatment on the emergence of such difficulties and the influence of moderator variables. A consensus seems to have emerged regarding the central characteristics of SBPs: similarity to adult sexual behavior versus normal childhood sexual behavior like genital exploration, greater frequency or duration than developmentally expected, often occurs between children of significantly divergent ages/developmental abilities and/or use of physical or psychological coercion, and often refractory to redirection or other typical parenting practices (Bonner & Silovsky, 2004; Hall, Mathews, Pearce, Sarlo-Garvey, & Gavin 1996; Pearce, 2001; Ryan, 2000).

Children exhibiting SPBs have an elevated history of sexual abuse (Bonner, Walker, & Berliner, 2000; Gray, Pithers, Busconi, & Houchens, 1999; Hall, Mathews, & Pearce, 1998; Johnson, 1988, 1989). Despite this significant association, the link is not perfect: not every child who presents with SBPs has a history of sexual abuse. Silovsky and Niec (2002) reported that 62% of preschoolers with SBPs did not have substantiated histories of sexual abuse. These findings and data presented by Kendall-Tackett and colleagues (1993) and Friedrich and colleagues (2001) indicate that sexual abuse does not invariably lead to sexual behaviors or SBPs, and that there must be other factors that influence their development.

For those children with histories of sexual abuse and SBPs, specific characteristics of the sexual abuse may serve as important moderators of impact. Hall and colleagues (1998) found sexual arousal of the child during sexual abuse and the perpetrator's use of sadism differentiated those 3- to 7-year-old children who exhibited developmentally inappropriate sexual behavior to others from those whose sexual behavior was self-directed (e.g., excessive masturbation). A typology of this sample revealed that the sexual abuse of those youngsters who exhibited planned, coercive, interpersonal sexual behavior was marked by discomfort, self-stimulation and arousal, and a high degree of participation by the child (Hall, Mathews, & Pearce, 2002).

Although Silovsky and Niec (2002) found that a majority of preschoolers with SBPs did not have a history of sexual abuse, a substantial number of children in their sample had been physically abused (47%) and/or had witnessed interparental violence (58%). These findings are consistent with those of other studies that have demonstrated that many children with SBPs have histories of physical abuse, neglect, and exposure to family violence (Bonner et al., 2000; Gray et al., 1999; Hall et al., 1998, 2002; Pithers, Gray, Busconi, & Houchens, 1998b). The impact of these adverse environmental events, including maltreatment, are mediated by other aspects of family functioning: impaired attachment between parent and child (Pithers, Gray, Busconi, & Houchens, 1998a; Pithers et al., 1998b), poor parental supervision and monitoring of child behavior (Wieckowski, Hartsoe, Mayer, & Shortz, 1998), higher rates of parental psychopathology, including PTSD (Hall et al., 1998), parental and family histories of sexual and physical abuse and domestic violence (Bonner et al., 2000; Pithers et al., 1998a), economic stress (Pithers et al., 1998a), and fewer social supports for parents (Hall et al., 1998; Pithers et al., 1998a).

Children with SBPs also present with a number of comorbid conditions. Substantial proportions of school-age children with SBPs have learning and school behavior problems and higher rates of depression, anxiety, conduct disorders, and oppositional defiant disorders than controls (Bonner et al., 2000; Gray et al., 1999; Pithers et al., 1998b). Silovsky and Niec (2002) reported similar findings for preschoolers with SBPs; they scored in the clinical range on the CBCL Externalizing Scale and in the borderline range on the Internalizing Scale. Their verbal abilities were in the low average range. As we argue in the next chapter, some of these variables represent important moderators. For example, low verbal abilities may increase the probability that such children may be more prone to express feelings behaviorally rather than using words to articulate their emotions (Burke, Crenshaw, Greene, Schlosser, & Strocchia-Rivera, 1989). Clinicians may have to modify their interventions to accommodate children with receptive or expressive language difficulties.

INTERNALIZING PROBLEMS

Internalizing problems, including PTSD, other anxiety-related symptoms, and depression, are further manifestations of disturbances in self-regulation and are associated with various types of maltreatment.

PTSD and Other Anxiety Problems

The characteristics and etiology of PTSD have received considerable attention in the literature. Although initial work focused on adult survivors of traumatic events, there is now a significant body of work examining children with PTSD, including those who were maltreated. Furthermore, a significant portion of the treatment outcome literature in the area of child maltreatment has focused on PTSD. Clearly, it is a significant problem that clinicians are often asked to assess and treat.

We recommend that the reader consult with the fourth edition of the *Diagnostic and Statistical Manual of Mental Disorders* (DSM-IV; American Psychiatric Association, 1994) for a complete description of the PTSD diagnostic criteria. In summary, a diagnosis of PTSD requires the presence of three broad sets of criteria (adapted from American Psychiatric Association, 1994, pp. 427–428).

- The person experienced, witnessed, or was confronted with an event that involved actual or threatened death or serious injury, or a threat to the physical integrity of the self and others.
- The traumatic event is persistently *reexperienced* through a recurrent and intrusive distressing recollection of the event. Young children may express themes or aspects of the trauma through repetitive play. The event may also be reexperienced through distressing dreams, a sense of reliving the experience, illusions, hallucinations, and dissociative flashbacks, intense psychological distress through exposure to internal or external cues that symbolize or resemble an aspect of the traumatic event, and physiological reactivity on exposure to internal or external cues.
- The individual engages in persistent *avoidance* of stimuli associated with the trauma and experiences a numbing of general responsiveness, such as efforts to avoid thoughts, feelings, activities, places, or people associated with the trauma. Individuals with PTSD also may be unable to recall important aspects of the trauma and exhibit a restricted range of affect.
- The individual experiences persistent symptoms of increased *arousal*, such as difficulty falling or staying asleep, irritability or outbursts of anger, difficulty in concentrating, hypervigilance, or an exaggerated startle reaction.

The literature consistently demonstrates that maltreated children are at significant risk for developing PTSD, although similar data pertaining to the association between maltreatment and externalizing behavior problems indicate that there is considerable diversity of outcome. Emery and Luamann-Billings (1998) reported that one-quarter to one-half of physically abused and sexually abused children have documented PTSD. Incidence rates may be higher in clinically referred samples of maltreated children: 42–90% in sexual abuse samples, 50–100% in child witnesses of domestic violence, and as high as 50% in physical abuse samples (see De Bellis, 2001, for a review). Rates are lower in nonclinical, nonreferred maltreated children: 39% in a nonreferred abuse or neglect sample and 36% in nonreferred sexually abused youngsters (De Bellis, 2001). Widom (1999) found childhood victims of physical and sexual abuse as well as neglect to be at increased risk for developing a lifetime history of PTSD when assessed prospectively in young adulthood.

The fact that a significant proportion of maltreated children do not develop PTSD leads us again to consider moderator factors. Pretrauma factors include previous psychiatric history, previous exposure to PTSD (especially child abuse), poor family functioning, a prior history of poor social supports, familial genetic history of psychiatric disorders, and being female (Dalgleish, 2004; De Bellis, 2001). Regarding trauma factors, the risk for PTSD increases when physical abuse is more severe and chronic (Kiser, Heston, Millsap, & Pruitt, 1991) and when sexual abuse occurs in a close relationship (McLeer, Deblinger, Henry, & Orvaschel, 1992) or involves threats, coercion, or guilt on the part of the child (Wolfe, Sas, & Wekerle, 1994). Dalgleish (2004) and De Bellis (2001) have identified the following posttrauma factors that influence PTSD: type of support the survivor receives, continued life events such as a change of school, repeated threats and fear of the perpetrator, and survivors' interpretations of the trauma (e.g., attributions about their responsibility for the assaults and appraisals of the nature/severity of their symptoms). Attributions are especially important for child outcome, and we review this topic in detail in Chapter 2 when we discuss mechanisms of impact.

Two of the factors identified above deserve more attention. We mentioned that the risk for PTSD increases when sexual abuse occurs in the context of a close relationship. This has particular relevance to maltreated children. Unlike youngsters traumatized by a natural disaster or a terrorist attack, maltreated children are subjected to trauma with a significant interpersonal component, especially when the perpetrator is someone whom they know well or even love. Sexual or physical assault by a stranger is a very rare event. This interpersonal element is often responsible for the emergence of other psychopathology in addition to the PTSD symptoms, such as feelings of betrayal and loss. Parents or caregivers may also react to their traumatized, maltreated children based on their unique perceptions and feelings about the interpersonal assault, especially if they have similar histories or were responsible for or complicit with the maltreatment (Chapter 3 reviews this area). To put it very simply, maltreated children with PTSD may exhibit a more complex clinical presentation compared to children who have been exposed to noninterpersonal trauma (De Bellis, 2001; Feeny, Foa, Treadwell, & March, 2004). This is consistent with the finding that PTSD prevalence rates for interpersonal trauma in all age groups are greater than for noninterpersonal trauma and range from 30 to 50% (De Bellis, 2001).

We also noted that the incidence of PTSD increases when the trauma is experienced over a period of time. This variable has played a central role in Terr's (1991) differentiation of childhood trauma into two types, each associated with somewhat different outcomes. Type I disorders, which follow from unanticipated single events, are characterized by full, detailed memories of the event, "omens" or attempts to develop a reason for the trauma or how it could have been averted, and misperceptions. The last includes misidentifications, visual hallucinations, and peculiar time distortions after a single, intense, unexpected shock.

Type II disorders follow from long-standing or repeated exposure to extreme external events. One primary characteristic of type II disorders is the child's attempts to preserve and protect the self from painful feelings, memories, and experiences engendered by the trauma. Terr (1991) identified three major characteristics of type II disorders. First, rage is common. Second, denial and psychic numbing occur as an accommodation to extreme, long-standing, and repeated traumatic situations, including maltreatment. In an extreme form, denial and psychic numbing may be manifested in children who forget whole segments of their childhood. These defensive operations are reflected in a reluctance to talk about themselves, a failure to define or acknowledge feelings, and a hesitancy to say anything about their ordeals. Terr suggests that the child's relative indifference to pain and lack of empathy for others may be further examples of denial and psychic numbing. Third, children accommodate or cope with this repeated experience through self-hypnosis and dissociation, thereby allowing themselves to escape mentally, as reflected in bodily anesthesia, feelings of invisibility, and amnesia for certain childhood periods. In their extreme form, these behaviors may culminate in dissociative disorders.

Other manifestations of anxiety include somatoform disorders. Haugaard (2004c) offers the following definition of somatoform disorders:

> A somatoform disorder can be diagnosed when a child has a physical complaint and an appropriate medical examination reveals no organic basis for the complaint or when a child with an identified organically based disorder has symptoms that are much more severe than would be expected. (p. 169)

Higher rates of somatization problems are associated with severe forms of child sexual abuse (Garralda, 1996; Kinzl, Traweger, & Biebl, 1995). Haugaard (2004c) speculates that severely abused children may be more prone to express feelings through physical symptoms because of the link between emotional trauma and physical trauma and pain. Their physical complaints may have been reinforced because they might have been abused less frequently when they were sick. We also speculate that maltreated children quickly learn to avoid directly expressing strong feelings or distress (similar to children with an avoidant attachment organization) because of caregivers' abusive or neglectful reactions. Rather, they suppress their feelings, which are eventually expressed via somatic complaints.

Researchers have also examined the presence of other indicators of anxiety, although this work is not as extensive as the research on formal diagnostic categories. Rather than using diagnoses such as PTSD and somatoform disorders, these studies incorporated more general measures of anxiety, such as the CBCL or the Trauma Symptom Checklist for Children (TSCC) (Briere, 1996). Despite these differences in measures, the same findings emerge: maltreated children exhibit more anxiety than nonmaltreated children. Ethier and colleagues (2004) reported that child victims of chronic maltreatment (physical abuse and neglect) had higher scores on the Anxious/Depressed scale of the CBCL. Witnessing violence was a significant predictor of anxiety as measured by the TSCC. Similar to the results they obtained for externalizing behavior, Newton and colleagues (2000) found that the number of changes in residence was associated with an increase in internalizing behaviors at an 18-month follow-up.

Depression

Maltreated children are also at risk for developing depressive disorders. Kendall-Tackett and colleagues (1993) calculated that across six studies, 28% of sexually abused children under 18 years of age showed evidence of depression. More recent research has borne out this association. Johnston and colleagues (2002) reported that direct physical abuse was a significant predictor of depression. Caregivers' level of depression moderated this relationship.

Maltreated children are also at risk for suicide. Of more than 1,000 8-year-old children identified as having been maltreated or being at risk for maltreatment, 9.9% reported suicidal ideation (Thompson et al., 2005). Maltreated children were about twice as likely to report suicidal ideation than those who were at risk. Severity of physical abuse, chronicity of maltreatment, and the presence of multiple types of maltreatment were also significantly associated with suicidal ideation. Other moderator variables included the level of the children's psychological distress, substance abuse, and poor problem solving. Witnessed violence was an especially strong risk factor for suicide (Thompson et al., 2005). Evans, Hawton, and Rodham (2005) found that physically and sexually abused adolescents are also more likely to experience suicidal thoughts and behaviors, with low self-esteem potentiating the risk for suicide.

DEVELOPMENT OF THE AUTONOMOUS SELF AND SELF-ESTEEM

Development of an autonomous self is another early stage-salient developmental issue confronting the young child. The child's experience of caretaking and subsequent development of attachment patterns have particular relevance for the emergence of the self. The young child who receives good care internalizes these experiences and develops a sense of self as worthy, lovable, and deserving of this care and love (Bowlby, 1973). Caregiving that is sensitive to the child's idiosyncratic needs reinforces a greater awareness of self. Furthermore, the young child who is securely attached to a caregiver can use that person as a secure base from which to explore the environment. This potentiates feelings of autonomy and independence. In turn, these feelings lead to an even greater differentiation of self from others and to enhanced self-esteem and self-confidence.

Internal State Language

Internal state language has been regarded as one component of the autonomous self. Internal state words "refer primarily to those words that have explicit reference to internal states ("mad," "happy") rather than words that have implicit connotations of emotion, motivation, or intention" (Beeghly & Cicchetti, 1994, p. 6). Bretherton and Beeghly (1982) showed that by the age of 28 months, most middle-class children master verbal labels for perception (i.e., the five senses), physiological states, goals, intentions, and ability. More than half discuss basic feelings (e.g., anger, sadness), whereas only a few talk about their own thought processes. The use of this internal state language for themselves and others reflects a growing awareness of the self as distinct from others. Internal state language allows young children not only to verbally communicate their feelings but also to clarify misunderstandings with others. The ability to talk about internal states promotes behavioral and affective self-regulation in interpersonal situations: rather than hitting another child, a youngster can express anger or frustration through words.

Maltreated and nonmaltreated 30-month-old toddlers did not differ significantly in receptive vocabulary but differed in their internal state language (Cicchetti & Beegly, 1987). The former used proportionately fewer internal state words, showed less differentiation and attributional focus, and were more context bound in the use of internal state language. Maltreated children were less likely to talk about negative affects (e.g., hate) or physiological states (e.g., hunger, thirst). In contrast, the internal state language of nonmaltreated children from a lower socioeconomic status was very similar to that of middle-class nonmaltreated children. Beeghly and Cicchetti (1994) suggest that maltreated children who attempt to talk about their internal states, especially their negative feelings, may provoke maternal disapproval and considerable anger, thereby increasing the risk of further maltreatment. Consequently, they avoid these discussions to minimize abuse and attenuate their anxiety.

Development of the Autonomous Self and Self-Esteem

Crittenden and DiLalla (1988) described a pattern of "compulsive compliance" in insecurely attached/maltreated children who passively complied with their mothers and did not openly express negative feelings. This behavior may be accompanied by ambiguous affect, masked facial expressions, rote verbal responses, and verbal–nonverbal incongruence. Compulsive compliance is consistent with older psychoanalytic notions of the development of the "false self" (Winnicott, 1965). To reduce anticipated conflict with the caregiver, the child learns to cut off, repress, or falsify the expression of feelings, particularly negative ones. The child then begins to exhibit false positive feelings but experiences few feelings of authenticity in regard to the self. This tendency is also similar to the concept of "other-directedness" described by Briere (1989, 1992). The maltreated child or adult is hypervigilant regarding the abuser's emotional demeanor or behavior. Sustained attention may be advantageous, inasmuch as it allows the individual to either avoid or placate the abuser before maltreatment occurs, but it exacts a significant cost from the developing child. The child is unaware of personal needs, feelings, and motivations, and the growth of self is seriously compromised.

Findings regarding the association between maltreatment and self-esteem are somewhat mixed, especially for sexually abused children. Tong and colleagues (1987) reported that sexually abused girls had significantly lower scores on the Piers–Harris Children's Self-Concept Scale than control girls, but there was no difference between sexually abused and control boys on this measure. Other studies using self-report measures have not found differences in the self-esteem of sexually abused children (Cohen & Mannarino, 1988).

The relationship between maltreatment and self-report of self-esteem is moderated by a number of variables. Studies of physically abused, neglected, and sexually abused children suggest that developmental level may play an important role. Black, Dubowitz, and Harrington (1994) reported that preschool children had elevated scores on measures of perceived competence and social acceptance, whereas school-age children had depressed scores. Black and colleagues (1994) speculated that perceiving themselves as more competent than they actually are might be adaptive for younger maltreated children because it protects them from profound feelings of personal inadequacy. However, by later elementary school, children can better compare themselves with others, thus undermining early efforts to preserve positive self-esteem. Furthermore, children may reconceptualize the meaning of their abusive experiences over time, which may result in different patterns of sequelae and adjustment as they grow older. Thus, self-esteem may suffer as they become more cognizant of the implications and meaning of their history of victimization.

Extreme Disturbances in Self-Definition: Dissociative Disorders

Maltreatment, especially severe abuse, is associated with extreme disturbances in self-definition and self-regulation, such as dissociative disorders. According to DSM-IV (American Psychiatric Association, 1994), the central feature of dissociative disorders is "a disruption in the usually integrated functions of consciousness, memory, identity, or perception of the environment" (p. 477). Types of dissociative disorders include dissociative amnesia—the inability to recall important personal information that cannot be attributed to normal forgetfulness—and dissociative identity disorder (DID, formerly multiple personality disorder), which involves the presence of two or more distinct personalities or identities, each of which take control over the person's behavior at different times (Haugaard, 2004a). Dissociation in children is manifested in disruptions in memory (e.g., having no memories of the trauma), disruptions in perception (e.g., confusion between reality and fantasy, "spacing out"), and disruptions in identity (e.g., DID) (MacFie, Cicchetti, & Toth, 2001).

Studies have shown consistently that maltreated children exhibit more dissociation than nonmaltreated children (see Haugaard, 2004a, and MacFie et al., 2001, for reviews). However, the relative contributions of physical abuse, sexual abuse, and neglect are somewhat unclear. Yeager and Lewis (1996) and MacFie and colleagues (2001) reported that neglect was less highly correlated with dissociation than physical and sexual abuse, whereas Ogawa, Sroufe, Weinfeld, Carlson, and Egeland (1997) found that neglect in infancy predicted dissociation in toddlers and preschoolers. Seventeen-year-old children who had disorganized attachments as infants and who experienced later trauma had the highest dissociation scores.

Haugaard (2004a) has identified the protective functions afforded by dissociation. Dissociation compartmentalizes and sequesters emotionally painful material out of conscious awareness and protects the child from overwhelming psychological and physical pain. The sense of self is altered so that a traumatic event is experienced as if "it's not really happening to me." In DID, the individual usually switches among a series of alter identities that personify specific capacities, functions, or experiences to protect against overwhelming trauma. Dissociation also interferes with memory encoding, resulting in no memory of the trauma. Frequent use of dissociation also interferes with other aspects of development. For example, dissociation in the classroom results in a failure to remember and integrate information, thereby contributing to academic underachievement or even failure. Children may not learn social skills if they dissociate in social situations (Haugaard, 2004a).

This protective function has been examined in several studies. Stovall and Craig (1990) compared the responses of three groups of 7- to 12-year-old girls on the Thematic Apperception Test (TAT). They found that mental representations of the physically abused and sexually abused girls did not differ but were significantly different from those of nonabused girls who came from a "distressed home environment." The abused girls were more likely to have negative unconscious perceptions of themselves and others, but their conscious perceptions of others were more positive.

LANGUAGE DEVELOPMENT

Between the ages of 24 and 36 months, the use of language emerges and becomes more differentiated. The available research suggests that maltreatment poses a substantial risk to the development of language competency in children.

Receptive and Expressive Language

As we have already seen, maltreated children use less internal state language than nonmaltreated children. Studies have examined other aspects of language development in preschool-age and school-age children. Coster, Gersten, Beeghly, and Cicchetti (1989) investigated differences in two groups of 31-month-old maltreated and nonmaltreated toddlers. Although there were no differences in receptive language between the groups, maltreated toddlers had less well developed expressive language. They used syntactically less complex language, scored lower on measures of expressive vocabulary, and showed deficits in discourse abilities—for example, using fewer descriptive phrases and sentences. The maltreated children also talked less about their own activities. They made fewer requests for information and fewer references to persons or events outside the immediate context.

Burke and colleagues (1989) demonstrated an association between expressive language deficits and physical aggression. Expressive language deficits were significantly more prevalent in physically aggressive, physically abused school-age children than in physically abused children who were not physically aggressive. Although expressive language abilities differed, these groups did not show any significant difference in general verbal ability. Katz (1992) reviewed the deleterious effects of neglect on language development. Both physically abused and neglected children evidenced language delays and disorders, but those of neglected children were more severe.

Play and Symbolic–Representational Development

Children's play can also reflect their symbolic and representational development. Play becomes more social and cognitively more symbolic over the preschool years, as evidenced by increasing dramatic play and games with rules. Alessandri (1991) compared the play behavior of 4- to 5-year-old maltreated children with that of nonmaltreated children of the same socioeconomic status. The maltreated group included children who had been physically abused, sexually abused, emotionally mistreated, and neglected. Maltreated children engaged in less play overall and more simple and repetitive play than nonmaltreated children. The former displayed a routine, stereotyped use of play materials, more frequently touched toys but did not directly manipulate them, and engaged in more pounding activities. Nonmaltreated children showed more frequent constructive play (learning to use materials, creating something), in which the play was sequentially organized and purposeful. Alessandri speculated that the more restricted and less elaborated play of maltreated children might be related to their insecure attachments, which undermine their use of the attachment relationship as a secure base from which to explore the environment, thereby contributing to developmental delays in their play. In a subsequent study, Alessandri (1992) found some indirect support for the presence of significant problems in the mother–child relationship. Maltreating mothers were more negative, less involved with their children, and used fewer physical and verbal strategies to direct their children's attention.

COGNITIVE DEVELOPMENT AND ADAPTATION TO SCHOOL

Intellectual and Academic Performance

In general, the literature indicates that maltreatment poses a risk to the child's cognitive development and academic performance. In early work, researchers investigated the cognitive functioning of physically abused children, especially its association with neurological damage. Martin, Beezley, Conway, and Kempe (1974) found that 40% of the physically abused children they studied were functioning within the range of mental retardation. The authors attributed these deficits to neurological impairments sustained in physical assaults by parents. Other earlier studies of physically abused and neglected children who were neurologically intact also reported significant differences in IQ scores between maltreated children and controls (e.g., Barahal, Waterman, & Martin, 1981; Pezzot, 1978).

Investigations of the cognitive functioning of school-age children support the notion that maltreatment poses a risk to academic performance. Physically abused children exhibit serious academic and socioemotional problems. They perform poorly on standardized tests of language and mathematical skills, receive low performance assessments by parents, and are more likely than nonmaltreated peers to have repeated one or more grades. Neglected children score far below the control group on standardized tests of language, reading, and mathematics. In contrast to physically abused children, neglected children do not display significant behavior problems in the classroom and do not differ from controls on any of the socioemotional measures over time (Kurtz, Gaudin, Wodarski, & Mowing, 1993). Kurtz and colleagues (1993) speculated that the characteristics of physically abused children, such as anger, distractibility, anxiety, and lack of self-control, seriously compromise their learning ability. Neglect, which may include a lack of encouragement for learning, little language stimulation, and unresponsiveness to the child's achievements, undermines school success and poses a direct threat to academic performance.

Kendall-Tackett and Eckenrode (1996) confirmed the deleterious effect of neglect on academic achievement; in addition, their data indicated that neglect may also be associated with behavior problems in the classroom. Neglect alone was equally as detrimental to grades and number of suspensions as neglect in combination with physical or sexual abuse. The combination of neglect and abuse had a particularly strong effect on the number of disciplinary referrals and grade repetitions, with abused and neglected junior high school students having the highest number of grade repetitions. Academic performance in all subjects dropped in junior high; neglect and neglect in combination with abuse exacerbated this decline.

In regard to sexually abused children, Trickett, McBride-Chang, and Putnam (1994) compared the classroom academic performance and behavior of 6- to 16-year-old sexually abused girls with those of a nonabused group. Sexual abuse was related to lower classroom ratings of social competence, lower competent-learner ratings, and lower academic performance. Sexually abused girls scored lower on a test of cognitive ability (Peabody Picture Vocabulary Test). These girls showed higher levels of anxious depression, bizarre destructiveness, and dissociative hyperactivity, which in turn were predictive of academic performance, than nonabused girls. Thus, the relationship between sexual abuse and academic functioning is complex and probably mediated by a number of socioemotional variables.

Researchers are now examining the effects of other types of maltreatment on cognitive development. Koenen, Moffitt, Caspi, Taylor, and Purcell (2003) reported a dose–response relationship between domestic violence and IQ: low domestic violence is associated with an average suppression of less than 1 IQ point, medium domestic violence with almost 5 points, and high domestic violence with 8 points. These effects were independent of the genetic effects on IQ and persisted even after they were controlled for direct maltreatment and children's emotional and behavior problems.

Nonorganic Failure-to-Thrive and Psychosocial Dwarfism

Other research has revealed the insidious effects of neglect, especially emotional neglect. Spitz (1945, 1946) reported an infant mortality rate of more than 33% in a sample of 91 institutionalized orphans, despite adequate physical care. The syndrome of nonorganic failure-to-thrive, in which children fail to grow and are apathetic and lethargic, has been described as a consequence of emotional neglect (Bullard, Glaser, Hagarty, & Pivchik, 1967; Garbarino, Guttman, & Seely, 1986). Besides showing compromised physical health and emotional and behavioral problems, many of these children evidence academic and intellectual delays. Oates, Peacock, and Forrest (1985) assessed 14 children who had been admitted to a hospital 12 years earlier and whose condition, in each case, had been diagnosed as failure-to-thrive. Their mean age was 13.4 years. As compared with a group of children matched for age, sex, social class, and ethnic group, the children with previous failure-to-thrive syndrome had significantly lower verbal IQ values on the Wechsler Intelligence Scale for Children—Revised (WISC-R) than the controls. Eight were more than 3 years behind their chronological age in reading ability, whereas only one control group member showed such a delay. Children who had suffered from failure-to-thrive also scored significantly lower on a verbal language development scale. In other follow-up studies, children with nonorganic failure-to-thrive syndrome have shown deficits in intellectual and academic functioning (e.g., Hufton & Gates, 1977). Polansky, Chalmers, Buttenwieser, and Williams (1981) also described the hostile, defiant behavior of young adolescents whose condition had been diagnosed as failure-to-thrive during infancy.

Other syndromes have been linked to severe neglect during childhood. Many years ago Powell and his colleagues (Powell, Brasel, & Blizzard, 1967; Powell, Brasel, Raiti, & Blizzard, 1967) published evidence linking abuse and neglect to psychosocial dwarfism, a syndrome characterized by short stature, intellectual deficits, and behavior problems. Money (1977; Money, Annecillo, & Kelly, 1983) described intellectual delays in such children. However, IQ level rises in those rescued from their abusive or neglectful environment, and increases in IQ are also correlated with increases in height (Money et al., 1983). Money and Annecillo (1976) found that the length of time spent away from the abusive or neglectful environment was the primary variable associated with an increase in IQ scores. A return to the maltreating environment was associated with a decrease in IQ that paralleled a deceleration of the rate of statural growth and puberty onset. Gardner (1972) suggested that the recovery of these children, including their intellectual functioning, may not be complete and that they may continue to evidence deficits in personality structure and intellect.

PEER RELATIONS

Establishing peer relations during preschool-age and school-age years is an important stage-salient developmental task. The successful negotiation of this task depends, in part, on the successful resolution of earlier tasks, including establishment of a secure attachment relationship with the primary caregiver and development of effective emotional and behavioral self-regulation. Failure to establish adaptive relationships with peers and others may interfere significantly with a child's ability to negotiate developmental tasks successfully in later life, leading to continued incompetence and maladaptation. Poor interpersonal relationships are not only strongly associated with concurrent psychiatric disorders in children, but they have predictive validity for future interpersonal difficulties as well (e.g., Garmezy & Streitman, 1974).

We have already described the significant association between maltreatment and physical aggression, but a few more comments can round out our discussion of this topic. Howes (Howes, 1984; Howes & Eldredge, 1985; Howes & Espinosa, 1985) demonstrated the importance of context for maltreated children's physical aggression. When interacting with a familiar peer, maltreated and comparison children behaved similarly, and on some dimensions, maltreated children were more socially competent than comparison children. However, this similarity disappeared when investigators examined their interactions with unfamiliar peers. In a free-play situation, comparison children tended to ignore unfamiliar children, whereas maltreated children tended to become physically aggressive with them, thereby compromising their ability to establish new peer friendships. Maltreated children responded aggressively to peer aggression, whereas nonmaltreated children exhibited either distress or resistance. Furthermore, physically abused children became aggressive when peers became emotionally distressed, but nonmaltreated children responded with prosocial behaviors.

Heightened aggression in peer interactions is not the only reaction maltreated children display. Other studies have reported patterns of withdrawal and avoidance (Dodge, Pettit, & Bates, 1994; Kaufman & Cicchetti, 1989). This may be especially characteristic of the social interactions of neglected children (Hoffman-Plotkin & Twentyman, 1984; Howes & Espinosa, 1985). Results of other studies reveal that maltreated children are less popular and more disliked than their classmates, and their relationships with other children are less likely to be reciprocal. They are more frequently rejected by peers they consider their friends, even their best friends, and they are likely to be negative when interacting with peers (Salzinger, Feldman, Hammer, & Rosario, 1993).

There have been few investigations of sexually abused children's peer relations. Manly and colleagues (1994) assessed the social competence of abused children between the ages of 5 and 11 years. Sexually abused children were rated as more socially competent than physically abused and physically neglected children. As well, the sexually abused group did not differ in social competence from the nonmaltreated group. Conflicting results were obtained by Hibbard and Hartman (1992), who reported that CBCL subscale profiles tended to show withdrawal and impairments in social interaction. The sexually abused children who first joined the Minnesota Mother–Child Interaction Project at age 6 years were socially withdrawn and unpopular, and their dependence on adults was striking.

In summary, maltreated children are at significant risk for the development of a number of problems, including insecure attachments and attachment-disordered behavior, externalizing and internalizing problems, and a compromised sense of self. Maltreatment has also been associated with lower cognitive functioning, poorer adaptation to school, deficiencies in language, and poor peer relationships. Despite being at increased risk for psychological and behavioral problems, maltreated children do not demonstrate a uniform response or reaction to abuse or neglect. Furthermore, there is considerable overlap in the characteristics of children exposed to different subtypes of maltreatment, and some children subjected to abuse or neglect experience only transient effects and others display no symptoms. The outcomes of maltreatment do not fall neatly into one diagnostic category and do not constitute a homogeneous syndrome that we can call "the maltreated child."

This diversity of outcome argues against the notion of a simple or linear connection or pathway between maltreatment and sequelae. The transactional model offers a way of conceptualizing the impact of maltreatment on children. Abuse and neglect, although significant risk factors for many serious problems, interact with other variables, which in turn moderate the impact of maltreatment on the developing child. Furthermore, the model contends that change is possible at many points in an individual's life, and that early toxic experiences do not invariably result in psychopathology. As we describe in Chapter 2, neuroscientists have also advocated such a position, arguing that critical periods in early childhood are atypical and exceptional (Thompson & Nelson, 2001). Indeed, it is on this basic premise of the possibility of change that this book is based. Although less complex conceptualizations are simpler to understand, we must move beyond them to attain a fuller and richer understanding of the lives and experiences of maltreated children. This increased knowledge can enhance our clinical work with these children and their families.

CHAPTER TWO

Mechanisms of Impact

PATHOGENIC PROCESSES

We now review some of the mechanisms responsible for the association between maltreatment and developmental outcomes described in Chapter 1. Although a discussion of these mechanisms and processes remains somewhat hypothetical and more research is needed to corroborate these tentative and incomplete ideas, we hope that it will assist clinicians in their attempts to understand the impact of maltreatment on young clients and to develop useful intervention strategies.

Two key questions form the basis of any clinical assessment. We take the first for granted: "What is the nature of this child's problems and are they clinically significant?" Answers to this question usually entail descriptions of behaviors and assignment of a formal diagnosis. In our experience, some clinicians do not devote as much attention to the second question, "Why is the child exhibiting these problems?," which can be further elaborated: "What are the variables and processes that have contributed to and are maintaining this behavior?" Shirk and Russell (1996) argue that developing interventions on the exclusive basis of a formal diagnosis (i.e., the answer to the first question) is inadequate. They identify a major problem with formal diagnostic systems like DSM-IV: in their attempts to be of use to clinicians of different theoretical orientations, DSM-IV authors largely omitted references to underlying, inferred pathogenic processes and instead focused on observable patterns of symptoms. However, there are multiple pathways to childhood psychopathology. Although children may share the same formal diagnosis, the underlying processes responsible for the overt symptoms may be very different. Identification and explication of these "pathogenic processes" is essential to the selection of effective treatment (Shirk & Russell, 1996). Citing Persons (1991), Shirk and Russell (1996) offer a medical analogy in support of their argument:

> Fever, body aches, and lack of energy, though frequently co-occurring, are insufficient to constitute a diagnostic syndrome. This familiar cluster of symptoms could result from either a viral or bacterial infection, or could be associated with other pathogenic processes. The diagnosis and, in turn, the treatment, depends on the determination of the underlying process. (pp. 146–147)

The same argument is applicable to maltreated children with behavior and emotional problems and is illustrated in the following two case examples.

Geoff is a 10-year-old boy who made his 6-year-old sister perform oral sex on him on several occasions before she disclosed this to her parents. He had used some psychological coercion, telling her he would not play with her if she refused to do this, but he employed no physical force or threats of violence. When confronted by his parents, Geoff immediately acknowledged his behavior, was highly distraught, and did not blame his sister and empathized with her fear. Although they assured Geoff that they loved him, his parents told him they would not tolerate this behavior and placed him under stringent supervision and monitoring. They quickly sought out professional assistance, and Geoff eventually told the psychologist that he had been sexually abused on multiple occasions by an adolescent babysitter. This older boy had forced Geoff to fellate him and had threatened to kill him if he disclosed these acts. A review of Geoff's history revealed that he had been doing well academically and socially and had never exhibited any behavior problems prior to the incidents with his sister. As well, the psychologist regarded his parents as excellent caregivers who were able to support Geoff and his sister. They felt a fair degree of guilt about not knowing about Geoff's sexual abuse history and what he had done to their daughter, and both they and Geoff readily agreed to participate in treatment.

Now consider another 10-year-old boy who was also referred because he had sexually abused his sister:

Sam's 8-year-old sister disclosed that he had forced her to perform oral sex on him despite her objections. She told her parents, but they dismissed the allegations. Eventually, she told her teacher, who referred the matter to child welfare authorities. Although they were somewhat cooperative with the investigating worker, the parents thought that Sam's behavior was "no big deal" and attributed it to the idea that "boys will be boys." Sam adamantly denied the sexual behavior and blamed his sister, claiming she was his parents' "pet" and was just trying to get him in trouble.

A review of Sam's and his family's history revealed many problems. Although he denied any history of direct sexual victimization, he had easy access to his father's extensive collection of adult pornography. A subsequent investigation revealed that this consisted of video and magazine images of women being violently sexually assaulted, including vaginal and oral rape. When confronted, Sam's parents acknowledged having had the pornography in the home for many years and were aware that Sam often looked at it. Although they admitted that this was not a healthy situation for their son, they had imposed no effective limits on him and had not disposed of the material. This attitude was consistent with several previous child welfare reports alleging that Sam had been neglected as an infant and toddler. His parents had refused intervention, and child welfare had not pursued these concerns in the courts. Sam had no real friends and presented as a guarded, aloof child who had immense difficulty in articulating his thoughts and feelings. His parents reluctantly agreed to have Sam participate in therapy, but only after the child welfare worker threatened them with his removal from the home.

At an overt level, the behavior exhibited by Geoff and Sam is the same: they both performed oral sex on a younger sister on several occasions. Moreover, both had been significantly exposed to sexual behavior. However, returning to our earlier consideration of pathogenic processes and moderator variables, significant differences are readily apparent. After completing a thorough evaluation of Geoff and his family, the psychologist was of the opinion that Geoff's behavior was reflective of several pathogenic processes. The sexual behavior with the sister reflected his attempts to attenuate his sense of powerlessness and vulnerability engendered by the adolescent's threats to kill him; rather than being a passive victim, Geoff now became the initiator. In fact, Geoff described a number of PTSD symptoms, including nightmares, difficulty in concentrating and sleeping, intrusive memories of the assaults, and constantly checking and monitoring the whereabouts of the adolescent perpetrator who lived on the same block (hypervigilance). These symptoms exacerbated his feelings of powerlessness and potentiated his need to demonstrate, via the sexual behavior with his sister, that he was now strong and in control. He also revealed he had experienced considerable sexual arousal during his own abuse, and had wanted to engage in this behavior because of the sexual excitement.

The psychologist determined that Geoff had secure attachments to both his mother and father. Although we describe the processes that underlie attachment in much more detail later, we note here that it is probable that this secure attachment was responsible for Geoff's expectation that his parents would not reject him and would be able to meet his needs, thereby facilitating his quick admission of guilt. His intact basic trust in other people rendered him a good candidate for a therapeutic relationship, and his sensitivity to others' feelings promoted an empathic appreciation of his sister's distress. Geoff talked articulately about salient issues, a skill reflective of the adaptive emotional and behavioral self-regulatory abilities engendered by his parents' long-standing application of clear and consistent expectations and limits and the excellent cognitive and verbal stimulation he received at home. The sexual abuse of his sister was not indicative of chronically poor behavioral self-regulation but, as we have seen, more a reaction to his own victimization. Finally, his parents' very appropriate responses postdisclosure (e.g., seeking out assistance, imposition of close monitoring and supervision, willingness to participate in therapy with Geoff) made a positive prognosis much more likely.

Although Sam had not been directly sexually abused like Geoff, he experienced strong feelings of sexual arousal and had begun to masturbate when looking at his father's pornography. He admitted to the psychologist that he had begun to have fantasies of engaging in the same sexual behavior while masturbating, especially about coercing girls to fellate him. Given his history of chronic neglect, it was not surprising that Sam had no confidence that his parents would meet his massive needs for nurturance and care. He had also generalized this expectation to others, which had resulted in a guarded, emotionally distant interpersonal style. Sam became especially angry when he thought his parents were paying more attention to his sister, whom he regarded as "their pet." Unfortunately, Sam began to fuse this hostility to his sister with the sexual aggression toward females modeled in his father's pornography. The fantasies developed to the point where he visualized orally raping his sister "to get back at her." Furthermore, residing with caregivers who rarely commented on their son's internal affective states or even verbally articulated their own feelings, combined with inconsistent and lax discipline, had significantly potentiated Sam's tendency to inappropriately externalize his feelings, including his anger toward his sister. This precluded the possibility that he could empathize with her feelings. Along with his parents' nonchalance and long-standing difficulties in imposing firm and consistent limits on Sam's behavior and their difficulty in meeting his needs, these pathogenic processes served to increase the risk that he would engage in the same behavior in the future.

If we had only focused on the sexual behavior and had not initiated a more refined evaluation of the underlying processes and variables contributing to these boys' difficulties, we might have recommended similar interventions. However, given this analysis, treatment selection and plans were derived from conceptualizations of the respective pathogenic processes and moderator variables. Of course, we must also consider what the literature on empirically supported therapies (ESTs) tells us about what works. As we argue in Chapter 4, integrating knowledge of ESTs and conceptualizations of the contributions of unique pathogenic processes to maltreated children's symptomatology is an essential component of developing effective treatment plans.

Returning to our case examples: Geoff might benefit from an approach that equips him with cognitive-behavioral strategies to control the inappropriate expression of his sexual arousal and to alleviate the PTSD symptoms (e.g., relapse prevention, exposure), while at the same time helping him modify his attributions of the meaning of his sexual abuse (cognitive restructuring), that is, that he is an inadequate child who is powerless to prevent any future assaults. Developmentally, he is well suited for these strategies, given his solid cognitive and verbal abilities and the ease with which he would establish a productive therapeutic relationship. Geoff's parents might benefit from assistance and guidance about how to help their children, such as the therapist's reinforcing their supervision of Geoff's behavior and guidance on how to repair the relationship between the siblings. However, because of their solid parenting skills, they would not require the same level of intervention that Sam's parents need.

Given our understanding of the processes and variables responsible for the problematic behavior, interventions with Sam and his family would be much more extensive. Basic interventions for this youngster would include helping him develop some rudimentary self-regulatory skills, especially those he could use to control his anger toward his sister. Indeed, assisting Sam to accurately identify his internal states and to use words, rather than actions, might well constitute preliminary steps. Immediately putting him into a traditional cognitive-behavioral program that emphasizes the verbal expression of feelings and cognitions might be counterproductive or even harmful. Sam probably would encounter real difficulty with such requisite skills because of his poor verbal abilities, thereby increasing his frustration and anger and eroding his self-esteem even more. Given his exposure to pornography, he requires intensive help to understand the deleterious effects of sexual abuse on others, and we may anticipate that this would be a long and protracted process, given his core deficits in empathy. As much of his anger stems from the insecure attachment with his parents and their inability to meet his needs, working with his parents would be a central component of intervention. Helping them establish a more secure attachment; teaching them to monitor, supervise, and set firm limits on Sam's sexual behavior; guiding them to encourage and support his attempts to verbalize his feelings; and helping them to appreciate what is wrong about their son's sexual behavior are just some of the major targets of intervention with these parents.

These two case examples reinforce the need for clinicians to go beyond simple descriptions of overt behavior to an explication of the pathogenic processes and moderator variables responsible for maltreated children's symptomatology. Such conceptualizations, along with knowledge of ESTs, guide treatment selection. The rest of this chapter describes the major mechanisms of impact.

INTERNAL WORKING MODELS AND INTERPERSONAL SCHEMAS: GENERAL CONSIDERATIONS AND SOCIAL INFORMATION-PROCESSING STYLES OF MALTREATED CHILDREN

We believe that Bowlby's (1969, 1973, 1980, 1982) concept of the internal working model (IWM) is central to an understanding of the association between maltreatment and developmental outcome and has special relevance for clinicians who work with maltreated youngsters.

Although we briefly mentioned the concept of IWMs in Chapter 1, we elaborate on this fundamental notion here before we discuss the ways in which IWMs may mediate the relationship between maltreatment and outcome. Through actual interactions and interchanges with the primary caregiver, children begin to acquire mental representations, or IWMs, of the parent–child relationship. The IWM has two primary components. The first comprises children's information about, expectations of, and feelings about other people (whether these individuals will be responsive, trustworthy, accessible, and caring or, to the contrary, unresponsive, untrustworthy, inaccessible, and uncaring). Children's corresponding representations of themselves and their own roles in these relationships (whether they are worthy and capable of obtaining the other's care or whether they are unworthy and incapable of obtaining adequate care) constitute the second component.

As well as expectations about the self and others derived from actual experiences, the IWM includes unconscious rules for processing attachment-related information and memories. It affects how the individual perceives, remembers, interprets, and reacts to these experiences (Salzinger, Feldman, Ng-Mak, Mojica, & Stockhammer, 2001; Sroufe et al., 1999; Toth, Cicchetti, MacFie, & Emde, 1997). According to this concept, early relationship experiences become internalized as mental representations and create anticipatory images that shape attitudes and reactions to, and perceptions of, individuals encountered in the future. The individual is provided with a basic context for subsequent transactions with the environment, especially social relationships. For instance, if a child experiences and mentally represents caregivers as available, nurturing, and trustworthy, this information contributes to the child's more general model of others as available and trustworthy. Furthermore, the child regards the self as competent and effective in relation to these other individuals and worthy of being treated in a sensitive and caring manner. Conversely, if experiences of their relationships with caregivers have been characterized by unavailability, uncertainty, and insensitivity, children may develop negative expectations of other caregiving relationships. They regard themselves as unworthy and incapable of obtaining adequate care from parental figures. Children abused for many years and from an early age may expect similar treatment in new relationships.

Clinicians who treat maltreated children will readily recognize this phenomenon. A child whose caregivers consistently ignored or denigrated expressions of distress and requests for help may generalize this set of expectations to new caregivers, such as foster parents. The IWM, an accurate representation of the original dyadic interactions played out on countless occasions, now mediates the child's response in the new environment: the child avoids expressing distress and resists overtures of assistance from foster parents. On those occasions when the foster parents try to help, the child may interpret such attempts in ways consistent with the original IWM. For example, the foster parent may be unable to respond immediately when the child is distressed, perhaps having to tend to another child who is hurt or sick. Even if the delay is only several minutes, which most children regard as unavoidable in such circumstances and as having nothing to do with the caregiver's caring for or commitment to the child, maltreated children misinterpret the caregiver's intention or motivation. They may regard the delayed response as yet another piece of evidence that caregivers are unreliable and insensitive, thereby consolidating the IWM and eliciting even more avoidance or anger in the child. Unfortunately, some caregivers respond negatively to these reactions, such as by personalizing the child's avoidance ("He shows no reaction when I try to help him. He wants nothing to do with me!"), and eventually reject the child. Such reactions consolidate and confirm these expectations, leading to a self-perpetuating cycle. Sroufe (1983) and Suess, Grossmann, and Sroufe (1992) demonstrated that children with avoidant attachment organizations not only expect rejection but also elicit this reaction from others.

These data are consistent with Bowlby's (1969, 1973) claim that there are multiple pathways or trajectories to normality and abnormality. Continuity occurs when the individual's experiences are consistent with the personal IWM. Maltreatment in infancy may engender an insecure attachment organization and set the child on a particular developmental pathway. Subsequent experiences, such as continued exposure to abuse and neglect and subsequent adaptations by the child, support the child's course down this pathway. Other experiences and circumstances, including those discrepant from the ones underlying the IWM, may deflect the individual's trajectory (Bowlby, 1988a). Although this theory posits that change remains possible, Bowlby (1973) maintained that it becomes more unlikely the longer the child follows a maladaptive pathway. As we shall see later, a central therapeutic task with many maltreated children is to generate this sense of discontinuity to modify a maladaptive IWM.

As we emphasized in Chapter 1, organized attachments (secure, avoidant, and ambivalent) are adaptive in the original child–caregiver relationships in which they developed. They protect the child from further maltreatment, regulate the child's stress, and maintain proximity to the caregiver. Problems arise when the child generalizes or transfers the strategy, along with the constituent perceptions, interpretations, and reactions, to new relationships wherein people have no intention of responding insensitively or abusively. The child is hardly a passive recipient of experience. Rather, he or she is an active constructor of reality who both creates experiences and differentially attends to diverse information in the social world. In describing the influence of Bowlby's concept of IWMs, Sroufe and colleagues (1999) state:

> While simple and straightforward, this is a profound idea. It means that children approach new situations with certain preconceptions, behavioral biases, and interpretive tendencies. Thus, context, even new circumstances and new arenas, are not independent of the child's history. (p. 5)

We can expand this notion by examining the concept of interpersonal schemas (IS). A schema in general is a way of mentally representing knowledge. According to Dalgleish (2004):

> The task of schemas is the organization of knowledge at different levels of abstraction. By dint of such organization schematic representations bring order to the chaos of a lifetime of myriad experiences through the coding of the commonalities and regularities of these experiences and the representation of them in the mind. (p. 232)

IS are expectations about others' probable responses to the self. Unlike IWMs, they refer to a broad range of relational patterns, rather than being tied to the caregiving or care-receiving patterns central to attachment theory (Shirk, 1998). However, like IWMs, IS affect the range of what can be perceived, how perceptions are interpreted, and how the person behaves in accordance with these models.

There is considerable support for the influence of maltreated children's expectations on their perceptions and attention to threat-related stimuli. Rieder and Cicchetti (1989) found that maltreated children were more hypervigilant to aggressive stimuli than were nonmaltreated children. The introduction of aggressive distractions into a practiced task disrupted performance of the former more than it did for the nonmaltreated children. In addition, maltreated children recalled a greater number of distracting aggressive stimuli than did nonmaltreated youngsters. More recent work by Pollak and colleagues (Pollak, Cicchetti, Hornung, & Reed, 2000; Pollak & Sinha, 2002; Pollak & Tolley-Schell, 2003) has extended these findings. They demonstrated that physically abused children overattend to angry facial expressions, require less visual information to detect the presence of angry facial expressions, and have difficulty disengaging their attention from angry facial cues.

As well as influencing what maltreated children perceive in social relationships, IS affect children's interpretations of social interactions. Downey, Feldman, Khuir, and Friedman (1994) reviewed evidence that abused children develop a predisposition to anticipate rejection in their relationships, a concept they called "rejection sensitivity." Salzinger and colleagues (2001) subsequently reported that physically abused 9- to 12-year-old children were less likely than nonabused youngsters to expect their classmates to choose them positively and, at the same time, more likely to behave aggressively and less likely to engage in prosocial behaviors. These negative social expectations also mediated the relationship between abuse and internalizing problems.

This is similar to Dodge's research on the social information-processing styles of physically abused children (Dodge, Bates, & Pettit, 1990; Dodge et al., 1994; Dodge, Pettit, & Bates, 1997). Physically abused, aggressive, school-age boys are biased in their interpretations of peers' behavior. They make attributions of malicious intent and hostility in ambiguous social situations when no such motives are present, fail to attend to relevant cues, and express more positive evaluations of aggressive behavior. These attributional biases and deficits in processing social information are associated with an increase in aggressive behavior toward peers, similar to that found in the children described by Salzinger and colleagues (2001). Unfortunately, the aggressive behavior elicits rejection and even aggressive responses from other children, thereby confirming the expectation of unsatisfying and hostile reactions from others. A clinical example illustrates the negative influence of such misperceptions and misattributions.

Child welfare authorities took Gary into care when he was 6 years old. He had been severely physically and psychologically abused, and neglected by a woman to whom Gary's mother had entrusted his care when he was a toddler. He was placed in a foster home and began school for the first time in a grade 1 classroom at a large elementary school. At recess Gary began to experience intense anxiety. He told his therapist he was frightened by the behavior of some of the other children on the playground. According to Gary, "They were screaming at me and chasing me, and they was gonna hurt me!" He had interpreted this behavior as evidence that they were going to assault him. His teacher had observed these incidents and reported that the other children were merely playing an enthusiastic game of tag and that some had happened to run in Gary's general direction. Although the children were indeed yelling, their affective tone was happy and positive. Gary had not only misinterpreted their intention (i.e., that they were pursuing him and were going to hurt him), but he had even misperceived their smiles and laughter.

The years of abuse and terror he suffered had severely compromised Gary's expectation of social relationships. His hypervigilance was adaptive and protective when he resided with his abusive caregiver. It enabled him to quickly perceive cues that preceded her assaults, such as her yelling at him, and he would then quickly leave the apartment to protect himself. The regularities of his past abuse, represented as IS, acted as a filter through which new experiences were processed. New information was selectively processed and assimilated into his existing schematic structure. Gary had generalized these expectations to the novel school environment, and his IS were not yet open to discrepant information about how people would treat him. He expected the same pattern of assaults and anticipated that he would be abused again. According to Crittenden (1992b), "Representational models can, thus, become a double-edged sword. They both speed the process through which infants respond adaptively to their environments and also skew the processing of future experience to fit existing models of experience" (p. 578). Research does indeed indicate that information processing is biased in favor of maintaining the status quo with respect to schema content (Dalgleish, 2004).

Shirk (1998) presented several models to explain the operation of IS and how they influence behavior. The preemptive processing model contends that IS sensitize children to negative aspects of social interactions, which in turn amplify negative emotional reactions and problematic behavioral responses. This is associated with the biased and deficient patterns of social information processing we have just described. Gary's response to other children's screaming and running toward him is a good example. He was primed to perceive and attribute negative intent to people's behavior to the exclusion of other perceptions and interpretations because his early history had preempted his realistic perception and interpretation of his social world. The schema-triggered affect model maintains that stressful interpersonal events activate problematic IS, which then elicit related emotions. There were occasions when Gary's foster father became somewhat frustrated with his oppositional and defiant behavior. Whereas most children take these interactions in stride, Gary assumed his foster father's mild expressions of frustration were precursors to assaults, which activated the IS that he would be abused once again.

Shirk (1998) also described several characteristics of maladaptive IS. As we have already argued, they are overgeneralized and decontextualized; that is, although they were adaptive in the original context, they are transposed to new social situations that are, in certain important respects, dissimilar to the original social interactions; in a way, such IS are archaic. Children generalize the IS without identifying the essential differences. IS are also chronically accessible. Low levels of emotional arousal or limited degrees of situational specificity easily evoke IS. Minor disruptions in social interactions (e.g., a very minor delay in responding to a child's distress) also activate the IS and the associated affect. Finally, Shirk described IS as rigid and as becoming increasingly solidified with repeated experience.

Although these internal models are open to change (as suggested by the term "working"), Bowlby (1980), Bretherton (1987), and Sroufe and colleagues (1999) maintain that models become so ingrained or overlearned that they begin operating outside awareness. In one sense, this is advantageous, as it economizes effort and makes people efficient processors of information in different situations and is consistent with recent notions of the "adaptive unconscious" that researchers have claimed we all possess. Wilson (2002) describes the adaptive unconscious:

> The mind operates most efficiently by relegating a good deal of high-level, sophisticated thinking to the unconscious, just as a modern jetliner is able to fly on automatic pilot with little or no input from the human, "unconscious" pilot. The adaptive unconscious does an excellent job of sizing up the world, warning people of danger, setting goals, and initiating action in a sophisticated and efficient manner. (pp. 6–7)

We refer the reader to Malcolm Gladwell's (2005) recent bestseller, *Blink: The Power of Thinking without Thinking*, for a highly readable and entertaining account of this phenomenon.

Returning to maltreated children: They may be efficient processors of information as they repeatedly subject interpersonal behaviors to the same interpretations. These children need not engage in the strenuous mental efforts associated with a more critical and thoughtful analysis of social information. Although efficient, rapid processing of social information may lead to inaccurate perceptions and interpretations of others' behaviors and intentions. Individuals adhere rigidly to these maladaptive assumptions and beliefs, even in the face of discrepant information, because they are stable and protect them from the surprise and disorganization that a reworking of these models would entail (McCrone, Egeland, Kalkoske, & Carlson, 1994). In other words, stable organization is counterbalanced by oversimplification and possible distortion.

McCrone and colleagues (1994) integrate the traditional notion of defense mechanisms with the idea of multiple working models, claiming that young maltreated children cannot integrate discrepant and incompatible information from different models. For example, a child beaten from infancy or toddlerhood may have developed painful and unpleasant memories and a subsequent model of parents as dangerous and rejecting figures. However, the parents may have told the child that they were carrying out beatings because they loved and cared for the child (i.e., "It's for your own good"). Such statements may have generated a memory far more tolerable to the child. Rather than acknowledging that the beatings reflect the parents' hostility or even hatred, the child retains them at an unconscious level to avoid confronting overwhelming anxiety and sadness. Other models, "My parents really do love me, and that's why they are punishing me like this," are much more tolerable. In an extreme form, the child may idealize the parents. This defensive strategy, although adaptive in the short term, leaves children with little awareness of their sadness, anger, and anxiety. This is one example of defensive exclusion, the process that prevents individuals from consciously experiencing their own feelings, noticing what is going on in their lives, or signaling a need for help. However, models and feelings excluded from consciousness still exert a potent and sometimes malevolent influence on the child's adaptation to the world. For example, McCrone and colleagues compared maltreated children's responses on a projective storytelling task with those of nonmaltreated children. Maltreated children's stories revealed a significantly greater tendency to attend selectively to, and elaborate on, negative aspects, especially aggression, of interpersonal relationships. This finding is consistent with the hypersensitivity of maltreated children to aggressive stimuli reported by Rieder and Cicchetti (1989) and Pollak and Tolley-Schell (2003) and the social information-processing biases reported by Dodge and colleagues (1997). Our earlier description of Gary's responses to social stimuli is also consistent with the notion that maltreated children have IWMs/IS operating outside awareness yet influencing responses to interpersonal situations.

These processes may explain findings that abused children frequently strike out at a peer who is exhibiting emotional distress (Howes & Espinosa, 1985; Main & George, 1985; Troy & Sroufe, 1987). A peer's distress may elicit mental images and memories of instances when the maltreated child was similarly distressed and attachment figures had rejected the youngster or had not met his or her needs. As these memories and images often are intolerable, the child may strike out at the peer who exhibits this distress to terminate it and thereby avoid personal feelings of anxiety and pain.

ATTACHMENT ORGANIZATION AND EMOTIONAL AND BEHAVIORAL SELF-REGULATION

Our review indicates that maltreated children are more likely than nonmaltreated ones to engage in more disruptive, withdrawn, and aggressive behaviors and fewer prosocial behaviors. These behaviors are suggestive of problems in self-regulation. Many factors contribute to competence in behavioral and emotional self-regulation, including the child's level of physiological arousal and his or her capacity to verbalize internal affective states (Buchsbaum, Toth, Clyman, Cicchetti, & Ernde, 1992). We have highlighted the link between disorganized attachment and the risk for psychopathology. At the level of emotion regulation, children with a disorganized attachment face unresolvable fear because the attachment figure is the source of the fear. Cassidy and Mohr (2001) hypothesize that such children have not learned effective coping skills to use to soothe and control their feelings and behavior in frightening situations, which leads to problems in emotional and behavioral self-regulation. Moreover, children with a disorganized attachment are prone to take control of aspects of the parent–child relationship during the preschool years (Main & Hesse, 1990). Although such a controlling interpersonal style helps maintain connection to the parent and attenuates anxiety arising from living in an unpredictable and chaotic world, the child's bossiness and dominance may alienate peers and lead to further rejection. Furthermore, given negative expectations of relationships, maltreated children may relate to others with a general lack of enthusiasm, confidence, and overall positive affective stance. Friendlier and more cooperative children are more highly regarded by their peers, whereas aggressive children tend to be rejected (Asher & Coie, 1990; Denham, McKinley, Couchoud, & Holt, 1990). The absence of this positive affective stance impedes the establishment and maintainance of positive peer relationships and further consolidates maltreated children's models of others as unreliable, unresponsive figures and of themselves as unworthy of friendship.

Other qualities of the attachment relationship have particular significance for the attainment of behavioral and affective self-regulation in young children. A principal task of infants' parents is to help them modulate their physiological arousal. Buchsbaum and colleagues (1992) describe some of the processes responsible for this development; for example, parents respond to particular affective displays by their child and discourage others. Parents also begin to teach children alternate ways of expressing feelings. These characteristics of parenting are, of course, consistent with those that promote a secure attachment. Parents who articulate an accurate and empathic perception and understanding of their children's internal states and corresponding needs facilitate their understanding of their minds and use of internal state language. Rather than acting out feelings such as anger in impulsive, destructive ways, the child slowly begins to learn to talk about them. Parents who pay little or no attention to their children's feelings or who cannot perceive these feelings accurately may seriously compromise the children's ability to develop adaptive self-regulatory capabilities.

A "goal-corrected partnership" in which a child increasingly takes the attachment figure's own motivations and plans into account is a major result of the child's establishment of a secure relationship with a primary caregiver (Bowlby, 1969). In this phase, which usually begins some time after the third birthday, verbal interchanges between child and parent are a principal means for the two to communicate their respective needs and successfully negotiate a plan that takes these into account. Several factors account for this developmental advance. A secure attachment between the child and parent, characterized by parental sensitivity to the child's feelings and internal states, plays a significant role in the parent's ability and willingness to engage in these discussions with the child. Furthermore, the parent's ability to meet a child's needs models a particular style of interaction and the child incorporates this sensitivity and an appreciation of the parent's and others' needs and perspectives into his or her interpersonal style. Consequently, the child's burgeoning language skills and developing ability to see the world through the perspective of another individual result in more effective communication between the child and parent. Rather than acting out these feelings and behavior in maladaptive ways, the child engages in dialogue, and the two can then negotiate conflicts and disagreements successfully. These parental qualities that promote secure attachment, such as sensitivity to the child's internal states, afford the young child an initial model of reciprocity and sharing. This model then generalizes to other relationships and contributes significantly to rewarding adaptive interchanges with others.

Pears and Fisher (2005) regard the emergence of the goal-corrected partnership as a critical period for "theory of mind development." Theory of mind is the ability to recognize that other people may hold different ideas, desires, and beliefs that may affect their behaviors (Dunn, 1995).

Pears and Fisher contend that maltreatment may impede the development of theory of mind, as power-assertive parenting practices, such as yelling or hitting, do little to give children information about the specific effects of their behavior. Rather than the parent's identifying and talking about how he or she feels, hitting conveys very little except that the parent is angry. We have also seen that the same may be true of an insecure attachment wherein children receive little or no information about their feelings or their parents'. Maltreated children's attributional biases and their failure to attend to all the relevant cues and stimuli in social situations may preclude them from reaching a more accurate understanding of others' feelings and intentions. Fonagy, Redfern, and Charman (1997) reported that children's insecure attachments were significantly associated with poor theory of mind capabilities, even when age, intelligence, and social maturity were controlled for. Maltreatment is also related to delays in the development of theory of mind (Cicchetti, Rogosch, Maughan, Toth, & Bruce, 2003), as is being in foster care (Pears & Fisher, 2005). Overall, maltreated children are at significant risk for difficulties in interpreting and empathizing with others' thoughts, beliefs, and feelings, which contributes to their social incompetence.

Children's developing capacity to identify their internal states is also a crucial step in the emergence of "reflective functioning" (Fonagy, 1991; Fonagy, Gergely, Jurist, & Target, 2002; Hughes, 2004; Kretchmar, Worsham, & Swenson, 2005). Within a secure attachment, parents communicate an accurate understanding of their child's mind, and the child eventually becomes able to identify and express his or her inner life. This is similar to the concept of insight (Kretchmar et al., 2005) and "allows individuals access to their defensive processes (e.g., avoiding intimacy) so that these defenses are not automatically perpetuated in relationships (Fonagy & Target, 1997)" (Kretchmar et al., 2005, pp. 32–33). Cassidy and Mohr (2001) assert that reflective functioning may moderate a child's responses to maltreatment as the capacity to self-reflect on one's mental states facilitates resolution of the maltreatment. Children who lack this ability are unlikely to resolve these experiences and are prone to develop the disorganized intrapsychic and interpersonal life and self-destructive behaviors characteristic of a borderline personality disorder.

Attachment Organization and the Secure-Base Phenomenon

There may be other ways that IWMs mediate a child's response to maltreatment. A key concept of attachment theory is that of the "secure base." A basic component of human nature is the urge to explore the environment, which is antithetical to attachment behavior (Bowlby, 1988b). However, if the child feels secure in the relationship with a caregiver, this person can be used as a secure base from which to explore and become acquainted with the world. Essentially, the child develops a mental representation of the caretaker as reliable and responsive, someone who will take care of the child if difficulties are encountered while exploring his or her world.

Experience with the physical and social environment is critical to an infant's and young child's cognitive, language, and social development. Studies by Aber and his colleagues (Aber & Allen, 1987; Aber, Allen, Carlson, & Cicchetti, 1989) have shown that maltreated preschoolers and school-age children (through physical neglect, emotional maltreatment, and physical abuse) exhibit increased dependence on others and decreased "effectance motivation"—that is, the child's motivation to deal competently with the environment for the intrinsic pleasure of mastery (Aber et al., 1989). High effectance motivation, low dependence, and high cognitive maturity constitute the "secure readiness factor" (Aber et al., 1989). Low secure readiness-to-learn is manifested by maltreated infants and toddlers. They have difficulty in balancing their feeling comfortable with adults while exploring new aspects of the environment, and this difficulty may be accompanied by cognitive deficits. Maltreated children also may not feel comfortable enough to engage in new social relationships, which may well compromise the development of their social skills.

An impaired ability to explore the environment is by no means the only factor associated with the academic and cognitive difficulties of maltreated children. Other features of the caretaking environment in which the abuse or neglect occurs play a contributory role. One to consider is inadequate cognitive stimulation. For example, Vondra, Barnett, and Cicchetti (1990) demonstrated that the receptive language abilities of physically abused/neglected preschoolers were related to the quality of the home environment, especially the physical condition of the home and the availability of toys. We have already reviewed the detrimental effects of a neglectful environment, including little stimulation, lack of encouragement for learning, and an unresponsive attitude to the child's intellectual efforts or achievements.

Attachment Organization and the Development of the Self

Perceptions and representations of the self and the self in relation to significant others form a central component of IWMs. Negative self-esteem and self-evaluation are consistent with the experiences of a child who has received inadequate care. A child may begin to regard him- or herself as ineffectual or powerless, either in eliciting adequate caretaking from others or in terminating maltreatment. This latter concept is analogous to Finkelhor and Browne's (1985) concept of powerlessness. Maltreated youngsters may experience a sense of powerlessness because of their inability to avoid or stop the physical and emotional invasion of their bodies and internal lives. Children feel a similar sense of inadequacy and lack of control over their worlds when they cannot effect changes in the neglectful and inattentive child-rearing practices of their parents. Of course, feelings of powerlessness may be exacerbated by the perpetrator's coercion and manipulation or by ineffective responses of parents or caregivers (e.g., denial, lack of protective action). Larger social systems (e.g., child welfare programs, the judicial system) may respond to children's disclosures in ways that also diminish the child's self-efficacy, for example, by requiring children to undergo multiple investigative interviews or court appearances.

We have examined the concept of defense mechanisms from the perspective of IWMs and attachment theory. Incompatible information from different models is kept apart by defenses such as projection, displacement, splitting, and dissociation. Although these defenses arise to help the child cope with the painful and overwhelming affects and cognitions arising from traumatic experiences, they lead to an unintegrated sense of self, including the emergence of dissociative disorders. We reviewed the evidence indicative of a link between early disorganized attachments and later dissociation (e.g., Ogawa et al., 1997). Liotti (1999) suggests that a child with a disorganized attachment is more vulnerable to altered or dissociative states because of the constant and contradictory actions of seeking and fleeing from the attachment figure. The growth of an autonomous self may also be stunted by the phenomenon of "other-directedness": to monitor the abuse or rejection they believe is inevitable in interpersonal relationships, maltreated individuals become hypervigilant and focus on the other person's emotional state to the exclusion of their own (Briere, 1992).

We believe attachment theory, particularly in its emphasis on IWMs, contributes much to our understanding of the association between maltreatment and developmental outcome. The theory's extensive empirical base and growing popularization in the media may lead some overzealous proponents to rely on it exclusively to explain every human problem or suffering. This would be a grave mistake. A secure attachment in infancy and toddlerhood does not necessarily ensure later competence. Conversely, although an insecure early attachment is a significant risk factor for the development of a later psychopathologic condition, a poor outcome is not inevitable. There are many pathways between maltreatment and later adaptation. We would be remiss if we failed to describe other factors, processes, and mechanisms that contribute to the emergence of maladaptive behavior and psychopathologic conditions. It is to these conceptualizations we now turn.

CONDITIONING THEORIES

Mowrer (1960) proposed a two-factor (classical and instrumental conditioning) learning theory to explain the development of anxiety and avoidance that is directly relevant for our understanding of the development of PTSD. In this paradigm, a previously neutral stimulus becomes associated with an unconditioned stimulus that innately evokes discomfort or fear. Applying this paradigm to maltreatment, the abuse or maltreatment is the unconditioned stimulus that evokes fear, whereas other aspects of the situation (e.g., perpetrator, environmental context) represent the neutral stimulus. The neutral stimulus then acquires aversive properties such that its presence elicits anxiety. It now becomes a conditioned stimulus for fear responses (see Figure 2.1).

In a case of child sexual abuse, the fears the child experienced as a direct consequence of the sexual abuse could be associated with the perpetrator or environmental stimuli. The child would then experience feelings of fear and anxiety in the presence of these stimuli, particularly in situations most similar to those in which the abuse occurred (e.g., being alone with the perpetrator or being in a room where the abuse occurred). Over time

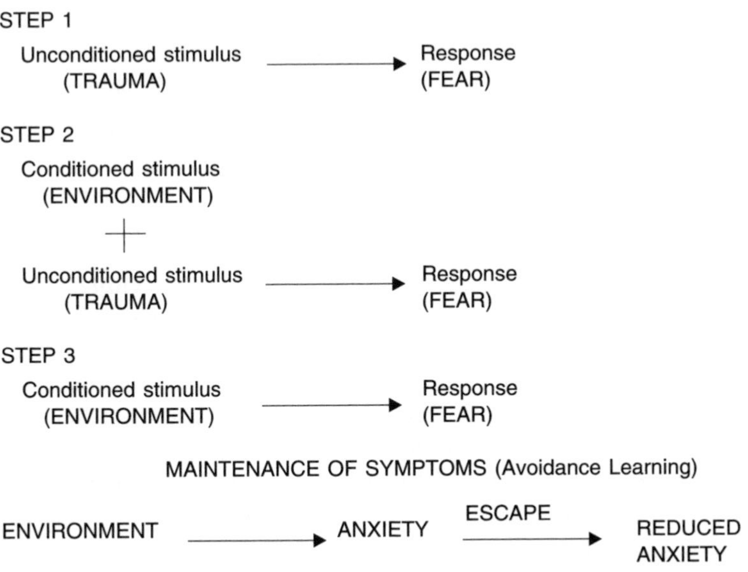

FIGURE 2.1. Development and maintenance of symptoms.

the child's fear could, through generalization, produce anxiety in the presence of persons (e.g., other males) or other stimuli (e.g., physical surroundings, sights, sounds, smells) similar to those associated with the abuse. Through higher order conditioning, these more recently conditioned cues for anxiety could themselves become paired with other previously neutral stimuli, producing still more cues for anxiety and leading to feelings of pervasive anxiety.

The second factor of Mowrer's (1960) model postulates that avoidance or escape responses, which decrease or end the discomfort that arises in the presence of the conditioned stimuli, are reinforced when this discomfort or anxiety decreases. Wachtel (1973) argues that defenses such as repression can be understood as a learned process of avoiding thoughts and events associated with anxiety. By not thinking of the abuse, the maltreated child minimizes his or her own discomfort, and these avoidant behaviors or thoughts are reinforced as the individual learns to redirect attention from the cues or signals associated with fear. In effect, repression is conceptualized in terms of avoidance learning. This defensive maneuver has some harmful consequences. If a child's avoidance of thoughts or discussions about the maltreatment is reinforced, the child never learns at what point, if any, fears are no longer justified or adaptive. By not examining or talking about the maltreatment, the child minimizes discomfort but also eliminates the possibility of exposure to the cues and affects associated with these fears. Therefore, the anxiety does not extinguish. Furthermore, the child is unable to examine other central issues critically, such as whether the maltreatment was deserved. Thus, the seemingly protective reaction on the part of parents of telling children "to forget about what happened" is not beneficial.

ATTRIBUTION THEORY

The case for using Mowrer's theory to explain PTSD is compelling. It accounts for the addition of fear to trauma-related cues that previously were neutral. It also explains why individuals with PTSD avoid seemingly innocuous situations and how such avoidance persists despite its disruption of daily functioning (Foa, Steketee, & Rothbaum, 1989). However, Foa and colleagues (1989) also raise some objections. They note that Mowrer's two-stage theory does not explain other PTSD symptoms and ignores the etiological significance of the meaning ascribed to aversive events. For example, such an event may destroy or compromise formerly held basic concepts of safety and inviolability: one's world becomes less predictable and controllable. Citing evidence that perceived threat better predicts PTSD than does actual threat, Foa and colleagues argue that any model of the development of PTSD must incorporate the significance of the meaning of the event for the individual. This argument is consistent with phenomenology that "refers to the survivor's personal experiences and perceptions as an important criterion for therapeutic reactions, rather than sole reliance on theoretical notions that may or may not fit the survivor's experience" (Briere, 1992, p. 84).

Most conceptualizations of trauma have incorporated a phenomenological perspective. As Lewandowski and Baranoski (1994) note, the definition of a trauma as a sudden, untoward event depends on one's perspective. A meta-analytic review demonstrated that interpersonal violence (childhood sexual and physical abuse, rape, criminal assault, and domestic violence) has deleterious effects on children's and adults' psychological adjustment (Weaver & Clum, 1995). Subjective factors, such as general appraisal of the incident, self-blame, and perceived life threat, contributed twice as much to the magnitude of psychological distress as did objective factors (e.g., extent of physical injury, force, use of a weapon). Developmental differences also may play an important role in this process. For example, in cases of physical trauma like motor vehicle accidents, adults tend to define these events as the disruption of social order. They mark the end of the event by the return of order, that is, the arrival of help. Children may have a different perspective of what constitutes trauma in the same event. They may find rescue efforts even more frightening than the actual accident: they may be separated from their parents as they are transported in different ambulances or even admitted to different medical facilities. Their course in a hospital, replete with painful procedures, which may be especially confusing for young children, and continued separation from parents, exacerbates their fear.

Attribution theory offers a systematic way of understanding this concept of "meaning." Traditionally, attributions are an individual's explanation of the causes of events, but the area has been broadened to perceptions of how the abuse has affected oneself and others (appraisals). Attributions and appraisals are best conceptualized as moderators of the impact of maltreatment (Kolko & Feiring, 2002). Maltreatment can alter children's basic assumptions of the self, about why traumatic things happen, and about relationships, all of which may influence adjustment. They are not static variables that never change but are assumed to be accessible and modifiable (Kolko, Brown, & Berliner, 2002; Kolko & Feiring, 2002). As we describe in later chapters, modifying maladaptive attributions is often a central task of therapy. Before we review the literature on attributions, maltreatment, and outcome, some definitions are in order.

Attributions can be categorized on four dimensions. The internal–

external dimension refers to the cause of the event. Internal attributions refer to the self as a cause of the event, and external attributions refer to others or circumstances as causes. Stable–unstable refers to the temporal stability of the cause of the event. Stable attributions interpret the cause as permanent, and unstable attributions view it as temporary. Global–specific refers to whether things are the same or different across situations: global attributions interpret the cause of an event as occurring across different situations, whereas specific attributions interpret the cause of an event as relevant only to a specific situation. Finally, controllability refers to whether the individual perceives the event to be under his or her control.

What follows is a highly summarized account of the relationship between abuse-specific attributions and outcome, based on Valle and Silovsky's (2002) excellent review of the area. Given space limitations, we cannot discuss the empirical research in any detail. In addition to Valle and Silovsky's review, a number of other articles provide comprehensive coverage of this area (Cohen & Mannarino, 2002; Feiring, Taska, & Chen, 2002; Kolko et al., 2002; Kolko & Feiring, 2002; Runyon & Kenny, 2002).

Much of the research has investigated the impact of internal and external abuse-specific attributions on sexually abused children. The number of studies examining attributions of physically abused children is much smaller, and there seems to be no work on the attributions of children exposed to domestic violence or neglect. Internal attributions (i.e., blaming oneself) for sexual abuse are related to internalizing problems, low self-esteem, and depression, although the relationship to PTSD is somewhat unclear. For example, Feiring and colleagues (2002) reported that abuse-specific internal attributions, as measured by the Abuse Attribution Index (AAI; described in Chapter 4) were related to higher levels of PTSD, especially when accompanied by shame associated with the sexual abuse. However, Chaffin, Wherry, and Dykman (1997) found that children's internal attributions were associated only with specific types of PTSD symptoms, such as hyperarousal or reexperiencing. Furthermore, another study demonstrated that PTSD was related to sexually abused children's abuse-specific shame rather than to their internal attributions (Feiring, Taska, & Lewis, 1998). Other studies have confirmed the importance of shame and guilt for the development of PTSD in sexually abused children; Wolfe and colleagues (1994) reported that PTSD was not related to abuse-specific attributions, but was associated with children's guilt about the sexual abuse. Self-blame and guilt for physical abuse has also been associated with greater depression and more abuse-specific fears (Brown & Kolko, 1999). The majority of studies have reported no association between internal attributions for sexual abuse and externalizing behaviors, including sexual acting out.

Investigators have also examined the impact of attributions that blame the perpetrator (external attributions), although the small number of such studies makes it difficult to draw firm conclusions about overall trends. A significant association between external attributions and lower depression in sexually abused children and adolescents has been reported (Feiring et al., 2002). In contrast to internal attributions, research suggests that the combination of external attributions for sexual abuse and expressions of anger may be associated with children's externalizing problems (Chaffin et al., 1997). Children may also make other types of external attributions. They may believe other individuals were also culpable for the abuse. Youngsters who attributed sexual abuse to their mothers' lack of awareness exhibited more PTSD symptoms of intrusive thoughts, avoidance, and hyperarousal (Feiring et al., 2002).

Children who believe that they will be unable to control current or future episodes of sexual abuse (i.e., attributions of controllability) exhibit higher levels of depression, anxiety, and PTSD, whereas those who believe that they can exercise control show lower levels of symptoms, especially internalizing problems (Wolfe, Gentile, Michienzi, Sas, & Wolfe, 1991). Locus of control specifically refers to individuals' general expectations for control over future outcomes. Physically and sexually abused children with external locus of control (i.e., the belief that they will be unable to control future episodes of abuse) exhibit more depression, anxiety, hopelessness, externalizing problems, and lower self-esteem (Mannarino & Cohen, 1996b). External locus of control seems unrelated to children's SBPs (Mannarino & Cohen, 1996a).

A pessimistic explanatory style (i.e., internal, stable, and global attributions for negative events and external, unstable, and specific attributions for positive events) is linked to depression in children. The literature on sexual and physical abuse has also found a relationship between a pessimistic attributional style and increased levels of depression, anxiety, and low self-esteem (Brown & Kolko, 1999), but the relationship to PTSD is unclear.

Researchers have also investigated maltreatment's impact on other beliefs, such as children's view of the world as a malevolent, unpredictable, and threatening environment (e.g., "Others will hurt me and they cannot be trusted"). As compared with nonabused peers, physically abused children are more likely to hold these "dangerous world beliefs" (Freedenfeld, Ornduff, & Kelsey, 1995) and, similarly, sexually abused children evidence lower levels of interpersonal trust (Mannarino & Cohen, 1996a, 1996b). Dangerous world beliefs are related to higher levels of depression, anxiety, and PTSD, low self-esteem, and heightened interpersonal sensitivity (Mannarino & Cohen, 1996a, 1996b). This is reminiscent of the research we have already reviewed on physically abused children's tendency to develop hostile attributional biases and their contribution to interpersonal problems.

In addition to there being developmental differences between children's and adults' attributions for the same traumatic event, children's attributions and interpretations may change or emerge anew as they grow older and progress through different developmental stages. The following clinical example illustrates this point.

Eight-year-old Chris had been sexually abused by his father and his father's female partner. A central theme of therapy was Chris's feelings of powerlessness and vulnerability, reactions that seemed to reflect the perpetrators' physical coercion and threats (e.g., statements he would be killed if he did not participate in the activity or if he ever disclosed it). After a year of therapy, Chris's nightmares, somatic complaints, and intrusive thoughts and images of the abuse disappeared, and therapy was terminated with the consent of Chris and his mother.

At his request, Chris's mother again contacted the therapist when her son was 12 years old. Interviews at this second referral revealed that Chris, who had begun puberty and was now in junior high school, was worried about the implications of the actual sexual activity for his own emerging sexual identity. In particular, Chris was distraught that he had been sexually abused by a male and had shown some physiological response, such as sustaining an erection, during this activity. He had recently interpreted his sexual response as evidence that he was gay and was beginning to think the perpetrator must have known he had a homosexual orientation and therefore was sexually attracted to him. Consequently, Chris thought he was responsible for the sexual abuse, an internal attribution, which engendered a great deal of anxiety. A short course of therapy focused on helping Chris to critically examine this attribution and resulted in his realization that his sexual response was not atypical, not indicative of a homosexual orientation and, most important, that the perpetrators still bore responsibility for the sexual abuse. These cognitive changes were accompanied by a significant reduction in anxiety and a return to a more adaptive level of functioning.

Chris's experience demonstrates that maltreatment may have different meanings for children at different developmental stages, and that attributions can change. When he was 8, sexuality was not a primary focus, but it emerged when Chris began puberty. Being exposed to peer discussions in junior high school about homosexuality, including pejorative comments, further sensitized Chris to this issue. These factors engendered a different perspective and, eventually, Chris's attribution that he was responsible for the sexual assaults, which was accompanied by considerable distress and anxiety. Moreover, this clinical example again reinforces the central theme of this chapter: clinicians must identify and intervene with such mechanisms and pathogenic processes in order to help maltreated children recover.

PSYCHOBIOLOGICAL MECHANISMS

There has been a rapid expansion in research investigating the neurological and psychobiological correlates of child maltreatment, ranging from studies of trauma's impact on neurobiological stress systems and its relevance for PTSD (De Bellis, 2001, 2005; De Bellis, Keshavan, & Harenski, 2001), to the influence of genetic factors for the development of conduct disorders in physically abused children (Jaffee et al., 2004, 2005), and to neurodevelopmental deficits in children and youth who exhibit sexual aggression (Fago, 2003). Some of the more prominent findings reveal, for example, that maltreated children with PTSD had smaller magnetic resonance imaging–based brain structural measures of intracranial volume, cerebral volumes, and midsaggital corpus callosum areas, and larger lateral ventricles than controls. These changes correlate with PTSD symptoms of intrusive recollections, avoidance, hyperarousal, and dissociation and may indicate neuronal loss (see De Bellis, 2001, for a review). Maltreated children with PTSD show elevations in cortisol and dopamine as a result of stress, which in turn are associated with alterations in brain functioning, including stress response and behavioral and emotional regulation problems (De Bellis, 2005).

The subjects discussed in this literature seem far-removed from the everyday practice of most clinicians. Many nonmedical mental health professionals do not have sophisticated backgrounds in neurology, biology, or genetics. Consequently, the research seems obtuse and irrelevant. Although the literature is highly technical, we contend that a basic understanding of such topics is important. First, it extends our understanding of the impact of maltreatment to another level of analysis. The integration of brain science into the matrix of factors that influence outcomes associated with child maltreatment is entirely consistent with developmental psychopathology's transactional model (Nelson et al., 2002; Post & Weiss, 2002; Thompson & Nelson, 2001). The model compels us to regard neuro- and psychobiological factors as one of a set of multiple variables that contribute to human development, albeit without relying exclusively on biology or genetics to explain the diversity of outcome linked to maltreatment.

Second, the literature is relevant because it has important implications for clinical practice and broader public policy. Consider the following two assumptions. First, early adverse experiences inevitably lead to permanent and life-long changes in brain structure, anatomy, and physiology; second, critical periods exist, each representing a very narrow window of opportunity during which a particular experience must occur for further brain development. If one believes, for example, that attachment is "hard-wired" by the early preschool years and no further change can be expected, why would we even attempt to help school-age or older youngsters modify insecure attachments or resolve clinical syndromes like reactive attachment disorder? Furthermore, should we expend all of our professional and financial resources on early prevention programs that target infants and toddlers? Although such programs do have a lot of merit, we believe older children also deserve first-class services, especially when the evidence indicates that "critical periods may be exceptional, not typical, in brain development" (Thompson & Nelson, 2001, p. 9).

Terms like "neuronal loss" are ominous and may elicit images of brain-damaged children who have no hope of recovery—why even try to do therapy with such a youngster? However, there is considerable evidence that questions the simplistic notion that the brain becomes immutable and increasingly difficult to modify beyond the first few years of life, or that we were born with all the neurons we will ever have. New discoveries of continuing brain plasticity suggest that experiences that occur after infancy and the early preschool years may result in cortical reorganization (see De Bellis et al., 2001; Nelson & Bloom, 1997; Thompson & Nelson, 2001, for comprehensive reviews of the research on neural plasticity). For example, there is strong evidence of neurogenesis (the formation of new neurons) throughout much of the lifespan in the dentate region of the adult human hippocampus and possibly in the regions of the parietal and prefrontal cortex (Thompson & Nelson, 2001). Although there are certainly significant constraints on plasticity, such as the neuropathology that accompanies normal aging, the adult brain is more modifiable than originally thought. Supporting this perspective are findings that indicate that environmental experiences, including interpersonal ones, can modify psychobiological phenomena. Social support decreases heart rate and cortisol levels during stress (Thorsteinsson, James, & Gregg, 1998). Another investigation reported that both a behavioral treatment for obsessive–compulsive disorder and a pharmacological treatment yielded identical behavioral outcomes. A positron emission tomography scan revealed that the changes that occurred in the brain under both treatment conditions were also identical (Baxter et al., 1992; Schwartz, Stoessel, Baxter, Martin, & Phelps, 1996). Thompson and Nelson (2001) eloquently summarize these findings and their implications:

> Brain development can be facilitated not only during the first three years but also at other developmental stages. This is important news for adoptive and foster parents, child-care providers, and parents and teachers of children of all ages. . . . Eliminating early disadvantages is important, but the plasticity of brain development means that early deprivation and harm can be treated in later years, especially with carefully designed interventions. This is important news for therapists, educators and others concerned with aiding troubled children. Adult brains are developing. This is important news for all of us. (p. 12)

OTHER MECHANISMS

We have reviewed important mechanisms that contribute to the diverse array of symptoms associated with maltreatment from the perspective of attachment, conditioning, and attribution theories and have briefly described some of the relevant research. Space limitations preclude a detailed and comprehensive review of every pathogenic process, although several deserve brief mention here. For example, physically and sexually abused children and those who witness domestic violence are exposed to potent models, and they may adopt these coercive strategies in future interpersonal relationships, especially if others readily comply with their demands that are buttressed by physical or sexual aggression. We have also alluded to the sexual arousal and gratification some children may derive from engaging other youngsters in sexual behavior. Other children who are survivors of sexual abuse and develop sexualized behaviors may have learned that these behaviors can satisfy a variety of other needs. Finkelhor and Browne (1985) describe traumatic sexualization as "a process in which a child's sexuality (including both sexual feelings and sexual attitudes) is shaped in a developmentally inappropriate and interpersonally dysfunctional fashion as a result of the sexual abuse" (p. 531). The perpetrator rewards the child for sexual behavior through the exchange of affection, attention, privileges, or gifts. Consequently, the child learns to use sexual behavior to manipulate others to satisfy a variety of needs, such as obtaining favors or attention (Briere, 1992; Wolfe & Wolfe, 1988). As well as traumatic sexualization, Finkelhor and Browne (1985) describe three other *traumagenic factors*—powerlessness, betrayal, and stigmatization—that they contend are responsible for the diverse array of symptoms exhibited by sexually abused children (see Table 4.1 for lines of inquiry based on this model). Finkelhor and Browne's conceptualization of traumagenic dynamics is similar to the notion of pathogenic processes we described at the beginning of this chapter.

Mueller and Silverman (1989) believe that the maltreated child's reliance on identification with the aggressor may play a significant role in this process. Expecting more maltreatment, the child behaves aggressively to fend off the expected assault and to compensate for concomitant feelings of helplessness, inadequacy, and vulnerability. A maltreated child also may react aggressively and provocatively to elicit a similar response from the abusive adult. By successfully eliciting this response, the maltreated child gains a sense of predictability and control over events (i.e., aggressive interchanges or rejection) that he or she believes are inevitable. In a much earlier article, Littner (1960) used psychoanalytic concepts to make the same point: abused children tend to provoke abusive reactions from caregivers, including foster parents, as a way to gain control and mastery over a frightening and unpredictable world.

As we have emphasized throughout these first two chapters, we must remain cognizant that these variables and processes interact with others. A sexually abused child may start to exhibit highly sexualized behavior as a result of some of the pathogenic processes described earlier, but the response of parents is a crucial variable in determining its clinical progression. The next chapter describes the importance of family variables as pathogenic processes and how to evaluate them.

CHAPTER THREE

Family Assessment

Consistent with the transactional model of development described in the preceding chapters, clinicians should never assess or treat children in isolation from those other factors that are critical in shaping an individual's adaptation to maltreatment. The family has special relevance for a comprehensive understanding of the child's response to maltreatment. In this chapter we provide an overview of family assessment, and in Chapter 6 we discuss interventions with caregivers and families that support and maximize individual psychotherapy with the child. Before dealing directly with the topic of family assessment, we offer some considerations about clinical assessment in general that have guided our thinking and practice.

CLINICAL ASSESSMENT: UNDERLYING ASSUMPTIONS

Clinical Assessment Is the Foundation of Therapy

We believe strongly that treatment of a child or family should not be undertaken until the clinician has a good understanding of the problems and the factors that contributed to their emergence. Chapter 2 described the importance of identifying pathogenic processes and moderator variables for treatment planning. A failure to do so decreases the chances of effective interventions. There are other compelling reasons to initiate treatment only after completing an assessment. Treatments selected without an understanding of the pathogenic processes and moderator variables may not only be ineffective, they may be harmful. For example, encouraging an open discussion in the family about a child's sexual abuse may be met with resistance by parents who have their own victimization history or cultural values that prohibit these conversations. Initiating such interventions with no prior knowledge of the important characteristics of family functioning may provoke the family's anger and resentment, eventually leading to premature termination. Consequently, the child is denied much-needed services and his or her problems may become even worse. We have also seen situations in which therapists have not conducted comprehensive assessments and then intervened in ways that significantly damaged their clients, such as insisting that they provide a full and detailed account of their history of victimization. Clinicians used these approaches with no appreciation of clients' brittle and fragile defensive structures or any knowledge of their history of psychiatric admissions associated with therapy that quickly (and prematurely) elicited painful feelings and recollections. Conversely, the lack of a comprehensive assessment may result in the therapist's failure to identify and capitalize on the strengths of a particular child or family.

Treatment should not begin until the clinician has formulated a set of treatment recommendations, derived from the assessment, that have been accepted by parents or caregivers. A guiding ethical principle of all mental health professions is that of informed consent. Legal guardians of maltreated children must have as full an understanding as possible of the professional's opinion about the problem, the basis and rationale for the treatment recommendations, and any contraindications. It is only when these conditions have been met that informed consent for treatment can be given. How can clients or guardians give informed consent if they do not understand the reasons for a proposed treatment plan?

Although critically important prior to the start of treatment, assessment plays an important role throughout the course of intervention. We should assess children's progress in therapy at regular intervals. Evaluations range from brief, weekly contacts with the child's parents or caregivers who provide informal reports about the child's functioning, to readministrations of formal assessment instruments. Reassessments are especially important for long-term therapy wherein it is often difficult to keep treatment goals in clear focus. Clinicians conducting long-term treatment should review regularly their clients' progress to make any necessary modifications in the treatment plan or to determine the appropriateness of termination.

Assessments Must Be Comprehensive

Given the wide diversity of outcomes arising from maltreatment, the large number of potential pathogenic processes and moderator variables that affect a child's response, and the complexity of the ensuing interactions, clinicians must conduct comprehensive assessments in order to identify the child's response to the abuse or neglect and formulate a specific treatment plan to meet the child's and family's unique needs. To evaluate maltreatment's impact on a child, a clinical assessment should address the following questions:

1. What is the nature of the problem?
2. Is it a problem that requires action?
3. What are the processes and factors causing and maintaining the problem?
4. What action, if any, is needed and by which members of the family or other significant people in the child's life?
5. Who can best carry out the intervention?
6. What is the prognosis for change?

Comprehensiveness includes three dimensions. First, assessments are ecological. Children do not develop in vacuums but in families that, in turn, fit into a larger societal and cultural context. Clinical assessments of maltreated children must evaluate the impact of parents' or caregivers' historical and current influence as well as the influence of larger societal forces (e.g., poverty).

Second, comprehensive assessments focus on a broad domain of child behavior. In Chapter 1, we described the great variability of children's responses to maltreatment and how many domains of functioning can be affected. The clinician should be prepared to evaluate numerous and diverse facets of a child's behavior and functioning. Besides being problem areas that require intervention, these domains of functioning may be moderators of the child's response to maltreatment. We have already seen that good academic achievement and intelligence may function as compensatory factors for some children who have undergone traumatic experiences. Similarly, maltreatment may affect many different aspects of family functioning. A child's victimization may elicit so much distress in parents that the care they provide is seriously compromised. There may also be situational changes (e.g., losing the income of an offending parent who must leave the home) that directly and indirectly affect the child and his or her caregivers. These changes play important, moderating roles in helping or hindering the child's attempts to cope with the maltreatment and are legitimate targets of intervention, as are problems that predated the maltreatment, such as an attention deficit disorder. Saunders, Berliner, and Hanson (2004) cogently summarized the importance of this approach:

> Assessments of abused children must be *abuse-informed*, but not exclusively abuse-focused. That is, the assessment should evaluate not only the

potential problems that are the direct effects of abuse, but also pre-existing and concomitant difficulties as well. (p. 25)

Third, comprehensive assessments of the child and family employ multimethods and multisources and are based in multisettings (Budd, Felix, Poindexter, Naik-Polan, & Sloss, 2002; Haugaard, 2004b; Kirby & Hardesty, 1998; Saunders et al., 2004). Relying on any one evaluation format or modality is foolish. No one assessment strategy or test is infallible or renders all the information needed about a child or family. In this chapter and the next, we argue for adopting a multimethod approach that incorporates data from different assessment methods and places the highest confidence in those findings that recur across different methods. Moreover, the clinician must attempt to gather information about the child and the family's functioning from different sources. Teachers may have a different and indeed valuable perspective on a child's functioning. In addition to offering information associated within their traditional domains of cognitive and academic functioning, they can often comment knowledgeably on other areas such as peer relations or symptoms of anxiety. Similarly, functioning may vary across different environments with significant implications for intervention. For example, the clinician may discover that the child does well at school, which points to strengths that can be capitalized on in treatment. Likewise, the family may show difficulties only in certain environmental contexts, such as when confronted by authority figures. Clinicians must be cognizant of the influence of contextual and environmental differences and be prepared to evaluate children in different settings.

Although these recommendations smack of common sense, it is surprising, and alarming, how frequently clinicians fail to implement them. Budd and colleagues (2002) analyzed 207 clinical assessments of children in child protection cases and found that clinicians failed to obtain information from caregivers in nearly one-half of the evaluations and rarely contacted teachers or day care providers. Assessments usually consisted of a single office visit and incorporated limited background information, and the majority reported no information about children's strengths and weaknesses in areas such as a child's relationships with caregivers or academic performance.

Distinction between Clinical and Forensic/Legal Assessments

Clinical assessments should be conducted only after child protective services or police have completed their investigations. Although there is a certain amount of overlap, the purposes of these two types of assessments differ. The purpose of a forensic/legal assessment is to determine whether the child was maltreated and, if so, to ascertain the identity of the perpetrator. Other issues include establishing the specific details of the maltreatment (e.g., what was done to the child, when, where, presence of threats or coercion). Conducting these assessments requires specific training and skills. Leading or suggestive questioning is strictly contraindicated as it may contaminate evidence and jeopardize the chances of successful court prosecution. However, clinicians sometimes use suggestive or leading questions in a clinical assessment to confirm or refute working hypotheses about the maltreatment's impact on the child and to obtain further information. Clinicians should not undertake forensic/legal investigations unless they have been properly trained and have confirmed that the assessment's mandate is indeed a legal/forensic one.

Clinical Assessments Should Have a Therapeutic Component

Although clinical assessments should not be construed as formal treatment, they can still have a therapeutic component. Assessment is the first step in establishing a collaborative alliance with parents or caregivers. The clinician acknowledges the parents' observations, feelings, and perceptions, respects their concerns, identifies them as the most important influences in the child's life, and asserts that their role in any subsequent treatment intervention is critical to its success. Although this part of the assessment does not constitute treatment per se, it creates a therapeutic atmosphere in which the clinician respects parents' perspectives and empathizes with their concerns and worries. Chapter 4 discusses the therapeutic components of the assessment process for maltreated children.

Assessments Must Be Culturally Sensitive

The assessment and intervention techniques we describe here are based on a consideration of relevant theory and empirical findings. They also reflect our own cultural heritage. The emphasis we place on the verbalization of feelings and beliefs associated with victimization is congruent with the notion held by most white, middle-class North Americans, that it is good to talk about affective and personal issues. However, therapists must guard against applying this assumption indiscriminately in working with maltreated children and their families from different cultural backgrounds (Budd et al., 2002; Cohen, Deblinger, Mannarino, & de Arellano, 2001). For example, some cultures may not condone explicit discussions of sexuality between children and people outside the family, or with adults of different gender (Bowman, 1989). Although descriptions of cultural norms and traditions may constitute useful guides for interactions, clinicians must avoid stereotyping the members of a cultural group. There is enough diversity, even in homogeneous groups, to make it necessary to assess the specific relevance and importance of cultural traditions for an individual child and family. We cannot assume that every member of a particular group will ascribe the same importance to its traditions and teachings. It may well be that some of the techniques and strategies we describe in this book are inappropriate for children from various cultural backgrounds, including formal measures that do not have normative data for certain cultural groups (Garb, Wood, & Nezworski, 2000). Clinicians must evaluate their utility and appropriateness for children from diverse backgrounds, modify them if necessary, and discard those that will not be helpful. Obvious examples include the judicious choice of formal psychological assessment instruments (some of which may not have been normed for the particular ethnic or racial group to which the child belongs) and the sensitive appreciation of the specific meaning of body language, eye contact, loudness and manner of speech, and tone of voice (Canino, 1988; Gutierrez, 1989). A failure to inquire about specific cultural traditions and the family's adherence to them often leads to treatment recommendations that are mismatched to the family's and the child's context.

Children and their parents are often the best sources of information about their cultural traditions and what constitutes appropriate interventions. In our experience, a sincere interest in the family's culture and a willingness to learn about its traditions convey a genuine respect that usually facilitates a useful exchange of information. Many families are willing to share knowledge of their culture with a therapist who asks for their help and guidance. Clinicians can prepare themselves for meeting a child and family from a different cultural background by reading relevant material or talking with other individuals from the same cultural group. By doing so, they can devise some preliminary guidelines and formulate tentative hypotheses regarding the relevance of cultural variables to the sequelae of the maltreatment and for possible treatment approaches. However, as useful as these general guidelines might be, therapists must inquire about the specific meaning and relevance of cultural traditions for a given child and family and then make appropriate adjustments in assessment or intervention strategies.

As we describe in a later section of this chapter, the early involvement of parents or other legal guardians in the assessment is absolutely necessary. They not only have to give informed consent for the child to participate and bring the child to the sessions, but also must convey a positive and cooperative attitude. Children residing with caregivers who demean the clinician or the assessment process are less likely to actively participate. If parents think this is a useless or even harmful exercise, why would their children open up and share personal information? Establishing a collaborative alliance with parents and caregivers is even more important when they and their children are members of cultural groups whose values, attitudes, and expectations of professional assistance are significantly different from the clinician's. In some situations clinicians must seek endorsement of their involvement from community leaders as well from parents. The following unique case example illustrates the complexity of such clinical work.

A child welfare worker referred a number of sexually abused school-age children to an urban child abuse program. The children all resided in a rural Hutterite colony. The Hutterite Brethern is a religious group originating in 1528 during the Reformation (MacDonald, 1985). They underwent considerable persecution and began to immigrate to North America in the late 19th and early 20th centuries, settling in western Canada and the United States. They are publicly identified by their plain dress and communal living on large agricultural tracts, which provide for 60–160 persons. All material things are held in common; all earnings are held communally, and funding and necessities are distributed according to a person's needs. Hutterites believe that there is a conflict between the spiritual world of God's order and hierarchy, and the carnal world of human creation. The dangers of submitting to this carnal, secular world are reflected in the myriad social problems affecting contemporary society. Consequently, they have kept their German dialect and historic patterns of dress and organization. They are also pacifists.

After completing this preliminary research about Hutterite beliefs and society, members of the treatment team decided that they needed to meet with the parents of the abused children in order to gain a better appreciation of their concerns about the sexual abuse and its impact and, just as important, their fears or worries about allowing their children to meet with non-Hutterite professionals who did not necessarily share their core beliefs. The treatment team also invited the head of the colony, given his powerful and influential role in the community. His endorsement of the children's and families' involvement was critically important to the clinicians' being allowed access to the children and to establishing positive and cooperative relationships with their parents.

Several themes emerged in this initial meeting. The clinicians explained that they were most interested in the Hutterites' beliefs and way of life and asked the parents and the colony's head to give them an overview. They stressed that this information was critically important, as they wanted to work with them and their children in ways consistent with these beliefs and values. This request and the genuine interest shown by the clinicians began to build rapport, especially when the adults spoke of their particular expectations for the clinicians' involvement, all of which were embedded in their religious tenets. For example, they directly told the treatment team that they did not want its members to impose their own religious beliefs on their children, a request the clinicians honored throughout their involvement with the colony. Parents also expected that the male clinicians would see the boys and female clinicians would be involved with the girls, with a clear separation between the two groups. Again, this was quite consistent with the colony's organizational structure regarding gender, such as having males and females eat at separate tables in the communal dining hall, and was especially important if sexual issues were going to be discussed. Furthermore, the clinicians were told that the use of instructional videos was unacceptable (the colony did not have or condone television). The clinicians provided an overview of how they would approach the initial assessments, the kinds of topics they would like to pursue with the children, and parents' involvement in this stage, such as being available for interviews regarding their children's functioning and history. Parents and the head of the colony provided explicit permission for the clinicians to raise the issue of the sexual abuse with the children, although they were worried that the clinicians would go into great detail about sexual matters, a practice at odds with their own. Finally, the members of the treatment team stated they would be happy to conduct sessions at the colony. They believed this would alleviate some of the parents' and children's anxiety and possibly increase their sense of control over the process. Although it entailed a considerable drive each way, this gesture was of real significance as it demonstrated the clinicians' sensitivity to the parents' concerns. At the end of this extensive meeting, all the parents gave their consent for the assessment to proceed; the colony head was equally supportive of the clinicians' involvement.

Assessments Should Strive to Use Empirically Supported Measures

Consistent with the EST literature, we should attempt to use valid and reliable measures of behavioral and emotional problems commonly exhibited by maltreated children. Such measures provide a standardized and structured approach and can be administered over time to assess progress (Saunders et al., 2004). Chapter 4 describes a number of these measures. Some have been developed specifically for assessing abuse-specific problems, such as the TSCC (Briere, 1996), whereas others are more general measures of children's behavioral and emotional functioning, such as the Child Behavior Checklist for Ages 6–18 (CBC/6–18; Achenbach & Rescorla, 2001). Although Chapter 4 does not constitute an exhaustive review, neither is it restricted to empirically supported assessment measures. Most interviews are not structured or standardized, but they are an invaluable means of eliciting important information from children about the details of maltreatment and, just as important, their idiosyncratic feelings and beliefs about what has happened to them. Clinical researchers and scientists are also striving to develop measures of aspects of maltreated children's functioning that have previously been ignored (e.g., attachment organizations of school-age children) and have made some gains, but there is still much work to be done. As clinicians are confronted daily with assessment questions for which there may be few, if any, empirically supported measures, we describe measures that have not yet received empirical support but may hold promise in future investigations. The use of such measures follows from our understanding that multimethods and multisources are absolutely critical to ensure converging validity for our findings and conclusions.

ASSESSMENT OF PARENTAL AND FAMILY FUNCTIONING

Reasons for Assessing Parental and Family Functioning

One obvious difference between child and adult therapy is that children are brought to assessment and therapy appointments by adults, especially if they are young. If parents or caregivers are hesitant about, or opposed to, clinical services for the child, they often fail to attend. If they do bring the child, they may still undermine or sabotage the clinician's efforts via disparaging remarks about the clinician or the clinical process or they may communicate a negative attitude more passively, such as through a lack of enthusiasm or reluctance to attend appointments. Although we discuss working with parents in much more detail in Chapter 6, it is important to note here that involving parents or caregivers in the beginning of the assessment phase conveys a strong signal to them that their information and participation are important. It is the beginning of the development of a collaborative alliance between the clinician and parent or caregiver, a relationship that may be especially significant for those adults who played a direct role in the maltreatment of their child. Their involvement may afford them some relief from guilt and anxiety as they collaborate to help their child. We also believe that successfully engaging parents in the assessment process transmits a positive message to the child: despite past parenting difficulties, parents are willing to make the effort to become involved on their child's behalf. Of course, some parents are not able or willing to follow through with either the assessment or subsequent therapy.

A proportion of the maltreated children whom clinicians see do not live with their parents but reside in foster homes or group homes with other caregivers. It is just as important to involve these caregivers in the assessment and therapeutic phases, although their level of involvement may differ from that of natural parents. Unfortunately, some mental health professionals regard foster parents merely as individuals who clothe, feed, and house the child and transport the youngster to and from therapy sessions. This condescending attitude is often associated with a failure to obtain the foster parents' often insightful and valuable knowledge of the children in their care. The clinician sees the child for only 1–2 hours per week, whereas a foster parent lives with the child and is, in many ways, the real expert. Similarly, therapists must enlist foster parents as significant collaborators and allies in treatment, as they are often the primary agents of change. Failure to engage them in the therapeutic process usually ensures that therapeutic gains are not maximized and even raises the possibility that therapy will flounder or end prematurely. The same basic principle applies to relationships with group home staff members. They, too, are an invaluable source of information about the child's functioning and, like foster parents, must be included as collaborative partners in subsequent interventions.

Besides establishing a collaborative alliance with parents and caregivers, involving these individuals facilitates a much more comprehensive understanding of the child. In addition to providing information about the child's functioning and strengths and weaknesses, parent/caregiver involvement gives the clinician an appreciation of those historical and current potentiating and compensatory factors within the family that contribute to the child's level of adaptation. Identifying these factors is more than an intellectual exercise: identifying them and developing a formulation of how they operate suggest intervention targets. For example, the clinician must address inconsistent parenting that is currently exacerbating the child's aggressive response to maltreatment. Historical information about moderator variables is relevant for treatment planning. Long-term problems that predate the onset of maltreatment may require a different therapeutic approach than others that are more reflective of a family's situational reaction to maltreatment. Returning to our example of inconsistent parenting, a therapist may have to use specific interventions with parents who have always had problems in setting limits. Chronic difficulties, especially those that have continued despite the provision of ample and generous help in the past, may necessitate intensive interventions, such as in-home teaching of parenting skills. Blindly recommending a short-term parenting group for a chronically troubled, multiproblem family may lead to further failure and frustration for these parents, and it will do little to help their child. In contrast, a family with numerous strengths and resources, including good parenting skills, may not require the same intensity of treatment or level of commitment of professional resources. These parents may respond rapidly to an approach that validates their distress but also encourages them to place firm and consistent limits on their child's acting-out behavior.

Knowledge of parental and family functioning helps the clinician develop other aspects of a child's treatment plan, including basic decisions about whether the child should be treated individually and when treatment should begin. Information regarding past and current family functioning is a critical component in this decision-making process. For example, a principal focus of child psychotherapy involves teaching children more effective ways to articulate feelings, such as sadness or anger. However, these changes may be terribly provocative for parents unused to hearing their children talk so openly. They may be unable to tolerate overt emotional displays, thereby increasing their anger and elevating the risk that they will physically abuse the child. Instituting such a therapeutic program without information about the parent's or caregiver's ability to accept and manage these changes may place the child in significant danger. As past behavior is often the best predictor of future behavior, the therapist must carefully evaluate parents' previous responses to expressions of strong feelings by the child. The clinician should consider this historical perspective while evaluating their current ability to accept and support their child's affective expression.

Getting Started: Who Should Attend the Initial Interview?

Even before meeting the child and family, the clinician faces several decisions. One of the first is whom to invite to the initial interview. Some clinicians interview the entire family first and then parents or caregivers separately, whereas others prefer to see parents by themselves first. We do not believe that clinicians must adhere to rigid rules about this issue. However, there are several considerations to keep in mind. Children probably should not be present when parents are asked about their own history, which may possibly include personal victimization. Similarly, in-depth discussions about their reactions to the child's maltreatment may provoke parents' strong and intense feelings. Children exposed to this level of parental distress in the assessment phase may experience an exacerbation of their own anxiety. They may become even more concerned about their own well-being upon learning that a parent is so upset about what happened, even though they are probably already aware of their parents' feelings. Children may begin to feel that they have been irreparably damaged, or they may stop talking so as to alleviate parental pain and suffering. Consequently, we believe that at some point in the assessment phase, parents or caregivers need an opportunity to talk privately with the therapist about these very personal and sensitive issues. Generally, we prefer to conduct several initial interviews with parents or caregivers by themselves. These provide an opportunity to focus our attention on the caregivers' concerns and to start establishing a collaborative alliance with them.

However, some argue that excluding children, even in this very early stage, results in a less than comprehensive perspective on family interaction patterns. Therapists may be interested in observing children's reaction to their parents' distress about the victimization. Do the children, for instance, stop talking about what happened to them? Do they become upset themselves? Do they attempt to nurture and engage in caretaking behavior with the distressed parent? Parents may also blame children for the abuse or criticize their inability to have protected themselves. Given the risk that children may be retraumatized in joint sessions, one could argue they should be excluded from these sessions. Berlin (2002) counters this argument by contending that this is not a novel experience for these children and that they are probably exposed to inappropriate interactions daily. Although painful to observe, these sessions render valuable clinical information that can inform the basis of interventions that provide relief to the child. Again, the assessor must rely on clinical judgment and give priority to the child's short- and long-term best interests.

Orienting Parents and Caregivers to the Assessment

Before being questioned about relevant issues, parents or caregivers deserve an explanation about the purposes of the assessment process. Clinicians should briefly review the referral process that resulted in the parents' attendance at the first appointment, ask them for their understanding of the assessment's purposes, clarify any misunderstandings, and seek informed consent to proceed. Many parents are already defensive about their role in the child's difficulties and have not had positive relationships with professionals in the past. Their belief that the clinician will be determining their fitness as parents or conducting a forensic/legal investigation of the child's allegations of maltreatment can precipitate considerable anxiety. The clinician should make it clear that the purpose of the assessment is to evaluate the impact of the maltreatment on the child and to formulate some appropriate recommendations regarding intervention. A thorough discussion of the assessment's purpose helps attenuate parents' confusion and anxiety.

As mental health professionals, we often assume that our clients know what will happen in a typical assessment and are comfortable with what may actually be an alien process. Discussing the assessment process also alleviates parents' anxiety and makes them feel part of the whole endeavor. The therapist can explain the purpose of the first session, which includes obtaining the parents' account of the child's difficulties, developing a tentative plan for subsequent sessions, and addressing any parental concerns or questions. It is important to emphasize that we are most interested in the parents' account of what happened to the child, the maltreatment's effects on the child's functioning, and the subsequent reactions of the parents. By stressing that the parents have a wealth of information to offer, we can often alleviate some of their guilt and thereby reinforce the nascent collaborative alliance. A positive alliance between the clinician and parents also facilitates a positive attitude in the child about the assessment and in turn increases the chances that the child will cooperate in the evaluative process. Children already exposed to inconsistency between their parents will not benefit from a similar relationship between their parents and a clinician.

Because of the child's distress and their own difficulties in managing it, parents or other caregivers, including foster parents, often ask for advice during the first session. After only one or two assessment sessions, they may expect an opinion about their child's difficulties and what can be done. To promote realistic expectations about the limits of advice that can be given during the assessment phase, it is helpful to broach this subject in the first session even if the parents do not request immediate advice or assistance. Clinicians can empathize with parents' desire for solutions to alleviate their children's distress, but they should inform parents that they will offer suggestions when they have completed the assessment so that they can anchor recommendations on as comprehensive a picture of the child and family as possible. In addition, the clinician should encourage parents or caregivers to report any significant developments in the child's presentation or behavior during the assessment that might merit quick attention. Clearly, any child who becomes acutely suicidal or a danger to others during the assessment phase will need immediate crisis evaluation and intervention.

Finally, clinicians must alert parents and caregivers to the limits of confidentiality, including their obligation to report any incidents of abuse or neglect to child protective services. They should review policies regarding the release of information to other individuals.

We now present a model for evaluating parental and family functioning and its implications for the child's adjustment and subsequent intervention. Although we have divided the assessment phase into what seems discrete segments, clinical practice is often messier, with clinicians weaving back and forth among issues and returning to topics again in the future, all the while formulating, revising, and discarding working hypotheses.

Inquiry about the Child's History of Maltreatment

Although the clinician may already have some detailed referral information about the maltreatment, it is important to ask parents about their understanding of what happened to their child and their own feelings and reactions. Open-ended questions, such as "Please tell me what happened to your child," are opportunities for parents to provide their account with minimal interruptions. Clinicians can then follow up with more detailed inquiries. Relevant content information includes the type(s) of maltreatment, child's age at the onset of maltreatment, its duration and frequency, the perpetrator's identity and his or her relationship to the child, the use of physical or psychological coercion or threats, and the presence of any physical injuries or medical symptoms. In addition, the clinician should inquire about how the abuse or neglect was discovered or disclosed and the response of the protective or legal/justice system. See Table 1.1 in Chapter 1 and Table 3.2 in this chapter for an outline of the maltreatment characteristics that deserve careful inquiry.

The way parents convey the information may be just as valuable as their factual accounts. Open-ended questions that precede detailed inquiries offer considerable latitude to parents about what they choose to talk about, which may be a clue to an issue's salience. Do specific aspects of the child's maltreatment provoke especially strong feelings? Are emotional reactions so strong that narratives become disjointed or even incoherent? These and similar observations suggest hypotheses about parents' or caregivers' reactions, which can be pursued in more depth in subsequent interviews.

Initial interviews may reveal other important information. The clinician may see evidence of major parental psychopathology (e.g., depression, psychosis) when parents recount the maltreatment incident or other aspects of the child's or family's history. However, applying a psychiatric diagnosis such as a major depressive disorder to an individual, based solely on impressions derived from an account of the child's problems, is unwarranted. With this caveat in mind, the clinician may note these parental behaviors or characteristics as indicators for a more in-depth inquiry into the parents' own mental health issues later in the assessment.

Information regarding family relationships also starts to emerge in these first interviews. If the child has more than one parent or caregiver and both are present, do they present a fairly consistent picture of the history of maltreatment and their respective reactions, or do they have divergent perspectives? If they have differing perspectives, are they aware of these differences and, if so, how do they reconcile them? Do they undermine each other in the interview, and does one member of the dyad fight for control? Do their divergent perceptions of the child extend to inconsistency in the way they actually manage some of the child's behavior? If the whole family is present, the clinician must remain alert to these and other interactions that are relevant for the child's functioning and recovery from the maltreatment. We discuss family functioning at a later point in this chapter.

Child's Response to the Maltreatment

A central question of any clinical assessment of a maltreated child concerns the impact of the maltreatment on this youngster. Although clinicians will want to assess directly children's perceptions of the abuse or neglect and how it has affected their functioning, obtaining this information from parents or caregivers is critical. This is especially so for younger children who may not be able to give a detailed account of their behavior and their internal psychological processes such as attributions. Information from parents or caregivers enables the clinician to begin forming some working hypotheses about the child's response to the maltreatment and identifies those areas that require particular attention in the child assessment portion of the evaluation.

Table 3.1 illustrates a fairly standard outline of the information regarding presenting problems that the clinician may want to gather from parents. We emphasized in Chapter 1 that we can expect a broad array of symptoms in maltreated children, and some may even be asymptomatic. Given this diversity, clinicians should inquire specifically about the presence of symptoms of PTSD, sexualized behaviors, and the other problematic reactions we have described.

It is especially important to determine if there is an association between the onset of difficulties and the maltreatment. Parents may report that their sexually abused daughter has been showing attention and concentration difficulties in the classroom. It is further noted that the onset of the attention problems coincided with the onset of the sexual abuse. Moreover, a review of the girl's developmental history, especially her academic and behavioral functioning at school, indicated no problems with attention or concentration prior to her victimization. Rather than being symptomatic of a primary ADHD, the attention problems reflect her increased arousal and constitute one component of PTSD. This is an important differential diagnosis: interventions based on a PTSD formulation would differ from those based on a diagnosis of a primary ADHD.

TABLE 3.1. History of Presenting Problems

1. Behavioral description of the problem.
2. Onset (particularly in relation to onset of maltreatment).
3. Where in the child's environment are the problems manifested?
4. How frequently do the problems occur?
5. What precipitates the problems?
6. What makes the problems better or worse?
7. How do the problems create difficulties, and for whom?
8. Child's and family's feelings about the problems, and their explanations of the causes.
9. What attempts have been made to help (duration of efforts, consistency of efforts, outcome, feelings about past efforts)?
10. What are the goals in seeking help now?

Clinicians should ask parents for concrete and specific examples of children's problems and how they are manifested in different environments: at home, in school, in the neighborhood among friends, and in other contexts such as recreational activities. Parents may describe difficulties that predated the abuse or neglect. Rather than dismissing these difficulties, the clinician must inquire about them in the same detailed fashion employed for symptoms more closely associated with the maltreatment. Although some of these symptoms are not directly related to the abuse, they may serve as important moderators that merit therapeutic intervention.

Clinicians should supplement informal parental reports of the child's behavior with standardized measures. The CBCL/6–18 (Achenbach & Rescorla, 2001), the Child Behavior Checklist for Ages 1½–5 (CBCL/1½–5; Achenbach & Rescorla, 2000), and the Behavior Assessment System for Children: Second Edition (BASC-2; Reynolds & Kamphaus, 2004) are parent-completed checklists of child behavior. In Chapter 1 we reviewed the CSBI (Friedrich et al., 2001), a comprehensive, parent-completed report of children's sexual behavior. These instruments can be used for other purposes besides generating profiles of different behavioral dimensions compared with age-based and sex-based normative data. The clinician may request each of the caretakers to complete these instruments independently to determine the degree of consistency between their respective perspectives of the child's behavior. Consistent with one of our basic notions of assessing children's behavior in multisettings, it is often useful to ask foster parents, teachers, or others who have significant involvement with the child to complete these instruments, such as the Teacher Report Form (TRF) of the CBCL/6–18, which provides normative comparisons between the child and other youngsters in the school setting. We discuss the process of gathering information from collateral sources in more detail in Chapter 4.

Just as parents' descriptions of their children's maltreatment are not restricted solely to the factual content of what has happened to their offspring, their accounts of their children's reactions to the maltreatment may reflect their feelings about the child. Do they talk about the child's difficulties in a very hostile, angry tone of voice? Do they seem to have little, if any, understanding of why the child may be reacting in a particular way to the maltreatment? Do they describe the problem behavior as a manifestation of a "bad" child, or do they see the behavior as symptomatic of the child's distress and a reflection of his or her attempts to cope with overwhelming, traumatizing experiences? The clinician begins to wonder whether the emotions associated with this account are merely situational reactions to the child's problematic behavior, reflections of the parent's own issues about maltreatment and victimization, or indicators of chronic and ongoing problems in the parent–child relationship. These are all hypotheses that warrant exploration in subsequent sessions.

Child's Developmental History

Obtaining a detailed developmental history is an important endeavor. It puts the information about the child's response to the maltreatment and presenting problems in a broader context that allows one to more fully and accurately elucidate the association between maltreatment and outcome. The previous example of the importance of development history for the accurate differential diagnosis that the girl's attention problems were attributable to PTSD rather than ADHD reinforces the need to gather relevant historical information about a child's development.

Developmental variables can serve as potentiating or compensatory factors that moderate the association between maltreatment and outcome, and taking a comprehensive developmental history is an essential step in making this determination. For example, does the child present with developmental delays as a result of his or her mother's difficult pregnancy, labor, or delivery? Careful inquiry may have already revealed that these problems, such as cognitive and language delays, long preceded the sexual abuse. Even though they are not direct sequelae of the victimization, they may have real significance for the child's adaptation to the trauma and for treatment planning. Have cognitive delays contributed to distortions in the child's understanding of what has happened, and contributed to his or her distress and anxiety? Have language delays restricted the ability to articulate feelings about the abuse, thereby increasing the probability of externalizing, aggressive behaviors? How can we adapt frequently used intervention strategies, such as cognitive-behavioral therapy (CBT), to accommodate these developmental delays? Would CBT even be useful? Table 3.2 presents an outline of a typical developmental history.

Clinicians can interview parents to obtain this information or request them to complete one of the commonly used developmental history forms, such as the Aggregate Neurobehavioral Student Health and Educational Review (ANSER; Levine, 1996), and then review the completed form with them and ask any follow-up questions. A review of other collateral information (e.g., obstetrical records) sometimes yields valuable information that enriches our understanding of a child.

Parents' or caregivers' accounts of their children's developmental history may also reflect their own problem areas or strengths. Do they have difficulty remembering details, and is this a reflection of a lack of interest in the child, an example of the deleterious effects of chronic substance abuse, or an indication of serious cognitive delays? Unfortunately, it may be difficult or impossible to gather reliable and comprehensive developmental histories of some children in the care of child welfare. Biological parents may be unavailable or the whereabouts of records unknown.

TABLE 3.2. Developmental History of the Child

1. Pregnancy and delivery
   a. Was the pregnancy planned? (Was this child wanted?)
   b. Was this the mother's first pregnancy?
   c. Parents' feelings about the pregnancy and their impressions and feelings about the baby during pregnancy
   d. Did the mother have medical care and consultation during the pregnancy?
   e. Health of the mother during the pregnancy
      (1) Weight gain
      (2) Medications taken, including substance abuse (e.g., alcohol, drugs, tobacco)
      (3) Medical problems and treatments
   f. Was the child born preterm or postterm?
   g. Labor
      (1) Were both parents present?
      (2) Duration
      (3) Medications administered
      (4) Special procedures used
      (5) Was the baby healthy at birth?
      (6) Baby's weight and Apgar scores
      (7) Was the baby held and fed immediately?
      (8) What were the parents' feelings and thoughts on seeing the baby? Reactions to the child's gender?
      (9) How did other family members react? (e.g., husband/partner, siblings, extended family members)
      (10) Did the baby have any problems postdelivery? Did the baby require time in the intensive care nursery?
      (11) How long did the mother and child stay in the hospital?
      (11) How and when was the name selected?
      (12) Was the baby breastfed? Why or why not? How long was the baby breastfed?

2. Neonatal period and infancy
   a. Constitution and temperamental style (e.g., activity level, reaction to stimuli, general responsiveness, reactions to change and transitions)
   b. Growth patterns, including failure-to-thrive
   c. Establishment of eating, sleeping, and toilet routines; crying. How did parents cope with any problems in these areas?

3. Developmental milestones
   a. Parents' general memory regarding whether concerns were apparent
   b. Specifics regarding approximate age at first smile, sitting, walking, first words, good communication understandable by others outside the family, day and night toilet training achieved, sexual maturity and puberty

4. Early relationships and attachment history
   a. Who was (were) the child's primary caregiver(s) during infancy and toddlerhood?
   b. Were there separations of the child from a primary caregiver(s), and at what age did these occur? Reasons for and duration of separations?
   c. What were the child's reactions when separated from primary caregiver(s), and how did the child relate when reunited?

d. How well did the child differentiate among adults and demonstrate a clear preference for a particular caregiver?
e. What did the child do when hurt, tired, ill, or distressed? Did the child seek out comfort, and from whom?
f. Child's response to comforting when offered.
g. Did the child seek out affection in an indiscriminate manner?
h. Did the child show initial reticence around strangers, or did the child readily approach unfamiliar adults?
i. Did the child check back with the caregiver, especially in unfamiliar settings, or did the child wander off without purpose?
j. Did the child show affection spontaneously (e.g., initiate a hug, touch, or kiss)? Did the child respond reciprocally in interactions? Was the child clingy?

5. Stresses
   a. Physical illnesses/injuries (acute and/or chronic)
   b. Emotional (e.g., separation/divorce of parents, death of significant family members or pets, family moves, poverty, family violence, substance abuse, physical/mental illness in family members)
   c. History of maltreatment
      (1) Type of maltreatment
      (2) Age at onset
      (3) Duration
      (4) Perpetrators
      (5) Child's reaction (behavioral, emotional, physical) to the maltreatment
      (6) Response of the environment to the maltreatment (e.g., parents/caregivers, siblings, wider community [including teachers, legal/justice system])
      (7) Previous or concurrent treatment or other services to the child and family and their outcomes

6. Other placements
   a. Number of placements and duration; types of placement
   b. Reason(s) for each placement (e.g., maltreatment, breakdown in placement because of the child's behavior)
   c. Feelings and attitudes of previous caretakers toward the child
   d. Child's behavior in each placement (e.g., any significant difficulties? if so, obtain as full a description as possible)
   e. Were alternate child care arrangements used when parents worked? Who were the caregivers, and what was the child's response to them?

7. Nature of and response to discipline

8. School history
   a. Emotional reaction
   b. Progress at school
   c. Behavior with teachers and classmates
   d. Special class placements or other educational and psychological assistance

9. Hobbies, interests, sports, chores

10. Peer relationships
    a. Number of friendships
    b. Nature and intensity of friendships (e.g., has the child been detached or unduly dependent on peers? Did the child have to take all the initiative to establish and maintain peer relationships, or did other children take the initiative?)

(*continued*)

TABLE 3.2. (*continued*)

- c. Problem areas in relationships with peers (e.g., fighting, withdrawal, sexual behavior)
- d. Issues and attitudes about sexuality (e.g., sexual maturity, identification as a male or a female, sexual behaviors, sexual interest—age at first interest, sexual behaviors, dating habits, attitudes, and feelings about sexual behavior)

11. History of any other previous problems
    - a. Nature of the problem
    - b. Onset, frequency, duration
    - c. Assessment, treatment, or other services; outcome

Note. Adapted from Pearce and Pezzot-Pearce (1997) and Pezzot-Pearce and Pearce (2004).

Parental/Caregiver Reactions to the Maltreatment

One of the most consistent findings in the empirical literature is the association between children's adjustment following maltreatment and the support they receive from parents or caregivers (see Elliott and Carnes, 2001, for a comprehensive review). But what does "support" mean? It is a broad term that subsumes several different components. Everson, Hunter, Runyon, Edelsohn, and Coulter (1989) developed the Parental Reaction to Incest Disclosure Scale (PRIDS), which measures three components of parental support: emotional support (e.g., commitment to the child versus abandoning the child psychologically), belief in the child (e.g., making clear public statements of their belief versus totally denying that the abuse occurred), and action toward the perpetrator (e.g., actively demonstrating disapproval of the perpetrator's abusive behavior by effecting a separation or cooperating with the criminal prosecution versus choosing the perpetrator over the child).

Table 3.3 represents an attempt to summarize some of the key variables subsumed by the term "support". The table does not provide an exhaustive list; there may be other supportive attitudes or behaviors by caregivers and parents. Although they are based on the child sexual abuse literature, some of these variables may also be relevant for children exposed to other types of maltreatment. The child who has been physically abused, neglected, psychologically maltreated, or exposed to domestic violence will probably benefit from the same kind of emotional support, belief of the nonoffending parent in his or her allegations, and protection from the abusive or neglectful individual, as would sexually abused children. Furthermore, Chapter 6 describes in detail the importance of parents' management of their children's behavioral and emotional difficulties associated with the maltreatment. Table 3.3 may serve as a rough guide for clinicians who are attempting to help parents and caregivers develop ways of supporting their children postdisclosure.

TABLE 3.3. Components of Family Support (Postdisclosure)

1. Parent believes child
   - *For example*: acknowledges the maltreatment, believes in the child's account and does not dispute its truthfulness
2. Emotional support
   - *For example*: committed to the child, has not abandoned the child psychologically, does not blame the child, and ascribes responsibility to the perpetrator
3. Instrumental support
   - *For example*: ensures that the child receives appropriate medical/psychosocial interventions
4. Actions toward the perpetrator
   - *For example*: notifies the police and/or protective services and cooperates with subsequent investigations, protects the child from further abuse (e.g., makes the perpetrator leave the home, chooses the child over the perpetrator)
5. Provision of adequate parenting postdisclosure
   - *For example*: imposition of firm and consistent limits on the child's externalizing behaviors, adequate supervision and monitoring

Note. Adapted from Elliott and Carnes (2001), Everson et al. (1989), and Leifer et al. (1993).

Elliott and Carnes (2001) make some astute observations about the components that constitute support. Belief, support, and protection are overlapping constructs that sometimes are difficult to separate, although they are not synonymous. They state:

> For example, when first learning about an alleged incident of abuse, an enraged caregiver may threaten to injure the perpetrator. Although this response indicates belief in the child's allegations, the child may perceive the high level of emotionality as nonsupportive if it does not meet his or her current psychological needs. Clearly, a response that is perceived as supportive or protective to one person may not appear so to another. (p. 315)

Most studies have not examined separately the impact of these factors, especially maternal supportiveness and protection; they are usually examined as one variable. Consequently, it is difficult to draw any definitive opinions about the specific mechanisms of action or pathogenic processes that underlie such a broad construct. Support, belief, and protection are not static constructs but may change over time and vary across situations. A parent may be supportive in some ways (e.g., ensuring that the child receives medical attention) but unsupportive in others (e.g., refusing to talk with a distressed child) (Elliott & Carnes, 2001). Evidence also indicates that initial reactions may not predict belief, support, or protection afforded by a parent in the future (Salt, Myer, Coleman, & Sauzier, 1990). Furthermore, although maternal belief in children's disclosure is a strong predictor of maternal protectiveness, it does not necessarily ensure protection. Almost 20% of mothers who believed their children failed to take protective action (Heriot, 1996).

Many studies have demonstrated that greater parental support is associated with maltreated children's better outcomes. Tremblay, Hebert, and Piché (1999) found that both social support and coping strategies exerted a significant effect on the adjustment of child victims of sexual abuse, and these constituted direct instead of mediating effects. Parental support was the best single predictor of resiliency in sexually abused girls (Spaccarelli & Kim, 1995), and abused children with supportive caregivers were more likely to disclose sexual abuse and less likely to recant their allegations (Elliott & Briere, 1994). Leifer, Shapiro, and Kassem (1993) described three components of maternal support: overt protective actions, such as taking a daughter to the hospital or calling the police, belief in the daughter's account without disputing its truthfulness, and not blaming the daughter for being abused. The authors reported that 49% of the mothers provided an adequate response to their daughters' disclosures of sexual abuse as assessed by these three components. Those children whose mothers provided little support demonstrated poor functioning. Similarly, children of mothers who became angry and punitive had more behavior problems (Sauzier, Salt, & Calhoun, 1990).

What factors predict parental belief, support, and protection? What little relevant research exists is sparse, focuses on childhood sexual abuse, and typically involves mothers. Studies of the mother's relationship with the perpetrator as a predictor of her belief and the extent of her support/protection have yielded inconsistent results, as have the victim's age and gender (Elliott & Carnes, 2001). A number of studies have found no relationship between a maternal history of abuse and the responses to one's child (e.g., Deblinger, Stauffer, & Landsberg, 1994), although one study found that mothers with a sexual abuse history were described as more supportive by their sexually abused adolescent daughters than were mothers without such a history (Leifer et al., 1993).

Theoretically, nonoffending parents' psychological problems and distress may compromise the support they can offer their maltreated children, although very few studies have examined this relationship. It is not surprising that parents frequently experience distress following their children's disclosure. In addition to grave concerns about their children's physical and emotional well-being, parents undergo other stressful experiences: losses or changes in income and in their relationships with friends and family, employment disruption, changes of residence, and dependence on government programs (Massat & Lundy, 1998).

The empirical research confirms these impressions (Elliott & Carnes,

2001). Nonoffending parents of maltreated (Famularo, Fenton, Kinscherff, Ayoub, & Barnum, 1994) and sexually abused children (Kelley, 1990) showed symptoms of PTSD, and these higher elevations have been reported for both mothers and fathers (Burgess, Hartman, Kelley, Grant, & Gray, 1990). Parents' PTSD symptoms can persist for at least 2 years following disclosure of the sexual abuse (Kelley, 1990), and parents whose children testify in court are especially at risk for developing intrusive and avoidant PTSD symptoms (Burgess et al., 1990). A maternal history of childhood sexual abuse is associated with more general psychological distress (Deblinger et al., 1994) and PTSD symptoms (Timmons-Mitchell, Chandler-Holtz, & Semple, 1996, 1997) in mothers following their children's disclosure of sexual abuse than in nonoffending mothers without such a history. Mothers and fathers of sexually abused children are more likely to experience depression than are parents of nonclinical, nonabused youngsters (Kelley, 1990).

What follows is a summary of our clinical impressions of some of the salient aspects of parents and caregivers' feelings and reactions to their children's maltreatment and their relevance to children's adjustment. Although some of these observations are supported by the empirical literature, many await confirmation.

PARENTAL FEELINGS ABOUT THE SELF

Some parents or caregivers feel extremely guilty about their child's victimization. This is especially so if they have a personal history of maltreatment and had promised themselves that they would never allow anything similar to happen to their own children. They may feel inadequate as parents, are embarrassed to disclose their children's experiences because they expect criticism from others (Regehr, 1990), and may even develop symptoms of depression. Unfortunately, such guilt feelings may contribute to deterioration in their parenting skills. We have seen some parents who allowed their child to engage in out-of-control or excessive behavior postdisclosure because of excessive sympathy for the child. In the empirical literature, lax limits and a high degree of parental tolerance of negative and socially inappropriate behaviors have been linked to preschool- and school-age children's externalizing behaviors and poorer social competence (Cohen & Mannarino, 1996a, 1998a). We speculate that some parents' failure to set firm limits reflects an attempt to alleviate a sense of guilt for what the child has experienced. Poor limit setting may also reflect long-standing parenting difficulties that predated the onset of the maltreatment. Depressed parents may encounter particular difficulty in monitoring, supervising, holding clear expectations, and placing firm and consistent limits on their children, as they have little energy for such tasks. Vegetative symptoms such as poor eating and sleeping leave them even more fatigued and unable to engage in the active parenting their children require.

At the other end of the spectrum, parents may become overprotective and severely restrict their children's activities to ensure that the abuse never recurs. This strategy may convey the implicit notion to children that they are powerless and unable to protect themselves from future dangers, possibly reinforcing a self-image as a victim. Restricting normal activities may also impede recovery by limiting the children's opportunities to be successful in age-appropriate activities (e.g., sports, extracurricular school activities, clubs) and to interact in healthy ways with peers.

We have already reported a link between a maternal history of childhood sexual abuse and mothers' general psychological distress and PTSD symptoms. These difficulties in turn may affect parenting, including aspects of the parent–child relationship not included in the belief, support, and protection components that constitute the great bulk of the studies to date. In one of the few studies to examine the relationship between a history of maltreatment and other aspects of parenting, Cole, Woolger, Power, and Smith (1992) found that adult female incest survivors reported significantly less confidence and a diminished sense of control as parents than other mothers. They also reported that they were less consistent and organized and made fewer demands on their children, which in turn impeded the emergence of their children's autonomy.

In general, a child's victimization experiences are capable of eliciting strong feelings in parents, such as sadness, anger, or anxiety and, as we have seen, clinical symptoms of PTSD and depression. The anxiety and fear engendered in most parents who discover that their child has been abused may be extremely potent for parents who have undergone similar traumatic episodes when they were younger. Their reactions may be significantly heightened if they have avoided recollections of their own experiences, along with the associated overwhelming, intense affect for many years. To cope with such pain and distress, parents engage in a number of defensive maneuvers that may have important implications for how they manage their children's reactions. Consistent with the short-term, adaptive function of avoidance in the PTSD model, parents may deny their child's abuse or neglect, or emotional or behavioral reactions, to avoid their own pain because these are powerful reminders of what happened to them as children. This leaves children questioning the validity of their perceptions of the maltreatment (e.g., "Did it really happen?") and the legitimacy of their feelings (e.g., "I guess it must not have been too bad because my parents never talk with me about it"). They cannot talk with parents about their feelings or the abuse, as parents may intentionally avoid such conversations or become so distraught that the children quickly curtail such discussions in order to protect their parents from more distress. Unfortunately, children may not receive the emotional support they require, such as parental statements that they still love their children, or statements that they were not responsible for the maltreatment, that allows them to modify their attributions. Utilizing Mowrer's (1960) two-factor model of PTSD as a conceptual basis, we can appreciate that children who are not exposed to the feared stimuli, because their parents are unable to talk with them about what happened, continue to suffer from anxiety that does not extinguish. Furthermore, their avoidance is strengthened as both they and their parents experience an attenuation of their anxiety because neither are exposed to cues associated with their respective histories of maltreatment. Parents may also deal with their own or their children's emotional reactions to the victimization in an intellectualized manner. This approach again leaves children feeling unsupported and reluctant to articulate or express strong emotions. In other instances, parents may become excessively preoccupied with issues related to their own victimization, having little time or energy to devote to their children. Consequently, children feel unsupported and abandoned or are exposed to inadequate parenting practices, such as poor supervision or inconsistent limit setting. Parents diagnosed with PTSD may revert to maladaptive ways of coping with the anxiety and distress. These maladaptions can include substance abuse, which can further impair their ability to give children special care postdisclosure (e.g., providing poor supervision and monitoring; being emotionally and psychologically unavailable and unable to respond sensitively to their children's distress). We have already reviewed Leifer and colleagues (1993), who found that substance abuse moderates the association between mothers' history of abuse and subsequent response to their children. Clinical depression may compromise parenting in similar ways. Children may also infer the meaning and significance of maltreatment from observing their parents' reactions. They may interpret their parents' PTSD or depression as incontrovertible proof that they have been damaged beyond repair.

Given the potential impact of parents' victimization history on their coping mechanisms and responses to their child's maltreatment, it is crucial to inquire about this variable, even though it has not yet been thoroughly investigated in the empirical literature. Clinicians should preface direct questioning about this issue by noting that a number of parents have such a history and adding that it often has important implications for their reactions to their children. If the child lives with a mother and a father, the clinician should ask both parents about this matter.

The clinician should gather enough information to form some tentative impressions about the significance of a parental victimization history.

The clinician can ask about the identity of the parent's perpetrator to determine if it is similar to the child's (e.g., a paternal figure), the type(s) of maltreatment the individual experienced, whether the parent ever disclosed the maltreatment and if others knew about it, and the response of his or her own parents or caregivers. It may be profitable to ask parents to describe how they coped with their maltreatment, how it affected their feelings and responses to their child's victimization, and what assistance or support they need now regarding their own history to help themselves and their offspring. We must be prudent when conducting this inquiry because it can sometimes provoke intense feelings. The inquiry should not go so far that parents' defensive structures are stripped away and their functioning deteriorates, such as in parenting and the ability to manage children's emotional distress and behavior problems. This caveat is especially important if there are no services in place to provide immediate and ongoing assistance to the adult.

Empathizing with and normalizing parents' distress can attenuate the sense of isolation and stigmatization that may accompany their disclosure of maltreatment. Clinicians should also draw parents' attention to the strength they displayed when acknowledging their own history and should reinforce the notion that in doing so, they have taken a significant step in helping their child. One component of the treatment plan might be a recommendation for such parents to participate in therapy to address those historical issues obstructing their ability to cope adaptively with the child's maltreatment. Commending parents for having talked about their victimization may render such a recommendation more palatable.

FEELINGS TOWARD THE CHILD

Although parents may believe their child's account of the maltreatment, some become angry with a child who did not stop or prevent the abuse or disclose it sooner. Our clinical experience suggests that this attitude is particularly prevalent in the reactions of fathers to their abused sons, especially those boys who have been sexually assaulted. These fathers may be anxious about their son's masculinity, fearful that the boy consented to the sexual activity, and harbor numerous concerns about the boy's sexual identity or preference. Other parents, especially those whose children have been sexually abused, may regard them as "spoiled goods" or see them as so damaged that any chance of recovery is slim. These reactions compound the child's sense of stigmatization and helplessness. Others outrightly disbelieve their child's allegations and accuse the youngster of fabrication. They blame the child for the perpetrator's being charged, convicted, or incarcerated, or for the resulting family disruption if the perpetrator is a family member. At its most extreme, this attitude is exemplified by the parent who chooses to support the alleged perpetrator rather than the child and insists that the child, not the perpetrator, leave the home. These sentiments can engender or compound the child's internal attributions of self-blame and feelings of betrayal and stigmatization.

FEELINGS TOWARD THE PERPETRATOR

Anger is, of course, a normal and expected reaction in any parent of a maltreated child. However, this may become so extreme that the parent begins to voice a desire to hurt or even kill the perpetrator. Such statements are not helpful for those children who were abused or neglected by somebody they know well and may even love. Many victimized children are ambivalent about their perpetrator and do not want the individual harmed. A parent's threats to harm or kill the perpetrator escalate the child's anxiety, especially when he or she is aware that such actions might result in that parent's incarceration or punishment. The child would then be deprived of parental availability and support at just the time when they are most needed. Furthermore, extreme displays of parental anger at the perpetrator serve as poor models of emotional and behavioral self-regulation and may lead the child to believe that his or her positive feelings are in some way deviant. Other parents feel extreme guilt about pressing charges and are unduly concerned about the welfare of the perpetrator or his or her family (Regehr, 1990). They may begin to question the validity of the child's disclosure, seriously compromising the support they offer the child. The situation can be magnified if others pressure parents to consider the perpetrator's welfare, especially when this individual is a relative and other members of the family ally themselves with the perpetrator.

FEELINGS TOWARD THE SYSTEM

Parental distress over a child's victimization may be heightened by fears and anxiety associated with an investigation and judicial proceedings (Regehr, 1990). Some parents are apprehensive about the impact of their child's testifying in court and feel they have little control over the investigatory and judicial process. Others believe that their own parenting capabilities are being questioned by representatives of the various systems, which adds to their distress. This reaction may be especially prevalent in families in which parents have been responsible for the child's maltreatment and have had extensive involvement with child protective or legal/justice systems. These parents may harbor considerable antipathy toward these systems and their representatives. Unfortunately, hostility and anger may be communicated directly to the child, who in turn begins to regard contact with staff of these agencies with similar suspicion and hostility. The child may generalize these attitudes and negative expectations to mental health professionals, which becomes a significant obstacle in establishing a therapeutic alliance between the child and clinician.

Parental Management of Children's Behavioral and Emotional Problems

The strategies parents use to help children overcome behavioral and emotional sequelae associated with their maltreatment are critically important for their subsequent adjustment (see Chapter 6 for a detailed review). When the clinician and parents were discussing the child's presenting problems, the clinician might have asked how they have handled the child's symptoms. If this area was not explored then, the clinician should now ask for a description of the specific strategies a parent used and is now using to manage these behaviors. For example, if the child displayed many anxiety-related problems, such as nightmares, how did the parent deal with them? Was this effective? What was the child's response? If nightmares are still a problem, has the parent changed strategies and has this been effective? Similarly, the clinician will want to know about the parent's response to any aggressive or sexualized behavior the child manifested. Inappropriate or ineffective strategies may well have exacerbated the child's symptomatology, whereas other practices may have proven to be extremely helpful in the child's adaptation to the maltreatment. Chapter 6 reviews specific interventions parents and caregivers can use to ameliorate these difficulties.

Other Aspects of Current Parental and Family Functioning

Previous sections reviewed in detail the importance of parental or caregiver reactions to children's maltreatment. Table 3.4 is a more comprehensive summary of the major variables to survey in the area of parental and family functioning, ranging from the individual and intrapsychic ones to broader areas such as financial status.

We offer a few brief comments here about these other relevant characteristics of parental and family functioning. A secure emotional attachment may serve as a compensatory factor for maltreated youngsters. They expect parents to quickly and sensitively respond to their distress. Consequently, they more readily seek out support and assistance than do children with an insecure attachment. Parents of children with secure attachments probably will not resent the time, effort, and energy required to help their children recover. A secure attachment may also contribute to a solid sense of self-esteem and self-efficacy, and adaptive emotional and behavioral self-

TABLE 3.4. Current Parental and Family Functioning

1. Parental functioning
   a. Presence of any identifiable psychiatric/psychological problems; substance abuse; health problems; current involvement in any treatment for these problems
   b. Quality of current relationships, including marital relationship; presence of problems (e.g., spousal violence, serious discord); efforts to seek assistance and current involvement
   c. Degree and quality of other social supports
   d. Current employment and financial status; stability and adequacy of living arrangements
2. Parenting ability
   a. A secure parent–child attachment
   b. The ability to perceive the child accurately and to recognize and meet the individual needs and characteristics of the child; appropriate expectations of the child
   c. Disciplinary style
   d. Impulse control (affective and behavioral self-regulation)
3. Family functioning[a]
   a. Structure and organization of the family: repetitive patterns of interaction (alliance, coalitions, subsystems; power hierarchy; separation of generations; boundaries between individuals; degree of individuality; cohesiveness; interdependency; enmeshment); clarity of roles and functions; rigidity and flexibility of system, openness to information
   b. Communication: clarity–ambiguity; directness–indirectness; consequences of verbal and nonverbal communication; metacommunication (rules about what can be said, by whom, to whom, and how), themes, preoccupations, avoidances
   c. Affect: emotional tone, expression, intensity, variation, rules about expression; comfort level with feelings, responsiveness
   d. Control and decision making: leadership style, flexibility, consistency, forms of reinforcement, cooperation, resistance, attitude to feedback
   e. Conflict resolution: method and style; management of differences and disagreement; areas of difficulty
   f. Developmental parameters: age appropriateness of expectations, roles, intergenerational issues; management of autonomy and individuation; fit between developmental tasks of adults and children

[a]Adapted from Broder and Hood (1983).

regulation, resulting in less distress and more adaptive coping mechanisms. Chapter 4 reviews specific ways to evaluate attachment.

The clinician must ask parents whether they have any current psychiatric or psychological problems that impair their functioning. A psychiatric diagnosis per se does not necessarily mean that an individual encounters significant difficulty with parenting, although it may represent a significant risk factor for compromised parenting. Consistent with the transactional model, many other variables mediate the relationship between the presence of a psychological or psychiatric disorder and an individual's functioning (e.g., provision of appropriate treatment, presence of social supports). Similarly, the significance of health problems, substance abuse, or problems with the law for a parent's functioning must be examined with reference to other variables. It behooves the clinician to gather specific information that explicates the relationship, if any, between these diagnoses or problems and a parent's ability to support the child's recovery.

The quality of a parent's current relationships is another important variable, including disharmony, discord, and violence. We have already discussed how parents' time, attention, and psychological resources that could be expended to help the child cope with the maltreatment are compromised or diverted to other problems. Conflict between partners may engender inconsistent approaches to child management, thereby compounding children's difficulties. Disagreements about how to handle other aspects of the maltreatment, such as whether to report the situation to the police, may also reflect long-standing conflicts between parents about childrearing.

Clinicians must inquire about the degree and quality of other social supports that are currently available to parents. This information should include not only the actual number of supports but also whether parents *perceive* them as supportive. What function do these supports play in parent's lives, and what kind of help or assistance do they provide? For instance, do parents have ready and easy access to alternate caregivers who will provide relief in caring for a maltreated child who is aggressive and defiant? Are there individuals with whom parents can talk and receive a sense of validation of, and support for, their feelings, or do they feel socially isolated? Are these natural social supports, or do parents rely exclusively on crisis nurseries, child welfare personnel, shelters, or professionals for support?

Social and cultural factors influence the parent's response to the child's maltreatment. A substantial proportion of children engage in sexualized behavior after being sexually assaulted. Social and religious values that strongly condemn any kind of sexual behavior in children may be associated with overpunitive and harsh parental responses, which may exacerbate the child's feelings of stigmatization, shame, and guilt (Gil & Johnson, 1993).

Parents' current employment and financial status can affect the quality of care they provide their children. Being unemployed and living in poverty may provoke strong feelings of inadequacy about themselves and their ability to provide for their families, especially if parents perceive the maltreatment as more proof of their badness as parents, and contribute to depression or hostility. Furthermore, a precarious financial situation may preclude parents from hiring caregivers to obtain a much-needed break from the sometimes intense demands of managing maltreated children's behavior, thereby heightening the parents' feelings of tension, anxiety, and frustration. Living in crowded, unsafe, or even dangerous environments increases stress in the child and other family members. In some countries, limited financial resources restrict the range of services and treatment options available to parents and children. Other parents may live in regions where treatment services are undeveloped. Besides identifying these areas of stress, a clinician must ask how parents handled these difficulties, paying particular attention to their successes in ameliorating them. These successes may highlight strengths in the parents and family and may serve as a basis for effective interventions in any subsequent treatment plan.

Finally, evaluation of the family system can provide important information about how the family has adapted to the child's maltreatment. For example, a family in which parents exhibit little leadership or executive functioning may be at risk for failing to provide the child with the high degree of consistency and structure needed after a disclosure of sexual abuse, which in turn is linked to the child's heightened distress and anxiety. Information about these aspects of family functioning not only helps to identify the presence of important moderator variables but also suggests important intervention targets.

Of course, most clinicians who treat abused and neglected children do not have sufficient time, and sometimes the prerequisite skills and training, to initiate comprehensive assessments of parents. Moreover, subjecting every parent or caregiver to such thorough assessments is impractical and unnecessary, especially as a number of parents function quite well. However, clinicians do meet caregivers who are having significant problems in parenting their maltreated children, coping with their own confusing and painful reactions, and managing the stress of residing in impoverished and sometimes dangerous communities. A number of sources describe the assessment of parenting capacity and the evaluation of the risk parents may pose to their children in terms of abuse and neglect (e.g., Pezzot-Pearce & Pearce, 2004; Schutz, Dixon, Lindenberger, & Ruther, 1989). We advise the reader to consult these references for more detailed and extensive discussions of such issues.

Parental and Family History

The parental and family history phase of information gathering provides yet more information about factors that have contributed to the child's current distress. Table 3.5 presents a summary of information the clinician may find relevant. This summary is based on the work of others (Broder & Hood, 1983; Wolfe, 1988; Wolfe & Wolfe, 1988), which the reader may consult for a more detailed discussion.

We have seen that parents' reactions to their children's victimization are important moderators of outcome. Numerous variables, including historical ones, affect parents' current abilities to respond in ways that will alleviate their children's distress and promote a return to a healthy developmental trajectory. Are parents' problems in responding sensitively and constructively reflective of acute situational reactions to the child's disclosure that will abate with time, or do they reflect chronic problems stemming from the parents' own histories of trauma and victimization or other psychological and psychiatric disorders that predated the child's maltreatment? Do current difficulties in talking with the child about the maltreatment reflect long-standing problems in communication and the sharing of feelings that have origins in a parent's own family?

History is also relevant to other factors that can moderate outcome. Have the parents always had difficulty in making friends, or is their current social isolation more an acute reaction to feelings of shame, guilt, and stigmatization elicited by the abuse? Do the family's current limited financial resources reflect chronic problems with educational attainment or employment, or is this situation just temporary, such as in the case of a parent who takes time off from work to devote more attention to a distressed child?

The history of a parent's significant relationships may also be relevant. A long-standing history of parental relationship problems, including spousal violence, may bode especially poorly for a maltreated child's subsequent adjustment to trauma. Consider a child who has witnessed considerable domestic violence and who now exhibits aggressive behavior with younger siblings. The nonoffending parent may be so preoccupied, exhausted, or traumatized by the violence and conflict that characterized an extensive history of brutalization that his or her attention has been deflected from the child, thereby resulting in lax supervision of the child's interactions with other youngsters or little energy to offer the needed emotional support to the child.

The actual parenting a child receives subsequent to the maltreatment has an enormous influence on adjustment. Again, historical information about parenting may be a rich source of relevant data. Had this child been exposed to inadequate or ineffectual parenting even before the onset of the maltreatment, or are the current problems a transient reaction to the sudden emergence of the child's symptoms in a family in which caregivers demonstrated good parenting previously and the child was abused by someone outside the immediate family? Such historical information contributes to treatment planning. Parents who demonstrate an acute, situational reaction and were functioning well before the maltreatment may respond positively to a short-term course of intervention. This approach, described in more detail in Chapter 6, entails getting parents into treatment quickly, rather

TABLE 3.5. Parental and Family History

1. Parental history
   a. Quality of relationship with parents/significant caregivers; relationship with siblings
   b. Description of family life during childhood: management of conflict and discipline; patterns of communication, including sharing of affection and feelings
   c. History of maltreatment in childhood and adolescence
   d. Quality of relationships with peers during childhood and adolescence
   e. Educational history
   f. Employment history
   g. Parental and family history of psychiatric/psychological problems, including efforts to seek assistance and outcome of professional involvement
   h. Problems with the law
   i. Other previous relevant life events (e.g., deaths, significant illnesses, financial problems)

2. Marital and family history
   a. Description of previous relationships or marriages, including any problems (e.g., spousal violence); reasons for termination of these relationships/marriages; problems regarding divorce or custody/access
   b. Current relationship/marriage—how the couple met and what attracted them to each other
   c. Length, stability, and quality of the relationship
   d. Presence of any previous problems in the relationship or family (e.g., spousal violence, substance abuse); lack of support regarding family responsibilities

3. Parenting history
   a. Planning for children (e.g., planned vs. unplanned pregnancies); pregnancies; births; adoptions; abortions or miscarriages
   b. Reactions to pregnancies; effect of pregnancies and arrival of children
   c. Brief description of physical, emotional, and behavioral problems of all children; previous attempts to seek help and outcome of these problems
   d. History of parenting difficulties; reasons; previous attempts to seek assistance and outcome of these difficulties
   e. History of maltreatment in the family; type of maltreatment, identity of perpetrator, time of onset, duration, and frequency; emotional and behavioral response of family members and involvement of other systems/agencies (e.g., child protective services, police)
   f. Placements of children (type of placement, reasons, reactions of parents and children)

than letting them linger on waiting lists and allowing their distress to become more entrenched. Interventions include giving parents emotional and practical support regarding their reactions to children's disclosures, information about abuse and children's typical reactions, practical guidance on managing their children's feelings and behaviors, and advice about collaborating with the other systems that frequently become involved. Another family, whose history reveals repeated incidents of child maltreatment and numerous long-term and refractory difficulties, probably requires a very different set of interventions.

Assessment Strategies

The main method of obtaining family information is through interviews with parents or caregivers. The clinician should reiterate the rationale for the very personal questions and can supplement parental reports by documentation from other agencies, such as child welfare reports or records of past involvement with helping agencies, including past therapy records.

Researchers have used several questionnaires and self-report measures to evaluate parents' reactions to their children's sexual abuse. We have already mentioned the PRIDS (Everson et al., 1989), which measures emotional support, belief in the child, and action toward the perpetrator. Cohen and Mannarino (1996a) used the Parent Emotional Reaction Questionnaire (PERQ) to evaluate parents' emotional reaction to their children's sexual abuse. It consists of 15 items that examine such reactions as fear, anger, guilt, embarrassment, and feeling upset. Cohen and Mannarino also designed the Parent Support Questionnaire (PSQ) to measure parental cognitions and perceptions of their own behaviors in response to their children's sexual abuse. It includes19 items that "examine the degree and kind of perceived parental support provided to the sexually abused child and the nature of the attributions that parents make regarding responsibility for abuse (i.e., who is to blame)" (Cohen & Mannarino, 1996a, pp. 1405–1406). Cohen and Mannarino report acceptable internal consistency and test–retest reliability for both their measures.

Given the heterogeneity of parents and families in which maltreatment has occurred, and given the broad array of contributing factors, including those related to parental and family functioning, the clinician should approach family assessment with reasonable expectations. It is unrealistic to expect to identify all the factors that influence the functioning of parents and family. However, the attempt to enrich our understanding of the potential influence of parental and family factors places the child's assessment in a much broader and more meaningful context.

CHAPTER FOUR

Assessment of the Child

In Chapter 3 we described our six underlying assumptions about clinical assessment. We would like to add one other assumption: *Clinical assessments of maltreated children must have a developmental focus.* This assumption is critically important for two reasons. First, knowledge of normal growth and development helps determine the significance of a particular behavior; that is, is the behavior or symptom a "problem" deserving attention, or is it expected of a child of that particular age? Consider a simple example: nighttime enuresis is common for 2-year-old children but much rarer for 12-year-olds. Unfortunately, such distinctions may not be so easily drawn for other behavior. For example, reports of normative data regarding children's sexual behavior are quite recent (e.g., Friedrich et al., 2001); previously, clinicians were hampered in determining the clinical significance of children's sexualized behavior. However, comparative frequency of the behavior alone is an insufficient consideration. The CSBI may indicate that the sexualized behaviors exhibited by a child are rare; that is, they are not displayed by the vast majority of the child's peers. However, clinicians must consider many other variables (e.g., use of physical or psychological coercion to gain the other child's compliance, lack of empathy for the other child's feelings) when deciding the clinical significance of a particular behavior or symptom. Although a solid knowledge and understanding of the comparative frequency of children's behavior does not provide the complete perspective, it is a necessary starting point from which clinicians can begin to evaluate the child's response to maltreatment.

Second, knowledge about a particular child's developmental level furnishes critical information that guides the choice and application of assessment strategies. Developmentally sensitive assessments are essential to obtaining useful information that can guide clinical decision making and planning. Clinicians must have a basic knowledge of the development of children's cognitive abilities, memory, and language to ensure that interviews and other assessment strategies are commensurate with their developmental levels and abilities.

PLANNING THE ASSESSMENT OF THE CHILD

After interviewing parents or significant caregivers, the clinician should have considerable information regarding their perceptions of the child's response to the maltreatment. The clinician should contact other significant people in the child's life to confirm parents' or caregivers' reports of the child's functioning. Some parents or caregivers, including those of maltreated children, are somewhat biased in their perceptions of the child. Everson and colleagues (1989) reported that among mothers who provided little or ambivalent support to their children, there was no significant correlation between their descriptions of their sexually abused children's psychological functioning on the CBCL and behavior ratings derived from a psychiatric interview. Of course, one cannot discount the possibility that teachers or day care staff may have their own biased perceptions. Direct observations of the child in the particular setting and a thorough history may help clarify discrepancies in reports. Collateral reports also provide an even broader description of the child's functioning in different settings. For example, a child who is having significant difficulties in a home with inconsistent expectations and limits may do much better in a classroom or day care center that provides a more structured environment.

After explaining the purpose of the call to the teacher or day care worker, the clinician can ask fairly open-ended questions about the child's functioning and then follow up with more specific inquiries to ensure that all relevant areas of functioning (e.g., intellectual and academic functioning, relationships with peers and adults, affective and behavioral self-regulation, self-esteem) have been reviewed. Teachers can complete broad-scale assessment instruments such as the TRF of the CBCL/6–18 or the BASC-2. Usually, clinicians want to talk to the teacher or day care worker again after completing the assessment to share observations, ask about areas of concern that became apparent during the assessment, and clarify any of the collateral's responses to the assessment instruments. These people play an important role in the child's recovery, and their involvement in the assessment process is a good way to establish a collaborative alliance.

Parents or other caregivers sometimes require some guidance to prepare the child for the assessment. If parents do not raise this issue, the clinician should broach it. It is best not to give direct guidance or suggestions immediately. We can learn more about parents' typical ways of dealing with the child by asking how they think the child should be prepared for the assessment and what they would like to tell the child about the first appointment. Some parents have no idea of what to say and have not considered this as a significant issue. Others are quite distraught about bringing their child to a mental health professional, especially for an evaluation of the impact of maltreatment. They are often overwhelmed by feelings of guilt, remorse, or shame and would prefer not to say anything about the assessment to the child. Still others fear having to be assertive in the face of their child's resistance to attending the first appointment.

The clinician can encourage parents or caregivers to give the child a brief but direct rationale for the assessment. They may tell the child that he or she is going to meet with the clinician and should tell the child the clinician's name. Parents should discuss the reasons for the assessment with the child, describing it as an opportunity to spend some time with a person who wants to talk with the child about the maltreatment (or whatever word may be appropriate). This person also wants to find out how the youngster thinks and feels about what happened. Some children respond well when the clinician is described as a "feeling doctor" as opposed to a medical or "body doctor." If the clinician works in a medical facility, parents can assure the child that no medical procedures will occur at this time (unless some are planned). Parents may also reassure the child by saying they have already met the clinician and by empathizing with the child's anxiety, fear, or anger. Regarding the timing of this discussion, parents should tell younger children about the appointment only a day or two before the actual meeting, as a longer wait often generates overwhelming anxiety. Older children (8 years and up) should be told several days prior to the appointment. This period provides them with an opportunity to ask more questions about the rationale for the assessment, the process, and any other concerns. However, clinicians should not rigidly apply these age guidelines and need to adapt them to children's idiosyncratic needs.

INTERVIEWING THE MALTREATED CHILD

As clinicians, we sometimes assume that children cannot or will not talk about the maltreatment they have undergone. We immediately rush them into the playroom with the expectation that this is the only way of gathering relevant information. However, although interviewing children takes training and experience, the therapist can use interviews to gather considerable information. Interviews also allow the clinician to do an informal evaluation of the child's verbal proficiency and the kinds of alternate assessment strategies that might be necessary. If clinicians make no attempt to talk with a child about the maltreatment and other issues, they may never learn if interviews are a developmentally appropriate format.

A detailed description of child development and its implications for assessment are beyond the scope of this book. We refer the reader to other works that include comprehensive accounts of the implications of developmental research for interviewing maltreated children (Garbarino, Stott, & Faculty of the Erikson Institute, 1989; Steward, Bussey, Goodman, & Saywitz, 1993). Some of this information, however, is incorporated in our discussion of practical assessment strategies.

Stage 1: Introduction

ORIENTING THE CHILD TO THE ASSESSMENT

Usually the clinician meets the child and parents or caregivers in a waiting or reception area. When greeting the child and introducing oneself, it is often useful to bend or crouch down to be more at the child's level. The clinician should then inform the child that they will be going to the clinician's office and that the parents or caregivers will be in the waiting room when the appointment is finished. Even at this very early point in the assessment process, the clinician can begin to gather information about the child. Does the child respond appropriately by acknowledging the clinician's presence (e.g., establishes eye contact, responds to the clinician's greeting, or shakes hands)? Was the family sitting together and interacting in the waiting room, or was one member, perhaps the child, sitting at a distance from other family members? How does the child separate from the parents? Does the child become anxious and insist that a parent accompany him or her to the clinician's office? Or does the child separate from the parents with no evidence of anxiety whatsoever and interact in an overfriendly manner? Is the child mute while walking to the office, or does he or she initiate or respond to social chitchat?

We should allow highly anxious children to have a parent or caregiver accompany them to the interview. Nothing is gained by insisting that a frightened, highly distressed child accompany you, by him- or herself, to your office. Such tactics may compromise the chances of forming a therapeutic alliance with the child and may reinforce the notion that adults are insensitive and unresponsive to the child's particular needs. After one or two sessions with the parent or caregiver present, usually the child allows that person to leave the session.

Once in the clinician's office, the clinician must orient the child to the assessment process. It is useful to say your name again and then ask for the child's understanding of why he or she has been brought to the session. Have the parents or caregivers prepared the child as planned? Some parents may have provided an explanation. However, the child may be too embarrassed or anxious to talk about the reasons, or may have many fantasies or misconceptions about the assessment. We have heard children explain that they have been brought to an outpatient program at a pediatric hospital because they were "sick" and needed "shots," or that they were "bad" children and the clinician would decide whether they should be taken away from their parents.

After determining the child's understanding of the assessment, the clinician must clarify its purpose. This is particularly important for those children who claim to have no idea of why they are there and for those who harbor misconceptions. Even when children have a clear understanding of the referral reasons, the clinician should confirm their accounts. We recommend strongly that the clinician talk directly about the assessment's purpose, that is, that the child is there because he or she has been maltreated in some way. The clinician can begin by saying, "Your parents [or foster parents or social worker, if appropriate] told me that somebody touched your private parts [when speaking with sexually abused children]." An equally straightforward approach should be taken with children who have been maltreated in other ways. Clinicians can acknowledge that the child has been hit (e.g., "Your dad has been hitting you"), neglected (e.g., "Your parents didn't give you enough food"), psychologically maltreated (e.g., "People yelled a lot at you and called you names"), or witnessed domestic violence (e.g. "You saw lots of fighting between your mom and dad"). The clinician should then clarify his or her role by saying, "I see other kids who have had the same kinds of things happen to them. My job is to find out how kids think and feel about these things and see if there is anything that I or other people can do to help kids feel better."

There are several reasons why we believe it important to raise the maltreatment issue at such an early phase. First, direct statements like these set the stage for establishing a therapeutic alliance with the child who now better understands the reasons for coming to see the clinician. Initially, children may not like it or agree with the referral, but at least they know why they are there. At this first meeting, the therapist begins to set some expectations—that is, the maltreatment will be a principal focus for both the clinician and the child. Second, by making statements such as "Your uncle touched your private parts" or "Your dad hit you" in a neutral, calm manner, the clinician begins modeling the direct expression of these sensitive and painful topics. This approach may be especially important for a child whose parents or caregivers have never talked directly about the maltreatment. Other parents may have become terribly distraught when their child disclosed maltreatment details. Often such children become reluctant to talk about the maltreatment in order to protect their parents from these painful feelings. Interacting with another adult who demonstrates a different way of handling these issues exposes the child to an adaptive model of behavioral and emotional self-regulation. This approach reassures the child that he or she can discuss the maltreatment with an adult who can tolerate the child's distress and will not fall apart. Third, the clinician begins to desensitize the youngster. The use of phrases that refer directly to the maltreatment exposes the child to this material so that anxiety can begin to abate. Fourth, by bringing up the subject of the maltreatment so directly and quickly, the clinician conveys an expectation that the child can eventually handle this topic. Finally, telling the child early on that the clinician has seen other children who have undergone similar experiences begins to counteract the child's sense of isolation and stigmatization. This can be done in a concrete way, especially for younger children. For instance, if drawings are displayed on a wall or bulletin board, the clinician can mention that they were made by children who had undergone similar experiences.

Rather than asking about the maltreatment, the clinician should inquire first about the child's feelings about the assessment, especially now that the child has a better understanding of its purpose. The clinician should empathize with feelings, such as anxiety or anger, and then provide the child with some control over initiating a discussion of the maltreatment (Friedrich, 1990). Some children immediately launch into a detailed discussion about what happened. However, most need further preparation and an opportunity to form a relationship with the clinician before they feel sufficiently comfortable to communicate their experiences, whether verbally or through other means. Adapting Friedrich's (1990, p. 151) suggestions about engendering a therapeutic component in the interview, the clinician might say, "You're right, it is hard to talk about this, especially with someone you've just met. Most kids want to get to know me better before we talk about what happened. Would you like us to talk about other things and do some other stuff before we talk about how you were touched [or whatever phrase might be appropriate for the specific type of maltreatment]?" If the child chooses to talk about other topics, the clinician can tell the child that he or she will raise the maltreatment in a future session when the youngster feels more at ease. Most children are relieved that they are not expected to divulge this information so soon.

Occasionally, we inadvertently replicate some elements of the original maltreatment in our clinical assessments. In response to the desperation of referral sources such as parents or child welfare staff, clinicians sometimes feel compelled to develop a quick formulation to explain the child's symptoms and identify possible courses of action (Budd et al., 2002). Consequently, we may put considerable pressure on the child to provide a full account of the maltreatment during the first few assessment sessions. To the child who has been exposed to previous coercive interaction patterns with adults, such as being physically or psychologically forced into sexual activity and into keeping it secret, such misguided attempts by the clinician may be yet another example of the untrustworthiness of adults. This coercive style confirms the child's IWM/IS of others as untrustworthy and insensitive and exacerbates feelings of powerlessness. Sometimes clinicians make false promises to persuade children to open up about the maltreatment. "If you tell, everything will be fine" or "Daddy won't go to jail" may have little basis in reality. For many maltreated children, their worlds fall apart after they disclose abuse or neglect. Families do not believe their allegations and are torn apart, the perpetrator is incarcerated, and the child is placed out of the home. The child feels let down again by clinicians whose promises quickly ring hollow, thereby reducing the likelihood of the child's active participation in the evaluation and an open discussion of the maltreatment.

We have to remember that like many adult clients, children coming to see a mental health professional are embarrassed, anxious, and sometimes overwhelmed by feelings of shame, guilt, and stigmatization. Assessments that respect these reactions and children's needs to have some control over the assessment process are more likely to actively engage them in the evaluation process. They begin to learn that some adults can identify and empathize with their feelings and will treat them with respect and consideration. For many chronically maltreated children, this is a novel experience that begins to modify their IWMs/IS of others as insensitive and uncaring and themselves as unworthy of respect.

Before beginning the interview, the clinician should clarify other aspects of the assessment. As many of these children reside in unpredictable, chaotic, and sometimes threatening environments, they anticipate the same adverse events during the first assessment session. Orienting the child to the structure of the assessment usually alleviates anxiety about what will happen and conveys a reassuring sense of predictability. The clinician should tell the child how he or she would like to be addressed (e.g., Doctor, Mr., first name) and where they will be spending the session. Using a clock for younger children, the clinician can show how much time they will spend together and tell the children that they will rejoin parents in the waiting room (or other previously designated locale) at the session's end. The clinician should also point out the availability of washroom facilities and that the child just needs to inform the clinician if he or she wishes to use them. Briefly previewing the assessment strategies may also reduce anxiety. The clinician can tell the child that they will be spending time together playing, talking, and doing some puzzles (if appropriate). By the end of the first session, the child should have some idea about how assessment sessions work.

INQUIRING ABOUT OTHER TOPICS

Now that the child is oriented to the assessment's purpose and structure, the clinician can begin to inquire about topics other than the maltreatment. This inquiry serves several purposes. First, it allows the clinician to establish some rapport with the child. The clinician can focus on the child's strengths by asking, "What are some things you do best?" These discussions are less threatening, enable children to talk more openly and easily, and may begin to counteract feelings of low self-esteem. Second, a child's responses and presentation in this interview phase may suggest unique strengths and weaknesses (e.g., self-esteem, verbal skills, intellectual status) that have moderated the maltreatment's impact. The child's responses also identify potential targets of intervention or alternate assessment strategies. For example, does the child display good attention and concentration, or is the behavior more consistent with a diagnosis of an attention deficit disorder? Can the child articulate ideas or feelings about a particular topic, or do poor verbal skills suggest the use of less verbally oriented assessment strategies?

Recreation and Interests. Previous interviews with the parents or caregivers may have given the clinician some good ideas about the child's strengths and interests. Inquiring about these areas often starts the process of building rapport. Most people, including children, are more likely to talk openly about the things they do well. Children's strengths may include hobbies, sports, pets, or even more mundane interests such as favorite television shows. The major goal is to get the child talking about personal strengths and interests and for the clinician to display genuine enthusiasm and curiosity. Rushing the child through this interview phase detracts from the rapport that can be established and may convey a lack of real interest by the clinician.

We need to emphasize that curiosity is a critical component of not only this phase of the assessment but of the entire evaluation (and subsequent therapy). Whether the child is talking about dance lessons, hockey, or the abuse he or she suffered, the clinician's principal job is the same: to understand as deeply as possible the child's thoughts and feelings associated with these experiences; that is, to enter the child's phenomenological world. Although this curiosity and empathic comments may well set a therapeutic tone for the interviews, your job at this stage is to understand the child, not to blindly recommend or implement interventions that may have little relationship to the pathogenic processes and moderator variables that remain to be identified and underlie his or her emotional or behavioral problems.

Conveying this interest is important in setting the right tone for the interviews. It is likely that children who perceive initial interest on the part of the clinician during discussions of recreational interests or other nonmaltreatment topics are more likely to talk openly about the abuse or neglect. This line of inquiry also allows the clinician to see the child at his or her best and provides useful information about the child's abilities and interests, or lack thereof, particularly as compared with those of his or her peer group.

School. Our review of the impact of maltreatment indicates that many maltreated children have significant academic, social, or behavior problems at school. Focusing on the child's problems in adapting to school may be too threatening to the child, resulting in sparse and unelaborated responses. These constricted narratives reflect attempts to protect themselves from even greater threats to their self-esteem should they fully and openly acknowledge such problems. Consequently, the clinician should focus first on more positive aspects of school by asking what the child likes and does best there. Similarly, the clinician can ask the child to identify the people in school he or she likes most. Is there anything about school that seems to provide a sense of satisfaction or pride? More troublesome aspects can then be addressed by asking what the child dislikes about school and why these situations or relationships are problematic. Besides paying attention to the content of the responses, the clinician should listen closely to the underlying affective tone. For example, when describing a fairly dismal academic record, does the child sound genuinely sad or distressed? Does the child attempt to defend against such feelings by minimizing the difficulties and displaying little emotion?

Peer Relations. Children's descriptions of peer relationships yield important information regarding their ability to establish and maintain healthy relationships, as well as characteristics of IWMs/IS. The clinician may want to begin this inquiry by asking about the depth and nature of the child's peer relationships. Does he or she have no friends, one friend, or many friends, or does the child claim friendship with nearly everyone? If the child has a best friend, what specific activities do they do together, how often do they have contact, and what do they like about each other? When disagreements arise, how do they settle conflicts? Does the child have conflicts with other children, and, if so, why do these problems arise? Some children blame others for their peer difficulties, assuming little, if any, responsibility. Have peers ever disappointed the child, and how frequently has this happened? The child's responses may reveal an expectation that others, including children of the same age, are unreliable, untrustworthy, and quite threatening figures. Alternatively, does the child describe him- or herself in fairly negative ways? Does the child convey an expectation that no one will ever want to be his or her friend because of these negative characteristics? Asking children to describe the "perfect friend" may reveal similar themes.

Family Relationships. First, clinicians can ask children to describe the composition of their families, including pets, and encourage them to describe pleasant family relationships. They can describe the fun they have together as a family unit, with mother and father separately, and with siblings, and identify what they like most about living with their families. Does the child provide an account with specific details of these positive aspects, or is the account vague and devoid of detail? Although other factors such as verbal skills can certainly play a role here, the clinician might start speculating about the veracity of a child's glowing descriptions if details are few. The clinician must also assess whether the child's affect is congruent with descriptions of these positive relationships and note whether the positive relationships are with parents, as would be expected in younger children in particular, or whether they are with extended family members, friends, or even pets.

After inquiring about these more positive aspects, the clinician can ask about some of the more troublesome characteristics of family life. Are there any changes the child would like his or her parents or family to undergo? Sometimes asking the child to pretend that he or she has a "magic wand" and can change parents or family in any way helps a younger child to respond with sufficient detail. What kinds of changes would he or she like to see in each parent or significant caregivers, siblings, and the family as a unit? At this point, maltreated children sometimes begin talking about their abuse or neglect or about other aspects of parenting, such as not receiving sufficient emotional attention. If the clinician believes the child can now cope with a more detailed inquiry about the maltreatment (discussed in a later section of this chapter), he or she can ask whether the child is now ready to talk about it. If the child responds affirmatively, the clinician can proceed with this line of questioning.

Other more general inquiries include the expression of feelings by family members. For instance, who gets angry in the family, what do they get angry about, and how do they express their anger? Who in the family becomes sad, and how can the child tell if someone is sad? Such questions may elicit material regarding the maltreatment.

Plans for the Future. The therapist should preface the following questions by saying that he or she appreciates that most people change their minds about what they would like to do in the future as they grow up. Again, it might be best to start with more neutral inquiries: What kinds of activities or job would the child like to do as an adult, and what is the specific appeal of each? The clinician can then ask the child about any thoughts regarding other aspects of adult life, especially relationships. Does the child expect to marry or have children? What would be the advantages and disadvantages of being married or having children? Again, the child's responses may provide some interesting information about expectations of relationships. Some children maintain adamantly that they will never have children because they are too much "trouble" and not worth the effort. Such attitudes may be a reflection of their parents' or caregivers' feelings.

General Health. The clinician should not forget to ask the child about general physical well-being and specific problems such as enuresis, encopresis, disturbed sleeping and eating habits, and somatic complaints such as abdominal pain. A child's general statement about not sleeping well may serve as a springboard for more specific inquiries, such as about any particular fears the child experiences when going to bed, intrusive or recurrent thoughts or preoccupations while attempting to fall asleep, and the presence of frightening dreams. These symptoms may indicate significant anxiety or even PTSD.

If the child has good verbal skills and becomes actively involved in this phase of the assessment process, the clinician generally spends a session discussing the aforementioned topics. At the end of the first session, the clinician should very briefly summarize for the child what has been learned, taking care to emphasize the child's strengths as well as identifying areas that are causing distress or difficulty. The clinician should also describe the next step in the assessment process, perhaps saying that the child will come back to talk further and do some other activities. Finally, the clinician might thank the child for attending and participating.

Returning to our example of the Hutterite children described in Chapter 3, this stage of the assessment is often particularly important for establishing rapport and building trust with children from different cultural groups.

Prior to contact with the children at the first assessment session held at the colony, the clinicians again met with the parents to review the purposes of this initial assessment session: to build rapport with the children and to start the process of identifying their feelings and thoughts about the sexual abuse and any clinically significant problems (parents were interviewed later that day to gather information about their respective children's functioning and any relevant history).

The male and female clinicians met with the boys and girls in same-sex groups and clarified why they were there and the process and structure of the assessment. The clinicians assumed the same stance with the children as they had initially taken with their parents: they were curious about their lives and beliefs and wanted to learn much more. Rather than talking about the abuse, lively discussions ensued in both groups, with the children recounting various aspects of life in the colony, including their school, jobs and chores, family life, and recreational activities. These discussions allowed the clinicians to start forming some initial impressions of their young clients. For example, they quickly learned that they had to pay particular attention to their use of language. The beginning speech of Hutterite children is a German dialect, and they become more fluent in English as they proceed through the colony's school (they attend "German school" for part of the day, where they receive instruction in reading German and writing German script, and "English school," where the teacher, who is usually a non-Hutterite from outside the colony, teaches the basics of the provincial curriculum). Some of the younger school-age children had a bit of difficulty in understanding the clinicians' vocabulary, and the older children needed to translate. The clinicians slowed their rate of speech, encouraged the children to ask the meaning of various words or phrases, and regularly checked with them to ascertain that they understood.

To build more rapport, the clinicians suggested that the children take them on a tour of the colony. Rather than the professionals assuming the "expert" role, the children had an opportunity to be experts. This was a real icebreaker: Even the 7- and 8-year-olds proved to be very knowledgeable about the agricultural operations of their community and took real pride in showing the clinicians the colony's impressive technological infrastructure. Again, the genuine enthusiasm and curiosity the clinicians displayed on the tour, and throughout the assessment, facilitated a positive relationship with the children. However, the curiosity was reciprocal. The children were just as interested in the clinicians as the clinicians were in them. This is understandable, given both groups' lack of exposure to one another. As they began to feel more comfortable, the children asked the clinicians about their lives and were especially interested in whether the clinicians had children, the sizes of their families, their children's ages, and what their children were like. Usually Hutterite families are large, and they were quite amazed that the clinicians' families were relatively small. The therapists' direct answers to these personal questions went a long way to consolidate rapport and set the stage for inquiry about the children's reactions and adjustment to the sexual abuse. Just as they were curious about other aspects of the children's lives, the clinicians conveyed the same sense of interest about the sexual abuse and the thoughts and feelings associated with it, thereby increasing chances that the children would talk openly about these issues.

Stage 2: Interviewing the Child about the Maltreatment

PREPARING THE CHILD AND BEGINNING THE INQUIRY

It is not a good idea to start an inquiry about the maltreatment near the end of an interview. Both the clinician and child need sufficient time to explore these issues gradually. Furthermore, strong feelings may be elicited in the child. Ending the interview without providing sufficient opportunity for the child to calm down, at least to a certain extent, does the child a real disservice. This is especially so if the child must return to an environment such as a classroom where the demands for sustained attention, concentration, and well-regulated behavior are quite stringent.

The clinician can initiate the discussion by saying something like, "I'd like to talk with you now about what happened when you were hit [or whatever phrase might be appropriate to the specific maltreatment]. I know some things about it, but it would sure help me if you could tell me more about it." The clinician should then reiterate the purpose of this discussion: "As I told you when we first met, I'm really interested in your feelings and ideas about what happened to you. This may help us think of some things we can do to help you and your family feel better about what happened." Children need this explicit rationale, especially those who believe that interactions with a professional will result in abusive or exploitative episodes. For example, a boy who has been sexually abused by an adult male may become anxious when a male therapist takes him into a private office and begins to talk about sexual matters. The perpetrator may have preceded the sexual assaults with similar private discussions of sexuality. Without a clear explanation of the rationale for these conversations, the child may misinterpret the clinician's actions in accordance with this expectation—that is, that adult males, especially those who talk in private about sex, cannot be trusted. After explaining the rationale, the clinician can ask if the child feels comfortable enough to begin talking about the maltreatment. If the child is ready, the clinician provides some further ground rules. The child should do it gradually, using whatever terminology or words are comfortable, and it is perfectly acceptable for the child, in response to the clinician's questions, to state that he or she does not want to answer a particular question, rather than saying, "I don't know." However, the clinician must also encourage the child to answer difficult questions and rely on "I don't know" only when absolutely necessary. The clinician should also inquire about any fears the child might have about the maltreatment or about describing it. It is important not to provide the child with any false reassurances that "everything is going to be OK."

To start this phase, ask the child to give an open-ended account of what happened. Rather than asking specific questions, give the child an opportunity to tell his or her story without interruption, apart from gentle encouragement like "Go on" or "What happened next?" A clinician's nonverbal signals of discomfort or anxiety may result in the child's prematurely terminating the description of the incidents to save the clinician from further discomfort. Managing one's personal reactions to these often horrific stories is critical; we discuss this issue in Chapter 12.

As in any clinical interview, the clinician must attend to the child's account on several different levels. The clinician must listen for the content. When compared with what the child told other people previously, are there any significant discrepancies? Are significant details omitted, or is the child now disclosing new information? Does the child provide a fairly elaborated and detailed account, or is it sparse and devoid of detail?

Besides listening to the content of the account, the clinician must attend closely to the process, or how the child describes what happened. The child's general emotional demeanor and any changes in the types of feelings and the manner in which they are expressed merit close attention. What kinds of feelings and emotions accompany the description? Can the child express feelings associated with the maltreatment, or does he or she attempt to constrict the affect and thereby provide a matter-of-fact account? Do particular segments provoke different emotional reactions? For instance, a child may become especially restless and fidgety, leaving the chair and moving about the room when anxious. Another child might "close down": he or she stops expressing any more feelings and terminates eye contact. Others may become oppositional and defiant to deflect attention from a particular aspect of the account. We have seen children who became sexually excited when talking about aspects of their sexual abuse. Children's thinking processes should also be carefully evaluated. Is their speech less coherent, do they evidence a deterioration in attention and concentration, or do they begin to provide tangential responses or comments as a function of anxiety associated with different aspects of their account of the maltreatment? Again, such reactions may provide clues about those aspects of the incidents that are particularly troublesome or distressing and information about the child's typical ways of handling the associated feelings, such as avoidance.

After the child provides an open-ended account of the maltreatment, the clinician may inquire about specific aspects of the incidents, including the emotional, cognitive, and behavioral sequelae. Finkelhor and Browne's

(1985) model of the traumagenic dynamics of child sexual abuse was developed to explain the impact of child sexual abuse. We believe that three of the factors—powerlessness, betrayal, and stigmatization—can be incorporated in interviews with children who have experienced other forms of maltreatment. The fourth factor, traumatic sexualization, is relevant to sexually abused children. Table 4.1 outlines these factors and some possible areas of inquiry. It is only a rough guide, and the clinician must adapt the vocabulary and structure of the questions to suit a child's developmental level. Interviewing the child who can talk about such issues in this systematic manner may provide the clinician with a rich source of data and deepens an understanding of the child's experience.

SEMISTRUCTURED AND STRUCTURED INTERVIEWS

Pynoos and Eth (1986) developed the Traumatic Event Interview Schedule, which can be used with maltreated children. After clinicians have established an expectation that the maltreatment needs to be described, they encourage the child to draw a picture of what happened and to tell a story about it. The interview then moves on to a more explicit discussion, with the therapist asking the child to review any sensory experiences (e.g., sensations, odors) connected with the maltreatment experience. The clinician promotes and encourages a full description of what happened and asks the child to identify the "worst moment" of the event.

ALLEVIATING ANXIETY

Raising the maltreatment issue generates considerable anxiety in many children, even if they have already provided an initial disclosure to representatives of a child welfare agency or police. Children become anxious for many reasons. As reviewed in Chapter 2, discussing maltreatment details or even being exposed to these stimuli via the clinician's questions can evoke anxiety. Some maltreated children have been threatened by the perpetrator or family members about disclosing the abuse. Threats range from further maltreatment, extreme or even life-threatening punishment, or the loss of love and emotional abandonment by the family. Others have been told that the perpetrator might have to leave the home or be incarcerated, or that no one would believe their accounts. Some maltreated children have been imbued with the notion that it is wrong to reveal personal family matters to others, especially if they have been threatened with the breakup of the family postdisclosure.

Other children become anxious when being interviewed about the maltreatment because of expectations about what others, including the cli-

TABLE 4.1. Areas of Inquiry Using Finkelhor and Browne's Traumagenic Dynamics

1. Traumatic sexualization (to be used for sexually abused children)
   a. Increased salience of sexual issues
      - Nature of the sexual abuse?
      - Pleasurable/reinforcing aspects of the abuse?
      - What kinds of sexual behavior does the child display now?
      - Frequency?
      - Onset?
      - Degree of pleasure/reinforcement?
      - Nature of sexual fantasies and feelings?
      - Frequency?
      - Onset?

   b. Confusion regarding sexual identity
      - Fears re future sexual desirability?
      - Fears of being gay?

   c. Confusion regarding sexual norms and standards
      - Is sex equated with affection?
      - Is sex used to obtain rewards and attention?

   d. Sexuality and anxiety
      - How did the child feel when being abused?
      - Worst fear?
      - How does the child feel now when thinking about the abuse or sexuality?
      - Does the child want to have sex in the future? Under what conditions?

   e. Fears regarding body integrity
      - Is the child fearful he or she was hurt or damaged, especially genitalia (e.g., sexually transmitted diseases, HIV)?
      - Fearful of implications for future sexual functioning?

2. Powerlessness
   a. Coercive aspects of the maltreatment
      - Degree of coercion (psychological/physical) used by the perpetrator?
      - Does the child perceive the aforementioned aspects as coercive?

   b. Helplessness
      - Could the child have done anything to stop the maltreatment?
      - Anticipated consequences of taking action?
      - Feelings re not being able to do anything to stop the maltreatment?
      - Anxiety?
      - Despair?
      - Depression?
      - Anger, identification with the aggressor?

   c. Perceived effectiveness/consequences of having taken action (e.g., disclosure)
      - Accidental versus purposeful disclosure?
      - If the disclosure was purposeful, what were the child's motives in disclosing?
      - Outcomes of the disclosure? (Did the maltreatment stop? Perpetrator incarcerated? Dissolution of the family?)

3. Betrayal
   a. Premaltreatment relationship with the perpetrator
      - Describe the relationship before the onset of the maltreatment. Positive and negative aspects?
      - Feelings toward the perpetrator?

   b. Feelings about the perpetrator after the onset of the maltreatment

TABLE 4.1. (*continued*)

- Extent of: loss? sadness? anger? hurt?
- How does the child express these feelings?
- Have these feelings been generalized to other people (e.g., can't trust any men)?
- Child's feelings re the future of the relationship? Does he or she want it to be reestablished (under what conditions)? Does he or she want the postmaltreatment relationship changed in any way?

c. Extent to which the child feels tricked or taken in by the perpetrator
- Was the child suspicious of the perpetrator? For how long? Why?
- How did the perpetrator involve the child in the maltreatment?

d. Environmental response to the child's disclosure
- What did others do or say when they heard the disclosure or were informed about it?
- Parents/caregivers
- Siblings
- Members of extended family
- Peers
- Other community members (e.g., teachers, church people)
- Response of the wider community?
- Legal/justice system
- Child welfare system
- Medical/mental health system
- Child's reactions to the above responses?

4. Stigmatization

a. Stigmatizing aspects of the maltreatment
- Child's perception of attitudes/feelings re the maltreatment conveyed by the perpetrator (e.g., shame, secrecy, disgust)?
- Child's perception of the reaction of others in acknowledging that the child was maltreated?
- Child's own attitudes/feelings re him- or herself?

Note. Adapted from Finkelhor and Browne (1985).

nician, might think of them. As we have seen, internal attributions may contribute to a negative self-image, which in turn is compounded by perpetrators or others who reinforce this notion via their claims that they are "bad" children who deserved the neglect, psychological maltreatment, or physical abuse or that they are "perverted" because they participated in sexual activity or "wanted it." When asked to reveal maltreatment details and the associated feelings and thoughts, many abused children believe their failings and weaknesses will be exposed if they do so, and that others will think of them in the same negative way they perceive themselves. Furthermore, acknowledging these negative self-perceptions is a great threat to a child's already shaky self-esteem and elicits even more anxiety. Friedrich (1990) notes that some sexually abused individuals fear that simply talking about the abuse will result in revictimization.

What can clinicians do to alleviate some of the anxiety? First, they should attempt to gauge the child's feelings about discussing the maltreatment before actually initiating such a conversation. They can ask the child what he or she thinks the discussion will be like and identify some of the easy and more difficult aspects. Asking, "What's the worst thing that could happen if you talk about this?" or, "What's the worst thing I or someone else could think about you?" helps the child to identify those fears. If the child identifies a negative reaction from other people or the clinician, the clinician can assure the child that he or she has heard the accounts of many other children and will not think negatively of the child. The clinician can use alternate media to ascertain the child's fears and anxieties, such as by asking the child to draw a picture of what would happen if the maltreatment was discussed and to depict how the child would feel or how others would react.

Second, the clinician should remain alert to any overt or covert manifestations of anxiety throughout these interviews. Labeling feelings by simple comments, such as "You look pretty upset right now," validating the normalcy of these feelings, and commenting on how other children have shown similar reactions in this context may attenuate the child's distress. The clinician should try to understand the basis for the child's anxiety and inquire further about particular fears or negative expectations that might underlie this response. By providing a deep sense of empathy and conveying the notion that the child is not necessarily crazy or disturbed for harboring these feelings, the clinician demonstrates that some adults can treat the child's worries with sensitivity and concern. This approach begins the process of modifying the child's negative IWMs of others and of the self as unworthy of this kind of response.

Third, the clinician must be patient and adopt a gradual approach when interviewing. Even though the clinician may have told the child that he or she will not think negatively of the child, some children, especially those with little trust in adults, may need to see concrete examples of this promise. They may gradually disclose information and their thoughts and feelings about the maltreatment while paying keen attention to the clinician's verbal and nonverbal responses. Children may also engage in provocative or oppositional behavior to determine the clinician's trustworthiness (i.e., whether the clinician will respond to such provocations abusively or adopt a firm yet respectful way to handle this behavior). The clinician can bring this dynamic into the open by commenting on the functions this behavior serves (i.e., it enables the child to determine, before he or she divulges sensitive information, whether the clinician can be trusted). Then the clinician might suggest some concrete ways by which to prove his or her trustworthiness. The following case illustrates this approach.

A 9-year-old boy who was severely sexually abused by his mother's boyfriend over many years was referred for clinical assessment. Historical information revealed that Darren had been subjected to other forms of maltreatment, including some physical neglect and abuse, in his very early years, and that his current behavior included numerous incidents of physical and sexual aggression. Darren's presentation in the initial assessment sessions suggested a youngster who had little, if any, trust in adults: he was reluctant to talk about his past and became defiant in an effort to determine whether the clinician would accept him when he behaved in this manner. The clinician empathized with Darren's fear of disclosing too much information too quickly but at the same time placed firm but nonabusive limits on his acting out. Darren agreed that he did not want to talk about the maltreatment because he expected the clinician, like so many other adults in his life, to discount his feelings and treat his account with contempt. He expected the clinician to reject or even hurt him if he became unruly in the assessment sessions. The clinician suggested to Darren that they develop a "trust meter." This was a chart on which Darren indicated whether the clinician had been trustworthy each session. The clinician and Darren developed some specific behavioral criteria that he could use in evaluating the clinician's reactions (e.g., not laughing at Darren's accounts of other problems or issues, paying attention to Darren as evidenced by not yawning, looking directly at Darren while he was talking, and not hitting him if he became defiant and oppositional). They also agreed that the clinician would have to prove his trustworthiness according to these and other criteria in five sessions before Darren would even start talking about the maltreatment. Fortunately, the clinician met these criteria, and Darren gradually began to talk about the abuse and neglect he had experienced.

As we can see, rushing the interview with a youngster like Darren or insisting he talk about his experiences would have just confirmed his view of others as insensitive, uncaring, and disrespectful of his needs. Clinicians must maintain realistic expectations about the amount of information that they can gather in any assessment. The goal is to obtain sufficient information to develop a working understanding of the child and a set of recommendations regarding interventions that, it is hoped, will be useful. Because the child may have a high level of anxiety or utilize defenses such as repression or dissociation, the clinician may have to enter into a therapeutic relationship with the child before more information is revealed. It is important to remember that a child may never verbally recall memories if he or she was very young and preverbal at the time of the maltreatment.

Fourth, the clinician should guard against giving false reassurances about the benefits of discussing the maltreatment. In the short term, some children probably feel worse after talking about these issues; they may remember more details of the maltreatment, and their defenses may not protect them fully from the onslaught of pain and distress associated with these recollections. The clinician should acknowledge that this is indeed a painful process and that many children do not immediately feel better after discussing such material more openly in the assessment phase. The clinician should emphasize that the assessment is just one part of a potentially longer process, which, over time, may afford the child some relief from pain.

PUTTING CLOSURE TO THE DISCUSSION ABOUT THE MALTREATMENT

At the end of the discussion about the maltreatment, the clinician must put some closure to it for the child. Briefly summarizing what has been learned and emphasizing the normalcy and understandable nature of the anxiety or other affects may alleviate some of the child's distress. The clinician can compliment the child for the courage he or she showed when talking about these painful issues and inquire whether the child has any more worries stemming from the discussion. Again, sending a highly distressed and disorganized child out of an interview into environments where behavioral and affective self-regulation skills are necessary for success (e.g., the classroom) can be harmful. The child's behavior may be so dysregulated after sessions that he or she is unable to cope with normal classroom routines and demands, which in turn elicits the anger of others and further erosion in self-esteem. The child may also become afraid of talking about the maltreatment in subsequent sessions because of the association between these discussions and a deterioration in behavior. Finally, the child should be informed about plans for subsequent assessment sessions.

Interviewing about Presenting Problems

Just as the clinician wants to gain an understanding of the child's perceptions of the maltreatment, so is it important to adopt the same kind of phenomenological approach to the assessment of the child's presenting problems. The child should be given an opportunity to talk in a more open-ended way about these problems. For example, the clinician may say, "You told me that you had been having some nightmares about what happened to you. Please tell me more about them." Subsequently, the clinician asks more specific questions about the problems, such as requesting a more detailed description of what the child actually does or feels and whether the child can identify any precipitants of these feelings or actions. The clinician also asks about the child's understanding of other people's concerns about these problems, the child's own desire to change them, what has helped in the past, and what might be useful now. The child's responses to these inquiries are affected not only by anxiety and a reluctance to speak openly about them, but by developmental variables. For example, very young children do not yet have the cognitive capacity to engage in introspection. Therefore, they will probably not be able to give an account of the precipitants associated with their problems. This fact again underscores the importance of gathering data via different modalities and from other sources.

The clinician should ask about other aspects of the problem behavior. If the child is physically aggressive toward others or engages them in inappropriate sexualized behavior, the clinician should ask about the other children's identities, how many children are involved, and whether the child can appreciate or understand their reactions. The last point may be especially important in understanding whether the child has an empathic appreciation of the effects of his or her behavior on others.

Children may show the same kind of anxiety and reluctance to talk openly about these problems as they did when they were asked about the maltreatment. Behavioral and interpersonal difficulties pose a real threat to their already low self-esteem, and public acknowledgment of these difficulties makes them feel even worse about themselves. They anticipate that others may regard them negatively if they talk openly about their problems, especially those that are particularly embarrassing (e.g., sexualized behavior, encopresis). They may expect parents to abandon them, send them away, or punish them severely. The clinician can use the same strategies to allay children's anxiety about discussing the presenting problems that were employed in interviews regarding the details of the maltreatment. We describe these strategies in more detail in relation to children who encounter difficulty in talking about SBPs.

The clinician who has conducted comprehensive interviews with children who are able and willing to talk about these issues has probably amassed a considerable amount of data. However, the clinician should attempt to confirm or refute some of his or her tentative hypotheses by using other modalities that do not rely so heavily on verbal skills. They are particularly applicable to children who do not have good verbal skills or those whose accounts may be significantly affected by other factors. It is to these assessment methods that we now turn.

PLAY ASSESSMENTS

The verbal skills of many children, especially young children, are limited. Moreover, our preceding review of the developmental outcomes of maltreatment indicates that the language of maltreated children is often compromised. Although we have maintained that clinicians should first try to talk with children to determine whether an interview will be a profitable assessment modality, many maltreated children cannot participate fully in such discussions. Moreover, many harbor real fears about openly discussing their experiences. Faced with these obstacles, clinicians must turn to other strategies to gather information.

A basic assumption of assessment and therapy is that both require a medium of exchange or communication between the client and clinician. Words and verbal interchanges serve this function for most adult clients. Play may serve this function for some child clients. Play provides an opportunity for them to communicate with others about important topics, such as internal, psychological events or experiences, and it may be a safer medium through which these issues can be addressed. By talking about the maltreatment to which a small doll was exposed, rather than about his or her own personal experiences, the child can communicate this information in a metaphorical and therefore safer manner. Similarly, by portraying a character in a play scene as extremely angry toward an abusive parent, the child feels less threatened than if he or she talked directly about the anger elicited by a parent's abusive actions. Engaging in play scenarios in which characters express sadness about never having the kind of parents they always wanted may be somewhat more tolerable than openly acknowledging such pain. In general, play allows children to deal with threatening or anxiety-provoking material as if it were someone else's problem, thereby placing much-needed psychological distance between themselves and the material.

We focused on two broad domains in our discussions of interviews with children: the content, or what the child said, and the process, or how the child said it. The same model can be applied to evaluating the play of maltreated children. The play may include examples of the child's own experiences of maltreatment, such as parental dolls who physically or sexually abuse, neglect, or psychologically maltreat child dolls or viciously fight in their presence. Thematic development in the play provides clues to relevant issues associated with the maltreatment. Play characters may express feelings about the maltreatment and exhibit responses reflective of the child's reactions, such as retaliating through physical aggression or adopting a very passive, victimlike stance.

Of particular interest is posttraumatic play (Terr, 1990). The child ritualistically constructs the same scenario, acting out a series of events that have the same outcome every time the play is enacted. Terr (1990) reported that by controlling the reenactment of this frightening and traumatic event, the child tries to gain a sense of mastery and empowerment over it. However, the rigid reenactment of the same ending (e.g., the child is physically abused and sent to the hospital) does not provide the child with any alternate resolution of this situation, thereby reinforcing a sense of helplessness and lack of control over an adverse situation. Furthermore, posttraumatic play is characterized by a lack of enjoyment or freedom of expression.

The process of the play, or the manner in which the child plays, is another valuable source of information. First, the child's relationship with the clinician in the play may yield information about the child's relationships with others. Does the child engage in solitary play and relegate the clinician to the periphery of the action? Does this style persist even when the clinician attempts to become more actively involved? Or is the child extremely dependent on the clinician—for example, asking for help in mundane tasks such as getting a toy from the cupboard or requesting that the clinician make most, if not all, of the decisions about what to do in the playroom? Does the child behave in a provocative and oppositional manner, such as refusing to clean up or even leave? These relationship patterns may reflect maladaptive ways in which the child interacts with other individuals.

Second, children's play may reflect their typical ways of handling difficult or painful material. For example, some children engage in compulsive play, in which they spend a great deal of time arranging the furniture in a dollhouse or insist upon using rulers when drawing. Such compulsive strategies may indicate underlying anxiety and a desperate attempt to control the overt expression of such feelings. As significant issues emerge in play and generate intense anxiety and conflict, a child may disrupt the play—for example, stopping the action and shifting to a new activity. At the other extreme are children who cannot manage their impulses and exhibit poor regulation of their behaviors and emotions when overstimulated by some of the material or themes. The impulsive, scattered play of some children may reflect other problems such as an attention deficit disorder.

The choice of play materials may be clinically significant. Are the child's choices appropriate to his or her age? Although immature choices may be manifestations of developmental delays, children may make the same choices because of significant emotional needs. But the actual use the child makes of these materials may be of greater significance than the particular things chosen. For instance, a 10-year-old physically neglected child may spend a great deal of time nurturing him- or herself by nursing on a baby bottle because such needs have never previously been met (Mills & Allan, 1992). Finally, the clinician should assess the degree of verbalization exhibited during the play. Does the child spontaneously verbalize while playing, and can he or she move from play to a verbal mode of interaction? The child who moves comfortably from using play to more direct verbal discussion of the issues exemplified in the play may evidence an ability and willingness to use both modalities for communication.

There are several ways of using play to gather more information about a child. Free play situations expose children to a minimum of directives from the clinician. In this type of play, some maltreated children quickly begin to reenact episodes from their own experiences of abuse and neglect. If the child does not communicate the feelings of the characters in the play about these experiences, the clinician can ask the characters how they feel and what they think about the maltreatment. The clinician might say, "I want to ask the little girl a question. How does she feel when her father hits her on the head like that?" The clinician can direct other inquiries via the metaphor of the play and in the third person to gather even more information along the lines of the traumagenic dynamics outlined in Table 4.1. The clinician should guard against asking too many questions too quickly, inasmuch as doing so may have a somewhat disruptive effect on the play's spontaneity.

Some children do not enact significant themes in play so as to avoid feeling anxiety and pain, just as they avoid the interview inquiries. Consequently, they gravitate toward certain activities. They may want to play endless board games that, after a relatively short time, provide little information. Rather than allowing this to continue, the clinician should take a more active role and depict situations or scenarios to which the child is asked to respond. There is a historical tradition for this approach. David Levy (1939) was a British psychoanalyst who promoted release therapy. He believed that the expression of feelings (catharsis) in certain situations is therapeutic. In order to elicit feelings associated with various traumas, Levy set up conditions or situations, such as play with small dolls, to resemble the situations in which the traumas occurred. Although we discuss the use of structured play therapy in subsequent chapters, this approach has real utility for assessment. The clinician might ask the child to "make up a story about a family," using small dolls. Sometimes this approach is all that is needed for the child to reenact maltreatment scenarios and to express associated thoughts and feelings. However, other children enact bland stories devoid of clinical content, which may reflect attempts to avoid painful material.

What can the clinician do in this situation? The clinician can take the lead and present play scenarios to which the child is invited to respond. Using small dolls, the clinician might introduce this approach by stating, "I'm going to act out a story for you using these dolls. All I want you to do right now is just sit back and watch and listen." Following this explanation, the clinician enacts scenarios in the doll play that are similar to the child's own maltreatment experiences. After the clinician depicts a scenario, he or she asks the child to respond by stating, "Show me what happens next," and then asks the child to show or express how the child character in the play feels about being maltreated. Questions that evaluate the child's beliefs about the maltreatment (e.g., "Why does [name of the doll] think she was hurt like this?") may be asked via the play. Clearly, though, the use of this approach, in which the clinician takes the initiative and presents these scenarios, is inappropriate for a forensic/legal interview. The use of this suggestive questioning should be used only after child protective and judicial authorities have investigated the child's allegations.

Buchsbaum and colleagues (1992) describe a narrative story stem technique that includes components similar to those in the directed-play assessment format just described. Using doll play, the interviewer begins a story (the story stem), which the child is asked to complete. According to Buchsbaum and colleagues, the content of maltreated children's stories included themes of interpersonal aggression, neglect, and some sexualized behavior, as well as their representational models. The doll play also revealed the use of defenses such as avoidance, idealization, and identification with the aggressor. The appendix accompanying the article by Buchsbaum and colleagues describes story stem narratives that may be of interest to the clinician who wishes to add this useful technique to an assessment repertoire. We describe in detail the use of story stems to assess children's attachment organizations later in this chapter.

Toys and equipment for play assessments do not have to be expensive or elaborate. Essential items include small bendable doll figurines, a dollhouse, puppets, domesticated and wild toy animals, assorted cars and trucks, a few table games to permit relief from emotionally laden activities, and art materials such as paper, crayons, felt pens, pencils, and paint.

PSYCHOLOGICAL TESTING

Psychological tests have been used for different purposes in the assessment of maltreated children. Professionals have employed them to evaluate allegations of child sexual abuse by examining how groups of sexually abused children perform on tests as compared with nonabused children. Given the negative findings of the ability of tests to discriminate between sexually abused and nonabused youngsters (e.g., Garb et al., 2000; Palmer et al., 2000), mental health professionals must be extremely cautious and judicious in the use of psychological testing to validate allegations of sexual abuse. Although we are not aware of any data on this issue pertaining to other forms of maltreatment, we suspect strongly that the same conclusions are applicable.

A second purpose of psychological testing of maltreated children is to gather more information about their response to the maltreatment and to identify those variables in children that influence the impact of such experiences. Given the limitations of this book, we cannot provide the reader with an exhaustive list of all the psychological tests that are clinically useful in assessing maltreated children. There are a number of sources that comprehensively review psychological measures that can be profitably used in the evaluation of maltreated children (Kirby & Hardesty, 1998; Mash & Terdal, 1997). What we do here is to alert the reader to the potential uses of these tests.

Cognitive and Academic Testing

Knowledge about a child's cognitive and academic functioning is important for several reasons. First, maltreatment may significantly impact cognitive and academic functioning. Second, intellectual functioning and academic achievement may serve as important moderators of the association between maltreatment and developmental outcome. Third, difficulties in the academic and cognitive areas merit clinician intervention. A maltreated child with significant academic delays will probably experience considerable frustration and even lower self-esteem, resulting in an exacerbation of symptoms. Fourth, knowledge of a child's strengths and weaknesses in these domains point to the use of particular therapeutic strategies. For example, a child with low verbal abilities and skills may not be an appropriate candidate for an approach that places heavy emphasis on verbal interchange.

A number of scales and tests may be used to evaluate a child's functioning. The Wechsler Intelligence Scale for Children–IV (WISC-IV; Wechsler, 2003) and Stanford–Binet Intelligence Scale—fifth edition (Roid, 2003) are widely used measures of cognitive functioning. The Vineland Adaptive Behavior Scales–2 (Sparrow, Balla, & Cicchetti, 2005) yield information about the child's developmental status and adaptive functioning. Academic achievement can be assessed through the administration of tests such as the Wide Range Achievement Test—third edition (WRAT-3; Wilkinson, 1993) or the Wechsler Individual Achievement Test–II (WIAT-II; Psychological Corporation, 2002). The clinician must also remember to evaluate or refer the child for consultation regarding other developmental problems, such as attention deficit disorders or speech/language delays. Similarly, problems such as sensory deficits, other neurological conditions, or fine and gross motor difficulties deserve a thorough investigation by qualified professionals. Fago (2003) identified a number of measures to evaluate the neuropsychological status of children and adolescents who engage in sexually aggressive behavior.

Child Self-Report Measures

In previous chapters we reviewed parental-report measures of children's behavior. Clinicians can use a number of child self-report measures to evaluate a wide range of symptoms and problems, including anxiety and fears, depression, and self-esteem. The Children's Manifest Anxiety Scale—Revised (CMAS-R; Reynolds & Richmond, 1978) and the State–Trait Anxiety Inventory for Children (STAIC; Spielberger, 1973) yield information about a child's level of anxiety, although again neither was specifically developed for use with maltreated children. Instruments such as the Piers–Harris Children's Self-Concept Scale—Second Edition (PHCSCS-2; Piers, Harris, & Herzberg, 2002) and the Perceived Competence Scale for Children (Harter, 1982) have been designed to assess children's self-esteem. The Children's Depression Inventory (CDI; Kovacs, 2003) is a commonly used measure of a child's level of depression.

The Fear Survey Schedule for Children–II (FSSC-II; Gullone & King, 1992) evaluates a child's specific fears and patterns across five areas but does not provide information about fears specifically related to maltreatment experiences such as sexual abuse. To remedy this situation, Wolfe and her colleagues (Wolfe, Gentile, & Wolfe, 1989) developed the Sexual Abuse Fear Evaluation (SAFE) subscale, a 27-item scale embedded in the FSSC-R. The SAFE subscale comprises two factors, the Sex-Associated Fear scale (e.g., watching people kiss on TV, talking or thinking about sex, being tickled) and the Interpersonal Discomfort scale (e.g., mean-looking people, people not believing me, being lied to by someone I trust). Briere (1996) developed the TSCC, a brief child self-report measure used to assess a number of dimensions related to trauma including anxiety, depression, sleep problems, dissociation, posttraumatic stress, and sexual problems. Other child-report measures that are abuse-specific have been published, and we review several of them in subsequent sections of this chapter.

Although self-report measures may provide some useful clinical information, there is danger in relying exclusively on them. As we have already noted, no single assessment modality or measure is infallible. A problem we have encountered with these measures is that some maltreated children respond in socially desirable ways, thereby rendering an underestimation of their problems. The same phenomenon has been reported in the literature; in Chapter 1 we described how some younger maltreated children deny problems that pose a real threat to their self-esteem. If clinicians begin to see an exaggeration of positive qualities in the self-report measures of a child who is, by the report of others, encountering significant problems, they should consider the possibility that the child is engaging in this defensive maneuver. This conclusion may be supported by other data, such as the child reporting, during the interview, that he or she has no problems whatsoever.

Projective Techniques

Projective assessment has a long history of use with disturbed children, particularly from a psychodynamic and psychoanalytic perspective. Unlike structured measures (e.g., self-report inventories and measures of intellectual and academic achievement), projective techniques present ambiguous perceptual stimuli. The child draws a picture, completes sentences, tells a story, or defines a visual image in amorphous stimuli such as ink blots, so that typical defenses against painful affects and cognitions associated with past experiences can be subverted. Although not every mental health professional has undergone the specialized training necessary to administer and interpret these measures, they offer the clinician another perspective on the maltreated child.

PROJECTIVE DRAWING

Drawings may be difficult for very young children to produce, inasmuch as they do not yet have the necessary visual–motor control. Similarly, somewhat older children with delayed visual–motor development may be unable to produce drawings. They may find the process so aversive that they refuse to draw or do so in a cursory manner. Moreover, one should remain aware that many of the following techniques do not have normative data and their validity and reliability as clinical instruments have not been established empirically. Clinicians should be extremely cautious about overinterpreting a figure's graphic representation, and especially about relying exclusively on the symbolism of drawings (Friedrich, 1990). Supplementing a drawing with an inquiry may serve as a catalyst to elicit more direct material. Drawings serve as a springboard for further interviewing, as we illustrate later with case material.

Draw-a-Person with Inquiry. Drawing human figures has long been a standard part of child assessment. We have found the following procedure helpful in assessing maltreated children. The child is instructed to draw a picture of a whole person and, after completing the picture, is asked to draw a picture of him- or herself. The clinician may have concerns about how the child views individuals of the opposite sex, and if the two drawings are of the same sex, the clinician can ask for a third drawing of a person of the opposite sex. After the child completes the drawings, the clinician asks the child a series of questions. Table 4.2 summarizes the inquiry developed by Dr. Bob Robinson of Alberta Children's Hospital a number of years ago. Some maltreated children begin to talk quite directly about their fears and anxieties, including those associated with their disclosures of the abuse. This is the case in the following example:

Nine-year-old Tom had alleged that he had been physically assaulted by an adult male, and presented with features of PTSD. His first drawing on the Draw-a-Person was that of the alleged perpetrator. Tom's responses to the inquiry about what this individual was thinking reflect his fear of further harm:

"Probably [thinking] of how to find me and what he'll do to me when he gets his hands on me. He knows I told."

Besides its content, clinicians must scrutinize the process of the drawing. Was the drawing done in a haphazard, quick manner that may reflect a child with poor self-esteem who has little confidence in his or her abilities? Alternatively, did the child adopt a meticulous, obsessive approach that reflected a lack of tolerance for any imperfection? When asked to do the task, did the child immediately protest, claiming that he or she couldn't do it?

TABLE 4.2. Draw-a-Person Inquiry

1. What is the person's name?
2. How old is ___________? (referring to the name the child has given the figure, including the child's own name in the drawing of the self)
3. What is ___________ doing?
4. What is ___________ thinking?
5. What would make ___________ feel:
   Happy?
      How would ___________ show it?
   Sad?
      How would ___________ show it?
   Angry?
      How would ___________ show it?
   Scared?
      How would ___________ show it?
   Worried?
      How would ___________ show it?
6. If ___________ could have three wishes, what would they be?
7. If ___________ could be any animal he or she wished to be, which would he or she most want to be? How come?
8. If ___________ could be any animal he or she wished to be, which would he or she least want to be? How come?
9. If ___________ were the only person on an island and could only have one person with him or her, who would he or she want to be there?

Note. Developed by Dr. Bob Robinson, Section of Psychology, Alberta Children's Hospital, Calgary, Alberta, Canada. Used by permission of the author.

Moreover, the child's language may be characterized by a lack of coherence and is thus difficult to follow. Children with weak verbal skills may show poor syntax and vocabulary and little elaboration of ideas or details.

Kinetic Family Drawing. Using this technique, the clinician asks the child to draw a picture of his or her family doing something together. Again, the content may reveal information pertinent to the child's perspective of the family. For instance, are family members actively engaged with one another, or are they disconnected from each other? Does the child depict him- or herself as on the periphery of the family? Do siblings receive more attention? The clinician should pursue these tentative hypotheses with follow-up questions (e.g., "You've drawn yourself away from everybody else in the family. I wonder why that is? How does it feel to be away from them?").

Sometimes the child's choice of which family to draw can be revealing. We have seen a number of maltreated children in foster homes who refuse to draw their natural families, preferring to depict their foster families. In response to our inquiries, some tell us that drawing their own families and thinking about them is too painful or that they now regard the foster families as their "real" families. As in the Draw-a-Person technique, the clinician can then ask questions like "Which person in the family gets the maddest?" "Which person gets the saddest?" "Which two people get along the best?" Sometimes when a child is asked to draw an ideal family, important clues emerge about the changes the youngster would like to see effected or the fantasies that she or he harbors about family life.

Draw the Maltreatment. Some children who cannot furnish a detailed verbal account of their maltreatment are much more able to draw episodes of their victimization. They may furnish considerable detail, and the clinician can inquire about what is happening in the picture. Addressing the child's self-depiction in the third person may be somewhat less threatening to the child, who then may be more able to answer questions about personal thoughts or feelings. Again, it is important to observe closely how the child does this drawing. Some adamantly refuse, reflecting their need to avoid the painful material. If they do participate, anxiety may impair their attention and concentration. They may also attempt to avoid the task by requesting a bathroom break or by asking extraneous questions. Children who approached the task of making other drawings in a more organized and thoughtful fashion may show a significant change when asked to draw a picture of their own victimization. Their anxiety may increase, resulting in a haphazard or chaotic picture.

Draw Your Feelings about the Maltreatment. Clinicians can now ask a child who did not depict personal reactions in the preceding drawing to draw how he or she looked or felt while being victimized and to identify the feelings this graphic depiction represents, another clue to the child's ability to express internal states verbally. Children's drawings often reflect themes of helplessness, inadequacy, and powerlessness. These are in contrast to the feelings of strength, power, or even identification with the aggressor that emerge when the clinician asks the child to draw how he or she would have liked to look during the maltreatment.

Draw Your Body. Some physically and sexually abused children may have been physically injured or harbor fears that their bodies were damaged by the abuse. These realities and fears may be accompanied by somatic complaints. Children's depictions of their bodies may provide important information relevant to this dimension.

Draw the Perpetrator. This drawing task can help the clinician understand how the child perceives the perpetrator, perhaps as a threatening or menacing figure. Other children depict the perpetrator more positively, reflecting underlying ambivalence about the relationship. Some adamantly refuse to draw the perpetrator at all because doing so provokes overwhelming anxiety. Asking the child to draw what should happen to the perpetrator provides the youngster with an opportunity to express ideas about this issue. Some are so angry that they want the perpetrator incarcerated for life or even executed. Others want the perpetrator to "get help."

Drawing of Dreams and Other Symptoms. Rather than talking about a frightening dream, a maltreated child may find it more tolerable to represent it graphically. This kind of drawing may serve as a springboard for the clinician to ask about other aspects of the dream, such as identifying "the worst part" of the dream, or what might have preceded or followed in the dream. This inquiry not only serves to evoke more content but also provides an opportunity for the child to begin to express some underlying affects and emotions associated with the maltreatment.

We have also asked children to draw selected aspects of their presenting problems. For example, asking children who are physically or sexually aggressive to draw a picture of the reactions of the children they have assaulted is one more way to gather information about the child's ability to appreciate the impact of his or her actions and the extent to which the child's feelings of empathy are developed.

PROJECTIVE STORYTELLING

The clinician has a considerable choice of projective storytelling tasks. The TAT, conceived by Murray (1938, 1943) and developed by Bellak (1993), is widely used with adults and some children. Bellak also developed the Children's Apperception Test (CAT) for youngsters ages 3–10 years. Clinicians may prefer a more recent measure, the Roberts Apperception Test for Children (RATC; McArthur & Roberts, 1982), because the pictures are more realistic, contemporary, and active (Friedrich, 1990). Caruso (1987) developed the Projective Story-Telling Test to evaluate maltreated children. Its pictures often elicit stories related to physical and sexual abuse. Friedrich (1990) notes that the child who is preoccupied with these issues is more likely to project them onto these cards than to respond to the more ambiguous stimuli of the CAT or TAT. Sometimes the stories are transparent reflections of important issues in a child's life.

Elliott was an 8-year-old boy referred for an assessment because of his impoverished social relationships. He experienced significant anxiety when he was not in close proximity to his foster mother, to the extent that he was unable to walk the short distance to and from school by himself. Elliott had been severely physically abused and neglected by his natural parents and then placed in a permanent foster home. The following story in response to card 4 of the CAT (a family of kangaroos on an outing) reveals his perception that the world is a dangerous, malevolent place where people are vulnerable to attack and reflects Elliott's reluctance to venture out in the world by himself:

> The kangaroo family is off to have a picnic in the woods. On their way they see smoke so they go off the road to investigate. When they go there they were frightened to investigate. They were so scared they didn't want to move. They were going to get shot by people, so they went all the way home and hid.

In an interesting study, McCrone and colleagues (1994) administered a projective storytelling task to grade 6 children enrolled in the Minnesota Mother–Child Interaction Project. The maltreatment group comprised 43 children who had been physically abused, sexually abused, or neglected or had parents who were psychologically unavailable. These children told stories in response to two cards from the Tasks of Emotional Development Test (Cohen & Weil, 1971) and two from the TAT. As compared with a group of 53 nonmaltreated children, the maltreated group evidenced significantly greater negative expectations of relationships as measured by their stories about these cards. They attended selectively to negative aspects of relationships portrayed in the cards, to the near exclusion of positive aspects. Defenses such as projection, introjection, displacement, splitting, and preoccupation were quite prevalent in the maltreated children's stories. Furthermore, maltreated children frequently told overelaborated stories characterized by unintegrated use of detail that added complexity, but not necessarily coherence, to the story. A smaller group of maltreated children, particularly the boys in the group, told impoverished stories that included little, if any, detail. McCrone and colleagues suggest that both the overelaborated and the impoverished styles were evidence of defensive exclusion, which diverts the individual's attention from a source of upset and involves the deactivation of internal processing. Although defensive exclusion minimizes distress, in new situations it limits children's attention to what is happening in relationships and prevents them from experiencing their feelings.

OBSERVATIONS OF THE CHILD

Sometimes the simple act of sitting quietly and watching a child behave or interact with others is a revealing exercise. Observing behavior while the child interacts with family members contributes to a comprehensive assessment and can occur in the waiting room, interview area or playroom, or at home. For example, cleanup is a common but useful natural observation time. Clinicians can compare the child's willingness to tidy up in response to their request in the playroom, with parental requests in the waiting room. It may also may be useful to observe the child in both unstructured (free play) and structured interaction with parents (Schutz et al., 1989). A parent and young child can participate in teaching tasks (e.g., matching shapes or puzzles) or cooperative tasks (e.g., building a house of blocks). The clinician might instruct a parent to teach an older child to sew on a button, to play checkers, or to engage in a cooperative task such as recreating a construction model. Schutz and colleagues (1989) provide a comprehensive list of observational targets: positive emotional warmth and attachment; differentiation of the child from the parent; accuracy of parental perceptions of the child's emotions, behavior, and verbalizations; reasonableness of expectations; and effectiveness of communication. The therapist must observe the child's responses closely and also evaluate parental responses in these domains.

Although time-consuming, observation in environments other than the clinician's office may be especially useful. Classroom observations may yield information about relationships with peers, the youngster's ability to manage academic and behavioral demands in a structured setting, and the quality of the child's relationship with important adults such as teachers. After completing observations, the clinician might confer with teachers to learn whether the child's behavior and presentation were typical and to clarify any remaining questions. Similarly, observations at a day care center or a babysitter's home are a source of useful information. Again, the clinician may have to speak with the caregiver to determine if the observed behavior is typical of the child in that setting.

Besides making observations of the child with parents and in other settings, the clinician should also note the youngster's mental status, as outlined in Table 4.3. The child's physical appearance, relationship with the clinician, behavior, cognition, perception, speech, affect, and insight and judgment should all be evaluated. The clinician should pay particular attention to those areas in which difficulties are apparent or the child seems to show an unusual response, as they may merit closer evaluation in subsequent sessions.

We devote the rest of the chapter to the evaluation of specific topics that are especially relevant for maltreated children: attachment disorders, attachment organization and patterns and IWMs/IS; PTSD; sexual behavior problems; dissociation; and children's attributions.

ASSESSMENT OF ATTACHMENT DISORDERS, ATTACHMENT PATTERNS, AND IWMs AND IS

This section of the chapter focuses on the assessment of three major domains: attachment disorders, attachment organizations and patterns, and pathogenic processes represented by IWMs/IS. Evaluating these domains may provide our best opportunity to obtain as comprehensive picture as possible of attachment's influence on maltreated children's development.

Attachment Disorders

In Chapters 1 and 2 we spent considerable time discussing insecure attachment as a risk factor for later psychopathology, but also mentioned that atypical attachment patterns can be considered as disorders, a concept we now describe in more detail. The concept of attachment as a disorder is not new. Bowlby (1944), Spitz (1946), and Goldfarb (1955) investigated the effects of "maternal deprivation" on children's development, work extended more recently by research teams examining the effects of institutionalization (e.g., MacLean, 2003). Although clinicians were well acquainted with the effects of early and profound relationship disturbances, diagnostic systems did not formally recognize that the disorder might result from disturbed or absent attachment relationships until the publication of the revised third edition of the *Diagnostic and Statistical Manual of Mental Disorders* (DSM-III-R; American Psychiatric Association, 1987; Greenberg, 1999). As we noted in Chapter 1, RAD, as defined by DSM-IV (American

TABLE 4.3. Mental Status Examination of the Child

1. Physical appearance
2. Relationship to the examiner
   a. Nature of the relationship; common presentations include:
      (1) Fearful and anxious
      (2) Closed and guarded, wary
      (3) Indiscriminate
      (4) Aggressive/sexualized
   b. Working alliance (extent of cooperation with the assessment)
   c. Social skills
3. Behavior
   a. Activity level
   b. Degree of organization (e.g., impulsive, compulsive, messy)
   c. Reactions to:
      (1) Limits
      (2) Failure
      (3) Challenges
4. Cognition
   a. Intelligence
   b. Attention and concentration
   c. Thought processes (e.g., organization, coherence)
   d. Problem-solving ability
   e. Thought content (major themes, general knowledge, delusions, etc.)
5. Perception
   a. Orientation in time, space, and person
   b. Short- and long-term memory
   c. Dissociation
6. Speech
   a. Vocabulary
   b. Syntax
   c. Articulation, fluency, and expressiveness
   d. Comprehension
   e. Specific disorders
7. Affect
   a. Emotional tone
   b. Range and intensity of affect
   c. Appropriateness to content
   d. Awareness and control of affect
8. Insight and judgment
   a. Regarding own problems, motives
   b. Regarding consequences of own behavior and actions

Psychiatric Association, 1994), distinguishes between two subtypes: excessively inhibited, hypervigilant, or highly ambivalent responses (inhibited subtype) and indiscriminate sociability or a lack of selectivity in the choice of attachment figures (disinhibited subtype). The age of onset is 5 years or younger, and there is the presumption that "pathogenic care" (i.e., persistent disregard of the child's basic emotional needs for comfort, stimulation, and affection; persistent disregard of the child's basic physical needs; or repeated changes of primary caregiver that prevent formation of stable attachments, e.g., frequent changes in foster care) is responsible for the disturbed behavior.

A number of criticisms have been leveled at RAD (Chaffin et al., 2006; Greenberg, 1999; Hanson & Spratt, 2000; Lieberman & Zeanah, 1995). Chaffin and colleagues (2006) describe RAD as "one of the least researched and most poorly understood disorders in the *DSM*. There is very little systematically gathered epidemiological information on RAS. . . . Similarly, the course of RAD is not well established. Long-term longitudinal data on the outcomes of children diagnosed with RAD have not been gathered (Hanson & Spratt, 2000)" (p. 80).

Greenberg (1999) also observes that "attachment disorders are by their very nature relational disorders, they do not fit very comfortably into nosological systems that characterize the disorder as person-centered" (p. 471). However, RAD focuses on the child's aberrant behavior rather than on the actual attachment relationship. A failure to recognize the relational aspects of attachment disorders disregards the fact that children often have multiple attachment relationships and may exhibit an attachment disorder with one caregiver but relate more positively to others. Greenberg also points out that the pathogenic conditions presumed to be etiological agents for disturbed social behavior are restricted to severe deprivation and maltreatment. "Pathogenic care" as defined by DSM-IV may not reflect some of the more subtle interactions between the child and caregiver associated with a disorganized attachment classification (Bronfman et al., n.d.). Moreover, a diagnosis of RAD cannot be made solely from a child's history of pathogenic care. As we reported in Chapter 1, a significant number of maltreated children show no developmental or mental health problems.

Historically, there has been a paucity of data pertaining to the reliability and validity of the diagnosis. Indeed, the use of untested diagnostic methods, such as broad diagnostic checklists, may easily lead to an overdiagnosis of RAD when it is not present and a failure to diagnose RAD correctly when it is present (Chaffin et al., 2006). These checklists include a wide array of childhood problems (e.g., fighting, aggressive behavior) that overlap with other disorders. These schemes raise a number of important questions: How many of these behaviors does a child require for a diagnosis of RAD, should some criteria be weighted more heavily than others, and are the behaviors (e.g., incessant chatter) valid indicators of an attachment disorder?

Given the easy accessibility of these checklists on the Internet, the risk of overdiagnosis (i.e., false-positive) is heightened even further. Consider the following scenario. Someone suggests a diagnosis of RAD to a parent or caregiver without any further elaboration or careful evaluation, or even direct contact with the child. The parent goes to the Internet and quickly finds what seems like a scientific checklist consisting of numerous behaviors. The parent then concludes that the RAD diagnosis is correct because the youngster does indeed exhibit several of the behaviors on the checklist. This scenario is especially worrisome if the parent has also been told that there is little hope for children with RAD, especially if they are older. Why expend a lot of effort and resources to help this child with RAD when the diagnosis implies little or no possibility of change?

Fortunately, diagnostic methods that incorporate questions more closely anchored to the diagnostic criteria of RAD have been developed and found to have stronger psychometric properties. Several studies of the effects of institutionalization have used the Disturbances of Attachment Interview (DAI; Smyke et al., 2002; Zeanah et al., 2002). Clinicians administer this semistructured interview to caregivers of young children, usually toddlers, who know the children well. The items are behaviorally based and coded on a scale of 0 (no evidence of any attachment disturbance) to 2 (evidence of behaviors consistent with attachment disorder). The first five items yield ratings of behavior relevant to the inhibited subtype (Smyke et al., 2002, p. 975):

1. How well does the child differentiate among adults and demonstrate a clear preference for a particular caregiver?
2. How much does a child seek comfort from a preferred caregiver?
3. How much does a child respond to comforting when it is offered?
4. Does the child respond reciprocally in interactions?
5. Does the child tend to regulate emotions well, showing age-expected levels of positive affect, or does the child tend to have higher than expected levels of irritability, sadness, or seriousness?

Although these items were developed for younger, preschool children, we believe they are relevant to the assessment of RAD in school-age children. However, we wonder whether the fifth question, regarding emotional regulation, might be particularly susceptible to overdiagnosis of RAD, given the frequency of emotional regulatory problems in childhood disorders, such as conduct disorders and oppositional defiant disorders. Furthermore, we agree with suggestions that clinicians explicitly ask parents about what the child does in situations in which he or she would be expected to demonstrate attachment behavior (O'Connor et al., 1999). Such a question could precede the second question and be posed as follows: "What does the child do when hurt or in pain?" Follow-up probes can ascertain the child's reactions in other situations in which the attachment system might be activated, such as when the child is frightened or upset.

Clinicians can assess behaviors indicative of the disinhibited subtype by using the first item (above) regarding whether the child differentiates among adults, plus three other items (Smyke et al., 2002, p. 975):

1. Does the child check back with the caregiver, especially in unfamiliar settings, or does the child wander off without purpose?
2. Does the child show initial reticence around strangers, or does the child readily approach unfamiliar adults?
3. Would the child readily go off with an unfamiliar adult?

Preliminary analyses of the DAI showed acceptable internal consistency and interrater reliability (Smyke et al., 2002). Zeanah and colleagues (2004) interviewed clinicians treating 94 maltreated toddlers in foster care in Louisiana regarding signs of RAD. The inhibited and indiscriminate subtypes could be reliably diagnosed with the DAI, and 17% of the sample was diagnosed with both types. Regarding the DAI's validity, Smyke and colleagues (2002) demonstrated that toddlers residing in a large institution in Bucharest, Romania, had significantly higher scores on both the DAI's RAD Inhibited and RAD Indiscriminate scales than those living in a unit designed to reduce the number of adults caring for each child, or toddlers living at home.

Although the DAI has been used with caregivers of younger children, clinicians may find the items useful when attempting to make a differential diagnosis of RAD in school-age children. The items are anchored to RAD's specific diagnostic criteria, and the preliminary data regarding reliability and validity are encouraging, at least for younger children. We hope this research will be extended to older youngsters to provide us with even more direction.

We now address what we consider one of the most important controversies: does a diagnosis of RAD tell us anything important about treatment? Does it inform us about what we should do to help these children? Even though it identifies etiological factors that must be present (i.e., "pathogenic care"), RAD is a good example of a diagnosis that says little about the underlying mechanisms or pathogenic processes responsible for these disturbed social relationships and what we should do to ameliorate them. As we emphasized earlier, we need to reach beyond the formal diagnosis to identify and elucidate pathogenic processes relevant to treatment.

Attachment Patterns, Organization, and Pathogenic Processes

In Chapter 1 we argued that assessing school-age children's attachment pattern via the strange situation is inappropriate, given its decreasing power to induce stress as children become more accustomed to and comfortable with separations. Moreover, there is a move to the "representational level" of attachment whereby school-age children express attachment patterns via words or play, although our preceding discussion indicates that their particular styles of interacting with attachment figures remain relevant.

Before we discuss assessment strategies for older school-age children, a few comments are in order regarding the use of separations and reunions for young school-age children, such as 5- and 6-year-olds for whom this strategy may still be appropriate. Gauthier, Fortin, and Jéliu (2004) and Slade (2004) employ brief separations from biological or foster parents to activate young children's attachment systems and then observe their modes of managing the ensuing distress, fear, and need for proximity. Both articles may be of interest to clinicians, because the separation–reunion procedures represent flexible adaptations of formal attachment assessments (i.e., the strange situation) to typical clinical environments. Most of us have not received the extensive training necessary to formally administer and interpret the strange situation, or others do not have access to facilities necessary to tape the interaction. Of course, clinicians must always be prudent about drawing conclusions from nonstandardized methods and must buttress hypotheses with data from other sources and derived from a variety of other methods. However, we believe the approaches described by Gauthier and colleagues (2004) and Slade (2004) represent workable and acceptable strategies to creatively and flexibly evaluate attachment constructs.

What should clinicians look for in these reunions? Gauthier and colleagues (2004) described several patterns of significance: clinging upon separation from parents or caregivers; joyful expression, ignoring, or withdrawal upon their return; seeking caregivers' proximity; sharing drawings or other productions; and avoiding gaze. Findings from empirical studies of young school-age children's behavior identified four main patterns of attachment derived from the first 5 minutes of reunion of 6-year-old children with their mothers (Main & Cassidy, 1988). Children judged *secure* responded to the mother's return in a confident, relaxed, and open manner. *Anxious–avoidant* children maintained a neutral coolness, including an avoidance of interaction with the mother. Children classified as *anxious–ambivalent* exhibited elements of avoidance, sadness, fear, and hostility and were clearly ambivalent about seeking proximity to the parent. Children classified as *disorganized–disoriented* in infancy took control in one of two ways when they were 6 years old. First, they took confrontational control and overtly rejected the mother in a punitive way ("controlling–punitive"; Lyons-Ruth, Alpern, & Repacholi, 1993, p. 583). In the second pattern, children attempted to care for or comfort the mother by providing helpful directions ("controlling–caregiving"; Lyons-Ruth et al., 1993, p. 583). The child at first appears as overbright and enthusiastic at reunions and seems to feel responsible for making the parent feel happy (Goldberg, 1991).

Boris and colleagues (2004) also designed a structured observational paradigm to evaluate attachment in preschool children. The clinician, who represents an unfamiliar adult to the child, plays an active role in this procedure, and approaches and picks up the child. The child's behavior with the unfamiliar adult is compared to his or her behavior with the familiar adult (i.e., parent or caregiver). For example, securely attached children should feel more comfortable when caregivers pick them up than when they are picked up by unfamiliar adults. Securely attached children will show some reticence, especially initially, when unfamiliar adults approach them; children with an insecure–disinhibited attachment organization will not show such reticence.

Categorizing children's attachment organizations via observations of their responses in separations and reunions leaves us with the same question as if we had applied a diagnosis of attachment disorder: What are the underlying pathogenic processes responsible, for example, for emotional constriction and reluctance to become involved in emotionally reciprocal relationships in a child with an avoidant classification? Chapter 2 discussed some of these mechanisms of impact in general, but how do we go about evaluating their potential importance for a given child's adjustment? Again, we argue that we must extend our evaluation beyond formal classifications, whether they are DSM-IV diagnoses or the attachment patterns that have received so much attention in the scientific literature. Slade (2004) expresses this perspective well:

> Indeed, child and adult attachment categories (and all their derivatives) have become, in a sense, the sacred cow(s) of attachment research. Certainly, these have been crucial to the scientific evolution of the field, and to the range of empirical validations that have carried the field forward immeasurably. At the same time, the focus on classification has reified and oversimplified the meaning and dynamic functions of attachment, resulting in an overemphasis on classification within the research domain and a failure to appreciate the complexity and depth of attachment processes as they are manifested within the clinical domain. . . . Attachment categories are simply ways of describing and organizing phenomena. From a clinical standpoint, it is these *phenomena* and the processes they represent that are the focus of our work, not the *categories*, per se. (p. 272)

A number of different strategies have been developed to assess the attachment organizations of older children from the representational perspective. We hope to demonstrate that although these measures may point to the most applicable attachment classification, they may also contain valuable information about attachment processes.

NARRATIVE STORY STEM TECHNIQUE

Earlier in this chapter we described the use of narrative story stems in which children complete stories using dolls. Bretherton, Ridgeway, and Cassidy (1990) developed five attachment-related story beginnings and then asked 3-year-old children to use the dolls to show and tell what would happen next. Bretherton and colleagues (pp. 300–305) described the administration details of the attachment story protocol, the required materials, and the content of the five story beginnings. This information may be particularly useful as a starting point from which clinicians can adapt the material for use with older children. For example, in the Departure story, the examiner depicts a mother doll and father doll facing a grandmother doll and two child dolls. The parents are going on a trip and say goodbye to the children, who remain at home with the grandmother. The examiner then asks the child to use the dolls to show what happens next. Solomon, George, and De Jong (1995) modified Bretherton and colleagues' doll-play story-completion task by encouraging 6-year-old children to select a doll to represent the self and to construct a pretend family. They provided subjects with a flat surface on which furniture was arranged into rooms, and used Bretherton and colleagues' Departure and Reunion scenarios as the story-completion tasks.

Solomon and colleagues (1995) reported that children with a secure attachment organization acknowledged the importance of the relationship with the mother in the doll play and described a warm, positive, direct, and supportive relationship with her. These children depicted the doll protagonist as accepted and valued despite flaws. Secure children were more likely to give "confident" stories, from which two major themes emerged. In the first, the "danger and rescue" story, the child telling the story introduced dangerous or frightening events originating outside the family, usually during the separation, but the situation was resolved safely by the reunion's end. The second theme was characterized by the child displaying confident, comfortable autonomy (e.g., the child makes an elaborate lunch). The characters expressed pleasure in the reunion, with an explicit acknowledgment that a separation had occurred.

Avoidant children dismissed the importance of the relationship, portrayed the doll protagonist as isolated or rejected, or sometimes gave no response to the story stem or did so only after several "I don't knows" or prompts. These children characteristically denied experiencing separation anxiety by negating, canceling, or "undoing" the separation itself (e.g., the child tried to accompany the parents on their trip). They also avoided the reunion or showed casual disinterest in the parents' return. A stereotypical depiction of household and babysitting activities and an empty, affectless quality characterized the stories' narrative structure.

Children with an ambivalent–resistant attachment organization were significantly more likely to give "busy" stories (Solomon et al., 1995, p. 454). They did not express fears directly about separation; rather, they reserved or displaced these fears and other negative feelings onto other story characters. The stories featured fun and pleasurable activities, and the overall quality was of a happy mood and busy activity. Reunion stories were characterized by delay and distraction. Reunions began but were never thoroughly completed because of obsessive and irrelevant actions by the child or other characters. These time-consuming and distracting activities constantly interrupted the story line (if one was detectable) and resulted in a digressive narrative structure.

Controlling children (i.e., those who had been disorganized–disoriented in infancy) were significantly more likely to give "frightened" stories consisting of two types: "chaotic" and "inhibited" (Solomon et al., 1995, p. 454). In the first, children enacted chaotic and dangerous events but, unlike the content of the stories of secure children, events were unresolved and led to the disintegration of the self and/or family. The behavior of parental figures or other adults was often frightening or abusive. The children in these stories were helpless to control their parents' behavior or the frightening events. Solomon and colleagues (1995, p. 454) described the narrative structure of these stories as "chaotic" and "flooded." Catastrophes arose without warning and dangerous people or events were vanquished, only to surface repeatedly. The children depicted punishments as abusive and unrelenting. "Inhibited" stories were markedly constricted, and the children appeared frightened in the testing situation. They seemed extremely uncomfortable with the task and did not want to enact the story. Children who were controlling gave odd responses that did not seem to make much sense or were disorganized, such as throwing a doll on the floor.

These different stories offer enticing clues about children's IWMs/IS. For example, disorganized–controlling children's chaotic stories reflect their view of the world as a malevolent, threatening environment wherein people cannot be trusted. Given such IWMs and broader IS, it is not surprising that these youngsters display little trust in others and have to exert some control over their world, often via aggressive, domineering, and controlling behaviors. They have little confidence that others, including primary attachment figures, will provide them with any sense of safety and security.

Toth and colleagues (1997) used the MacArthur Story Stem Battery (MSSB; Bretherton, Oppenheim, Buchsbaum, Emde, & the MacArthur Narrative Group, 1990), a derivative of Bretherton and colleagues' (1990) original story stems, to examine maternal and self-representations in 5-year-old physically abused, sexually abused, and neglected children and nonmaltreated comparison children. An added feature of this study was the inclusion of two variables to assess children's actual behavior during the administration of the story stems. "Controllingness" referred to the child's attempts to control the examiner or the situation, and "Relationship with the examiner" referred to the degree of enjoyment and eagerness evidenced by the child in response to the examiner's prompts to respond to the story stems (Toth et al., 1997, p. 788). Maltreated children's maternal and self-representations were more negative than nonmaltreated children's, their behavior was more controlling, and they exhibited a less positive relationship with the examiner. Physically abused children showed the most negative maternal representations, differing significantly from the sexually abused, neglected, and nonmaltreated groups. Physically abused youngsters also had more negative self-representations than nonmaltreated children. Sexually abused children showed more positive self-representations than neglected children, but both physically and sexually abused children exhibited more controllingness than nonmaltreated children; the latter were rated as having a more positive relationship with the examiner than the physically and sexually abused groups.

Although Toth and colleagues (1997) did not use the story stem responses to assign formal attachment classifications, they present a compelling case for the utility of data derived from story stems to understand maltreated children's representational models of others and the self. Given their histories of maltreatment, it is understandable why they would have more negative models and schemas of maternal figures (as potentially dangerous and insensitive caregivers) and themselves (as being unworthy of good care). Moreover, Toth and colleagues posited that maltreated children's controllingness and less positive relationship with the examiner reflected the generalization of these representational models and expectations to new situations and relationships. They also pointed out that this process may perpetuate their negative pattern of relationships, especially if their behavior elicits hostility or rejection that just confirms their IWMs/IS. This particular formulation suggests intervention strategies, such as those directed to assisting children to modify their maladaptive IWMs/IS (a primary pathogenic process), in order to facilitate healthier social relationships. Although directly targeting children and their internal processes would be important, this conceptualization also reinforces the need to intervene at other levels. Rejection and punitive responses to the child's negative behavior represent another set of pathogenic processes that, if unattended, will maintain or even amplify children's negative IWMs/IS. Consequently, clinicians must ensure that other people respond to the child's behavior in ways that start to modify the child's IMW/IS. The controllingness may be one symptom of a DSM-IV diagnosis of ODD or a disorganized–controlling attachment classification. We believe that neither the DSM-IV diagnosis nor formal attachment classification alone provides as much information relevant to intervention as incorporating a more fine-grained analysis of the associated pathogenic processes into the formulation.

Earlier in the chapter, we described other projective techniques, such as storytelling, that are useful in eliciting children's IWMs/IS. Other techniques include the Separation Anxiety Test (Hansburg, 1972; Klagsbrun & Bowlby, 1976; Shouldice & Stevenson-Hinde, 1992; Wright, Binney, & Smith, 1995), which features photographs of children undergoing separation from their parents. The examiner asks how the child in the picture feels about the separation and what this child would do. Although research has demonstrated associations between attachment classifications and the mental representations reflected in children's responses, there have been concerns about poor test–retest reliability (Wright et al., 1995) and validity (Bowers, Smith, & Binney, 1994). Other assessment measures include presenting a 6-year-old child with photographs of the child with his or her family and observing the youngster's reaction. Again, there seems to be a correspondence between these reactions and attachment classification (e.g., avoidant children avoid the picture, refuse to accept it, or actively turn away) (Main, Kaplan, & Cassidy, 1985).

The assumption underlying these indirect measures of attachment patterns is that children are unwilling or unable to talk about them (Target, Shmueli-Goetz, & Fonagy, 2002). This is similar to our earlier observation that clinicians sometimes employ more indirect assessment methods such as play, rather than taking time to talk to the children. Target and colleagues (2002) took a direct approach and developed the Child Attachment Interview (CAI) to assess attachment classification in 7- to 12-year-old children. Like the Adult Attachment Interview, it activates the attachment system by 14 questions plus probes (Table 4.4).

The CAI is scored on a number of dimensions to assess the child's overall current state of mind with respect to attachment: emotional openness, preoccupied anger, idealization, dismissal, self-organization, balance of positive/negative references to attachment figures, use of examples, resolution of conflicts, and overall coherence. The coding is based primarily on a linguistic analysis of the content and form of the attachment-related nar-

TABLE 4.4. Child Attachment Interview

1. Tell me who is in your family (lives with you in your house).
2. Tell me three words that describe yourself (examples).
3. Can you tell me three words that describe what it's like to be with your mom (examples)?
4. What happens when mom gets upset with you?
5. Can you tell me three words that describe what it's like to be with your dad (examples)?
6. What happens when your dad gets upset with you?
7. Can you tell about a time when you were upset and wanted help?
8. What happens when you're ill?
9. What happens when you hurt yourself?
10. Has anyone close to you ever died?
11. Is there anyone that you cared about who isn't around?
12. Have you ever been away from your parents for the night or for longer than a day?
13. Do your parents sometimes argue?
14. In what ways do you want/not want to be like your mom/dad?

Note. From Target et al. (2002, p. 94). Copyright 2002 by The Analytic Press. Reprinted by permission.

ratives, and the authors hope to develop a coding system that incorporates detailed behavioral information. Although this remains a work in progress, preliminary psychometric data look promising and it may prove to be a useful tool.

Clinicians can also informally interview children about their IWMs/IS. The following questions may elicit important information pertaining to these models, expectations, and possible pathogenic processes: What do you do if you're upset/hurt/sick/scared? Whom do you go to? When you ask them for help, what do you think they'll do? What have people done before when you asked them for help? Sometimes older school-age children show remarkable facility in verbally articulating their IWMs/IS:

Thirteen-year-old Linda's child welfare worker referred her for an evaluation, querying whether she was presenting with an attachment disorder. She had been subjected to extensive physical and psychological neglect and exposure to domestic violence, which eventually culminated in child welfare authorities apprehending her and her siblings. Linda's parents had chronic difficulties with alcohol abuse, which had severely compromised their caring for her when she was an infant and young child. Her parents subsequently separated, and Linda had some sporadic contact with her father. However, this contact was unpredictable, and he often failed to show up for scheduled visits.

Her foster mother told the clinician that Linda's social relationships vacillated between indiscriminate friendliness (e.g., hugging and initiating conversations with total strangers, sitting on people's laps) and a distant, aloof attitude with peers and adults alike, whereby she rebuffed overtures of friendliness, help, and support.

This ambivalence was also reflected in her descriptions of relationships. Linda told the clinician that she strongly desired to have close relationships with other people and in particular wanted a "big sister" whom she "could look up to." She portrayed this figure as someone with whom she could share her feelings, especially when upset. However, her desire for emotional closeness and intimacy was tempered by negative expectations of relationships. The clinician asked Linda what she did when she was sick, hurt, or upset, and she made the following statement: "I want to be in control and left alone. Sometimes I dream of living in the wilderness, all by myself, like a hobo. I don't like relying on others 'cause they always let you down. You have to do stuff yourself 'cause if you don't, they won't know what you need, or they won't keep their promises to help you."

Like many maltreated children, Linda anticipated rejection if she opened herself up to other people. Her IWM/IS that had their origin in the caretaking she received in her early years and her father's continued difficulty in fulfilling her desire for predictable contact. However, she craved attention, as evidenced by her indiscriminate friendliness. This pattern is consistent with Zeanah and colleagues' (2004) report that a significant proportion of children with an attachment disorder exhibit both the inhibited and disinhibited subtypes.

ASSESSMENT OF PTSD

Although PTSD is a syndrome commonly exhibited by maltreated children and clinicians must be able to make accurate differential diagnoses in order to provide the most effective treatment, it is only recently that clinical scientists have attempted to develop reliable and valid measures of PTSD in children. There are several self-report measures that clinicians may find useful (see Feeny et al., 2004, for a review). Pynoos and colleagues (1987) developed the Child Post-Traumatic Stress Disorder Reaction Index (CPTSD-RI) for children 8 years of age and older. Clinicians can administer this 20-item instrument as a self-report or in an interview format. It has been used for victims of violence, such as children exposed to genocide (Realmuto et al., 1992), but there seem to be few studies with maltreated children. Although the CPTSD-RI has satisfactory psychometric properties, Feeny and colleagues (2004) and Foa, Johnson, Feeny, and Treadwell (2001) describe several shortcomings. It does not include all the DSM symptoms of PTSD and thus cannot provide an accurate measure of PTSD diagnosis or severity. There are no items to evaluate trauma-related functional impairment, such as difficulty at school.

In response to these problems, Foa and colleagues (2001) developed the Child PTSD Symptom Scale (CPSS), a 17-item version of the Posttraumatic Diagnostic Scale (Foa, Cashman, Jaycox, & Perry, 1997), a well-validated measure for assessment of PTSD in adults. The original standardization sample consisted of 75 8- to 15-year-old children who had experienced the Northridge, California, earthquake in 1994. Although the CPSS has good convergent and discriminate validity, high reliability, and internal consistency, its use with abused and neglected children still requires scientific investigation. Foa and colleagues note that because none of these self-report questionnaires is entirely satisfactory, clinicians can use formal, structured interview schedules (e.g., Anxiety Disorders Interview Schedule for Children [ADIS-C], and the Anxiety Disorders Interview Schedule for Parents [ADIS-P]; Silverman & Nelles, 1988). However, these are prohibitively expensive and time-consuming, particularly when employed as screening measures in schools or community mental health clinics (Foa et al., 2001).

The Children's Impact of Traumatic Events Scale—Revised (CITES-R) includes subscales to assess the PTSD symptoms of intrusive thoughts, avoidance, hyperarousal, and sexual anxiety (Wolfe et al., 1991). We describe this measure in more detail in the section on the assessment of attributions. Briere's TSCC also includes a PTSD subscale (Briere, 1996).

Informal interviews of children and their parents or caregivers, especially with questions anchored to the DSM-IV diagnostic criteria, may yield useful data about whether a child's symptoms are consistent with PTSD. However, it has been our experience that some children, especially 5- to 8-year-olds, have difficulty answering some of the questions regarding their internal psychological states. Younger children can find general questions about symptoms, such as a foreshortened future or feelings of detachment from others, too abstract. Probably the best way of getting around such developmental limitations is by posing questions that incorporate concrete, relevant examples of these constructs. For example, clinicians can use the questions we described earlier about children's plans for the future (e.g., "What kind of job would you like to have when you're a grown-up?" "Do you think you'll get married? Have kids?"), to ascertain whether they have a sense of foreshortened future.

ASSESSMENT OF DISSOCIATIVE DISORDERS

As for all problems associated with maltreatment, and mental health problems in general in the school-age population, there are two main sources of information about childhood dissociative disorders: reports of observers (e.g., parents, other caregivers, teachers) and the self-reports of children themselves. Clinicians must carefully observe children's behavior to determine the presence of dissociation and to distinguish normal, age-appropriate dissociation from that used for coping with maltreatment. They can train parents, foster parents, child care workers, and teachers to monitor a child carefully and observe any range of behavior that suggests the presence of dissociation. Table 4.5 is an outline of behavioral targets to be observed for identifying the presence of dissociative identity disorder/multiple personality disorder (DID/MPD), as described by Lewis (1996, pp. 313–315), Lewis and Yeager (1994, pp. 732–734), and, more recently, by Haugaard (2004a). We strongly recommend these excellent reviews of the symptoms and behaviors characteristic of childhood dissociation disorders.

As indicated in Table 4.5, children who are dissociating may manifest a range of types and levels of intensity of behavior, although we do not yet have sufficient information regarding the exact number of behaviors or constellations of behaviors that warrant clinical intervention (Haugaard, 2004a). Lewis (1996) and Lewis and Yeager (1994) suggest that clinicians be alert to the possibility of dissociation if there is a family history of dissociative disorder and if the magnitude of different types of medical, behavioral, and psychological symptoms is high. A combination of perplexing forgetfulness, episodic trance states, mood fluctuation, and violent or self-injurious behavior may also be present. Symptoms may include observed changes in abilities, knowledge, preferences, and demeanor. Trancelike states may be present that are often labeled by others as daydreaming. These states involve spontaneous blank staring, with the child seeming unaware of surroundings. The child may experience amnesia for the duration of the episode; when it is over, the child resumes activity as if nothing had happened. The youngster also may deny performing actions that others observed. A diagnosis of dissociative identity disorder should be considered if the child displays one or more distinct personality states that periodically take full control of the child's behavior (Putnam, 1993), as illustrated in the following case:

Megan was a 9-year-old child placed in a residential treatment facility because of out-of-control and outrageous behavior in her home. According to Megan's mother, a stepfather had left the home when Megan was approximately 3 years old. He reportedly had been harsh and degrading with the child. Megan reported few memories of this man. Her behavior in the residence and at school was highly unpredictable, with no apparent precipitants to the marked shifts in her presentation. She often strongly denied her behavior and absolved herself of responsibility for her actions. Megan's presentation in the assessment was also confusing. During a period of play observation, Megan chose to play checkers

TABLE 4.5. Dissociative Symptoms in Childhood

1. Extreme fluctuations in moods, behavior, preferences (e.g., foods, games, or clothes), and demeanor; changes in language, accent, or voice quality; appearing completely confused by a task that was completed easily before; during psychological testing, dramatic changes in the child's responses to tests during a session or between sessions, or changes in the child's attitude toward testing from one session to another
2. Trancelike states: in fantasy world and oblivious to surroundings, including classroom activities; sometimes labeled as "daydreaming" or "spacing out"; frequent staring ahead with no particular focus
3. Amnesia for actions and events occurring during the absent time while in the trancelike state; missing blocks of time; may have no memories of a previous day, afternoon, or hour; may deny responsibility for actions during these times, and sometimes labeled pathological liar; waking and not being aware of how one got there; reports of changes in relationships with people that the child cannot explain (e.g., several relationships end suddenly and the child does not know why); people are angry with the child for reasons that are unknown to him or her
4. Vivid imaginary companionship extending beyond 6 or 7 years of age; companions are relatively continuously present and, while defending the child, maybe demeaning
5. Wide variety of physical complaints; medical records of numerous physician and hospital visits for symptoms that seem to defy medical explanation
6. Hysterical paralysis
7. Sleep disturbances and nightmares; sleepwalking; sudden losses of consciousness; tends to have undergone neurological evaluations for these symptoms; symptoms may have been diagnosed as a seizure disorder
8. Auditory hallucinations; in severely dissociated children the voices may give orders; symptoms sometimes diagnosed as schizophrenia
9. Inner hierarchies of entities who serve specific functions sometimes present; child is periodically called by other names, generally by people he or she does not recall meeting
10. Sometimes withdrawn and depressed but may present with severe behavioral problems, including unprovoked rages and violent behavior that seem to come from nowhere; commonly receives diagnosis of attention-deficit/hyperactivity disorder or sometimes of bipolar mood disorder; symptoms often diagnosed as conduct disorder

Note. Adapted from Haugaard (2004a), Lewis and Yeager (1994), and Lewis (1996).

but seemed confused and angry during the game. After making a move, she vehemently denied making it on her next turn and argued with the clinician to be allowed to change it. Initially this behavior seemed manipulative, but over time it was clear that Megan did not remember making the moves. Combined with many observations by other individuals, this behavior confirmed that Megan often dissociated. In later months, she demonstrated two distinct personality states that allowed her to cope with previous maltreatment and her expectations that others would degrade and humiliate her. Megan varied from appearing as a young and gentle girl to a tough adolescent who wore thick makeup and verbally and physically attacked others.

Administration of behavioral checklists to parents and caregivers can supplement their informal reports of children's behaviors. The principle that observations of a child's behavior are made by persons thoroughly familiar with the child underlies the Child Dissociative Checklist (CDC), a 20-item instrument (Putnam, Helmers, & Trickett, 1993). The adult circles a response on a 3-point scale that best describes the child's behavior on a given item over the past 12 months. The items tap several domains of dissociative behavior: dissociative amnesias; rapid shifts in demeanor; access to information, knowledge, abilities, and age-appropriateness of behavior; spontaneous trance states; hallucinations; identity alterations; and aggressive and sexual behavior. Malinosky-Rummell and Hoeir (1991) and Putnam and colleagues (1993) demonstrated that the CDC readily discriminates between normal and traumatized children. The vast majority (95%) of children with formally diagnosed dissociative disorders score 12 or higher, whereas only 1% of controls achieve this level. However, the CDC does not systematically inquire about the DSM-III-R/DSM-IV criteria for dissociative disorders. As with any assessment strategy, clinicians can incorporate it into a set of measures in order to attain as rich and accurate an understanding of the child as possible.

Clinicians can also ask children for their perceptions of whether they are experiencing any dissociative phenomena or symptoms. However, the very internal nature of dissociation may pose real challenges to young children who may not yet have the introspective skills to identify or articulate dissociative symptoms (Ogawa et al., 1997). Lewis and Yaeger (1994) and Lewis (1996) developed developmentally sensitive questions designed to reveal the presence of symptoms and behaviors of dissociation (see Table 4.6).

Lewis (1996) also described the development of the Bellevue Dissociative Disorders Interview for Children, an interview protocol that covers the major signs and symptoms of dissociative disorders. She noted that interviewers have freedom to move flexibly from one topic to another rather than having to adhere to a structured interview, a format many anxious children are unable to handle.

ASSESSMENT OF SBPs

Assessing children's SBPs relies on the same principles that underlie the evaluation of other problems: the assessment must focus on specific behaviors but must also evaluate the influence of comorbid conditions and moderator variables, such as the family' s response to the SBPs; it utilizes

TABLE 4.6. Questions Regarding Dissociative Symptoms

1. You know the way people can switch channels on a TV set? Well, some kids, if they are in trouble and need to be especially big or strong, or if they want to play around like a baby, can switch and become big and strong, or they can be little like a baby. Can you ever do that? (If the answer is "yes," ask: "When?" "What is it like?")
2. Many kids who have been through a lot or have been hurt are able to space out and go to a special place in their heads and not feel it. Can (could) you do that?
3. Many children who have been through a lot or who feel lonely can talk with someone in their heads. Can you do this? (If "yes," ask: "What does the voice sound like? Is it a man's voice? A woman? A child? An animal? Are there ever two voices talking to each other? Do they ever tell you what to do or not to do?")
4. Many children, when they are lonely and upset, have a make-believe friend or a toy they talk with. Can you do that?
5. Have you ever been told that you said or did something and you could swear you had not done it? (e.g., saying something? talking about something? hurting someone?)

Note. From Lewis (1996, pp. 313–316) and Lewis and Yeager (1994, p. 736). Copyright by Elsevier. Adapted by permission.

multisources and multimethods; and it is based on a developmental perspective. As such, there is nothing magical or terribly different about evaluations of SBPs, although the content is an area with which a number of clinicians may not have a great deal of familiarity. Given space limitations, the following section of this chapter can highlight only a few of the salient issues. We refer the reader to sources of more extensive and detailed information about assessing children with SBPs (e.g., Bonner, Walker, & Berliner, 2000; Gil & Johnson, 1993).

Developmental Perspective

We have emphasized that assessments have must a developmental focus. This tenet guides our selection of developmentally sensitive measures and informs us about the significance of the behavior. The latter is especially important in evaluating school-age children's SBPs. Chaffin and Bonner (1998) argue cogently that we must be particularly prudent about applying adolescent or adult models of sexual offending indiscriminately to preschool-age or school-age populations. This caveat extends even to the terms we use to describe these children. Young children repeatedly called "perpetrators" may begin to define their self-images and identities according to this term, along with the connotation that sexual perpetrators have an incurable and life-long condition (Pearce, 2001). This may raise the probability that they will begin to think of themselves as incapable of stopping the sexual behavior, thereby setting up a self-fulfilling prophecy. Does a 10-year-old boy who touched his 5-year-old brother's genitals in the bath on several occasions truly have an incurable and compulsive disorder?

Chaffin and Bonner (1998) question the utility of the "conventional wisdom" applied frequently to younger children with sexualized behavior—that is, the belief that sex-offender treatment is the only acceptable and effective approach; that denial must be broken; that treatment must be long-term and involve highly restrictive conditions; that deviant arousal and fantasies, grooming, and deceit are intrinsic features; and that the behaviors always involve an offense cycle or pattern that must be identified.

Interviewing Children about SBPs

Earlier we mentioned the CSBI (Friedrich et al., 2001), a 38-item standardized parent-report measure of the frequency of various types of 2- to 12-year-old children's sexual behaviors. Although the CSBI yields valuable information about the comparative frequency of various sexual behaviors, interviewing children about SBPs is another crucial step to gather information about the nature and clinical significance of sexual behaviors. Sexual problems are usually associated with a significant degree of shame, embarrassment, and stigmatization, and children, like adults, are extremely reluctant to openly talk about their difficulties. Exacerbating their reticence is ignorance about sexual terminology and their relative lack of experience in talking directly about sex, at least with adults. Their anxiety may escalate when they are brought to a clinic and expected to reveal details of their sexual behavior to a complete stranger. What can clinicians do to help children talk about SBPs?

Many of the same techniques we have already described to help children discuss details of the maltreatment are applicable here. Clarification of the assessment's purpose (e.g., "Your mom told me that you've been touching the private parts of other kids. I want to try to help figure out why you're doing that and what people can do to help") and a description of the evaluation's process and structure may attenuate the anxiety. Negotiating about the timing of the discussion about the SBPs and expending sufficient effort to establish rapport are often necessary before children will talk openly. Modeling the use of appropriate sexual terminology is especially important. Children who hear adults use immature or juvenile anatomical or sexual terms may infer that sex is such a sensitive issue that even adults cannot broach it directly. Although children may want to use their own terms, clinicians should use adult terms after clarifying their meaning with the child (Berliner, 1989).

It is our impression that given the shame and stigmatization attached to SBPs, children are more likely to deny or minimize them. Informing children that they are allowed to tell the clinician when they do not want to respond to a question, rather than lying, gives them a sense of control over what they say, which may reduce their resistance. Follow-up probes (e.g., "I wonder why that's such a hard question," "What would be the worst thing that could happen if you had really done those things to your sister?") facilitate conversations about sources of anxiety and reasons for denial. The clinician's empathic response (e.g., "You're really scared that I'm going to think you're weird because of those sexual things you did") and clarification of any misconceptions about the consequences of disclosing the SBPs further reduce anxiety, although children often require evidence that talking about the SBPs will not be catastrophic. For example, some children anticipate that disclosing such problems will elicit negative reactions from others, including the clinician. Gradually exposing the child to the questions, while at the same time directing him or her to observe closely the clinician's reactions, was used to good effect in assessment sessions with 9-year-old Darren, whom we described earlier in the chapter:

As well as having little trust that the clinician would respond sensitively to his account of the maltreatment, Darren expected similar responses to the sexual behavior he had been exhibiting with other children. In order to increase Darren's confidence that he would respond appropriately, the clinician proposed that he develop a series of questions about the SBP, writing each on a separate strip of paper. Each week Darren pulled one of the strips out of a container and then decided whether to answer the question. Again, Darren used the same criteria to evaluate the clinician's reaction to his answers (e.g., Did ____________ (the clinician) look angry or "grossed out"? Was he interested in what Darren was saying? Did he seem to understand how Darren felt about the sexual behavior?). Initially, Darren answered just one question per session, and sometimes refused to answer a particular one if he found it too threatening. After the fourth week, however, he volunteered to draw several questions from the container and he stopped refusing to answer questions. His anxiety had begun to extinguish as a result of being exposed to material directly relevant to his SBP and the clinician's supportive, empathic, and respectful reactions.

Appropriate confrontation may also be helpful. Confrontation does not mean yelling at children and berating them to confess; instead, it entails providing children with the evidence in a respectful manner, such as the other child's very specific descriptions of the sexual behavior, and then asking the child to respond.

Gil and Johnson (1993, pp. 155–167) presented a comprehensive list of areas to be included in interviews of children with SBPs. We have adapted this list and summarized areas of potential interest in Table 4.7.

We do not have sufficient space to describe each of these areas, but we would like to add some detail about evaluating the precipitants of the sexual behavior and the presence of sexual arousal and sexual fantasies. These two areas often pose challenges to clinicians. Most of us have had little experience with engaging children in explicit and direct conversations about sexuality, and we may feel some discomfort in initiating them. Developmental challenges are also significant obstacles to obtaining a full account. Most precipitants of SBPs, as well as arousal and fantasies, are private, internal events, and young school-age children, with their less sophisticated introspective and metacognitive skills, encounter difficulty in identifying and articulating them.

Identifying precipitants to a SBP is a basic feature of the adult model of sexual offending; that is, there are affective, cognitive, situational, and somatic cues and reactions that precede and precipitate unhealthy sexual behavior. Although clinical experience suggests that some children can, with the correct support and guidance, identify some of the precipitants, there is little scientific information about their exact role in SBPs of school-age children.

Adolescent and adult models also place considerable emphasis on sexual fantasies and arousal as precipitants in the genesis of sexual offending, but again we have little empirical information about the specific role of fantasies and arousal in school-age children's SBPs. Although some children do indeed report fantasies and arousal, they are by no means universal phenomena in preadolescent children with SBPs. However, it is still important to ask about sexual fantasies and arousal. These are among the experiences that children will rarely divulge spontaneously, and they usually describe them only when asked. But even then, they may not have the linguistic abilities to describe these experiences, and their feelings of shame and embarrassment may prevent them from talking openly. Gil and Johnson (1993) recommend that clinicians inquire about fantasies by saying:

> "Some kids tell me they day dream a lot. I think what they mean is that they sort of space out and think about things, like when you are at school and you are bored. Some kids say it is kind of like having a movie running in their head. Sometimes they are in the movie and sometimes not. Do you ever day dream? Some kids say they think about touching stuff in their day dreams. How about you? What things do you day dream about?" (p. 160)

Clinicians can encourage children to elaborate on fantasies—whether they have played them out, and where they learned about them. Gil and Johnson

TABLE 4.7. Interview Content for Children with Sexual Behavior Problems

1. Description of the sexual behavior:
   a. What were the sexual behaviors?
   b. Who were the other children? Were adults involved? Relationship to child?
   c. When did the behavior start?
   d. Frequency of the behavior?
   e. When did the behavior stop? Why?
   f. Was any coercion involved (physical, emotional, threats, secrets)?
   g. Does the child acknowledge the sexual behavior? Extent of denial or minimization? Is the child's report of the sexual behavior consistent with others' reports?
2. Precipitants of the behavior.
3. Degree of sexual arousal; presence of sexual fantasies.
4. Motivation for the behavior and feelings about sexuality.
5. Specific reasons for the behavior, for example, history of prior victimization, exposure to sexually explicit material (pornography).
6. Child's perceptions of sexuality in the home.
7. Child's perceptions of parents' reactions to the sexual behavior; reactions of others (e.g., teachers, relatives); child's understanding of why they might be concerned.
8. Child's feelings about the victim (e.g., empathy or appreciation of how the other child felt or reacted).
9. Child's willingness to acknowledge responsibility for the sexual behavior, or does the child attribute responsibility to others?
10. Child's reaction to the behavior (e.g., regret, remorse, guilt, shame).
11. Child's willingness to accept responsibility for the behavior.
12. Desire to change the behavior.
13. Child's thoughts re future; for example, does the child believe he or she is at risk for reengaging in sexual behavior in the future?

Note. Adapted from Gil and Johnson (1993).

(1993) suggest that clinicians ask directly if the children have ever seen these fantasies played out (e.g., in real life, on television, in pornographic videos, in magazines, or on Internet sites).

Basing an assessment about the significance of school-age children's SBPs solely on parents' reports about the type or frequency of such behavior is insufficient. We need to find out what the sexual behavior means to the child and why it might be so important (Berliner, 1989): Does the child ever think about sex? How does the youngster feel when he or she has sexual feelings? Do these bother the child? How does the child feel when thinking about another person having sex? Why do people have sex? When shouldn't people have sex?

A similar straightforward approach to assessing children's sexual arousal is probably best. Most will have no understanding whatsoever of the term "arousal," so clinicians have to describe what this means using developmentally sensitive language. They should initiate this discussion after reaching a basic agreement with the child about sexual terminology. Clinicians can mention that sometimes boys get erections (after ascertaining that the boy understands what this means or briefly clarifying the term) when they think about sex, which are accompanied by feelings of excitement. Asking children about sexual arousal that may have accompanied their thoughts about engaging in the sexual behavior may further clarify arousal's role as a precipitant, especially if the child began to masturbate while thinking about engaging in the sexual behavior or looking at sexually explicit material. Masturbating can intensify the child's arousal and reinforce the associated thoughts and fantasies (e.g., "Did you feel sexually excited when you were thinking of touching your sister?," "When you were thinking of touching her, did you start to touch your privates?," "How did that feel when you touched your privates?").

There are a few child-report measures that tap children's perceptions of sexual behavior. These include the TSCC (Briere, 1996) and the CITES-R (Wolfe et al., 1991). Although these are useful, especially as some highly anxious children may find completing a form about their sexual behavior and concerns less threatening than answering questions in a face-to-face interview, the clinician will probably have to supplement questionnaire responses with follow-up inquiries in order to reach a more comprehensive understanding of the significance of the SBPs. Chapter 9 discusses other strategies to help children identify precipitants to SBPs and physical aggression.

We must have reasonable expectations about the amount and specificity of the information children can offer. Developmental limitations or overriding feelings of shame and embarrassment may preclude them from giving a full account, or they may divulge information slowly throughout the course of treatment. A more reasonable hope is to gather sufficient information to develop working hypotheses that guide intervention, but with the full appreciation that we may have to revise these and our treatment plan as more information emerges.

ASSESSING ABUSE-RELATED ATTRIBUTIONS

In Chapter 2 we reviewed research demonstrating the significant yet complex set of relationships between attributions and outcome in response to maltreatment. It speaks to the importance of assessing children's abuse-related attributions in order to identify potentially influential pathogenic processes that may be appropriate targets of intervention.

Clinicians can pose open-ended questions to sexually abused children, such as, "Why do you think the touching problems happened?" (Feiring et al., 2002). However, children may not necessarily provide a full account of their attributions in response to these inquiries. Feiring and colleagues (2002) reported that very few of the 8- to 11-year-old and 12- to 15-year-old sexually abused children who were asked this question made internal attributions; external attributions that blamed the perpetrator were more common, along with responses that indicated they did not know why the abuse occurred. Children may be reluctant to express their perception that they were to blame if other people have reassured them that they were not responsible (Feiring et al., 2002). They may worry about others' reactions (e.g., disapproval, rejection) if they express a different opinion. The particular wording of open-ended questions can be another source of variability in children's responses. For example, a question such as "Who was to blame for the touching?" may also inhibit children from expressing internal attributions. The term "blame" may signify failure or moral transgressions, rather than simple causal responsibility, and children may deny internal attributions because blame is associated with these negative connotations (Dahlenberg & Jacobs, 1994; Feiring et al., 2002).

These concerns highlight the need to employ multimethods to assess maltreated children's attributions. Several child-report measures have been developed, with Feiring and colleagues (2002) pointing out that children may feel more comfortable identifying their real attributions by making a checkmark on a form than in a personal interview. As we mentioned earlier, Wolfe and colleagues (Wolfe et al., 1991) developed the CITES-R to gather information about a child's perceptions, attributions, and feelings about his or her sexual victimization. The CITES-R has nine subscales, six related to impact (betrayal, guilt, helplessness, intrusive thoughts, sexualization, and stigmatization) and three related to attributions about the abuse (internal versus external, global versus specific, and stable versus unstable). The child is asked to respond "very true," "somewhat true," or "not true" to 54 items. Feiring and colleagues modified the CITES-R and added 10 items to measure internal attributions of sexual abuse. The resulting scale, the Abuse Attribution Index (AAI), consists of 22 items. Nine measure internal global attributions (e.g., "This happened to me because I'm a bad person"), five tap into internal specific attributions (e.g., "This happened to me because of the way I was dressed"), and eight measure external attributions (e.g., "This happened because the perpetrator has a problem"). We reported in Chapter 2 that abuse-specific internal attributions as measured by the AAI were significantly associated with higher levels of PTSD, especially when accompanied by feelings of shame, although other studies have not found a relationship between internal attributions and PTSD.

Feiring and colleagues (2002, p. 30) used four items to assess feelings of shame:

1. "I feel ashamed because I think that people can tell from looking at me what happened."
2. "When I think about what happened I want to go away by myself and hide."
3. "I am ashamed because I feel I am the only one in my school who this has happened to."
4. "What happened to me makes me feel dirty."

Each of the items is rated on a 3-point scale: not true, sometimes true, and very true.

Mannarino, Cohen, and Berman (1994) developed the Children's Attributions and Perceptions Scale (CAPS) to assess the unique attributions and perceptions related to the victimization experiences of sexually abused youngsters. The scale consists of 18 items and four subscales: Feeling Different from Peers, Personal Attributions for Negative Events, Perceived Credibility, and Interpersonal Trust. Mannarino and colleagues point out that as the items do not make any reference to sexual abuse, the measure is not as abuse-specific as it could be. The scale is administered in an interview format, and children are instructed to respond based on a 5-point Likert scale. Seven- to 12-year-old sexually abused girls scored significantly higher than nonabused controls on the total CAPS and three subscales. This pattern reflected a greater sense of feeling different from peers, heightened self-blame for negative events, and reduced interpersonal trust (Mannarino et al., 1994).

The Children's Abuse-Specific Perceptions (CASP) Scale is designed to elicit maltreated children's attributions or perceptions of a specific abuse experience (Kolko et al., 2002). In the original sample, 47 physically or sexually abused children, ages 6–18 years, rated 16 items on behaviorally anchored 5-point scales. Kolko and colleagues (2002) reported that among the many findings, a diagnosis of PTSD was associated with greater endorsement of perceived victimization and of the need for consequences to the perpetrator. Sexually abused children were more likely to believe that the abuse was uncontrollable, intentional, and undeserved than physically abused youngsters. Sexually abused children were also more likely than physically abused children to have negative perceptions of abusers and a stronger belief that the offender had negative intent to abuse them. In a cogent analysis of these findings, Kolko and colleagues speculate that these differential attributions may reflect differences in the respective relationships between physically and sexually abused children and their offenders. There was a significantly higher proportion of biological relationships between perpetrators and physically abused children than between perpetrators and sexually abused children. Consequently, children whose biological relatives have physically abused them may be less inclined to perceive their offenders in a negative manner and more likely to minimize the consequences of the assaults. According to Kolko and colleagues:

> The functional purpose of the attributions may be to mitigate a harsh reality that threatens the fundamental assumption that children make about their parents. Abused children may have many non-abusive experiences with a biological parent, which serve as the template for interpreting parental behavior even when specific acts involve behavior the children recognize as unacceptable or wrong. Finally, because children will most often continue to have some level of relationship with biological parents and may desire to have these relationships, it is often more adaptive to have a less malignant view of the experience and their parents' motives. (p. 52)

This brief review has highlighted several methods of assessing children's attributions. Just as they have difficulty identifying the precipitants of their behavior, young children may find thinking about and reporting attributions to be a formidable challenge (Valle & Silovsky, 2002). Although open-ended questions represent opportunities for maltreated children to more fully explicate their attributions, especially if clinicians have established solid rapport with their young clients and have conveyed an accepting attitude that facilitates children's expression of their true attributions, clinicians should supplement their informal inquiries with standardized measures.

FORMULATION OF THE TREATMENT PLAN

After completing the assessment, the clinician will have amassed a vast amount of information. Integrating the data and formulating a treatment plan can be a daunting enterprise. It is crucial to maintain a focus on the child and his or her needs and to develop a conceptualization or formulation of the problem, especially with reference to relevant pathogenic processes. As we have seen, accurate identification and appreciation of pathogenic processes provide a richer understanding of maltreatment's impact than would a diagnosis alone, and point to viable interventions likely to benefit the child and the family.

Developing a treatment plan involves three major steps, which are outlined in Table 4.8. Before any interventions can be considered, the clinician must determine the clinical significance of the presenting problems. First, the clinician should review the findings derived from the assessment of the child and determine if effects arising from the maltreatment are situational reactions or reflective of more long-term developmental problems. As we have argued, a comprehensive history is invaluable in making this determination. Are the child's behaviors within normal developmental parameters, or are they significantly interfering with the child's developmental trajectory? Are the problems causing the child or others significant distress? The clinician must remain alert to the presence of other problems that are not necessarily the direct result of maltreatment, but may interfere with development and therefore merit intervention.

Once clinically significant problems are identified, the clinician may proceed to the second step in developing a treatment plan tailored to the specific child and family. Here the clinician must develop a conceptualization about the pathogenic processes contributing to the emergence and maintenance of clinically significant problems. Of course, there may be more than one mechanism operating, and moderator variables are interwoven with these pathogenic processes. The clinician must examine relevant information regarding the family members, as they may serve as important moderators of the maltreatment. The relevant domains include marital and family functioning, individual functioning of the parents, and parenting abilities and skills. Parental support of the child postmaltreatment requires particular attention. Finally, the clinician should consider broader environmental factors that may exacerbate the child's and family's response. These include extended family, peer, and community negative reactions to the child's maltreatment and broader ones such as poverty. The clinician should evaluate the appropriateness of past and current services provided to the child and family and their response to these interventions. It is important to remember that moderator variables also include strengths in the child and family that can be profitably used in therapy.

Step three, development of an intervention plan, begins once the clinician has developed a formulation of the problem. The prior identification of pathogenic processes serves as a major foundation for the plan. If the child initially shows symptoms of PTSD and the therapist adheres to the model that was hypothesized to underlie these symptoms in Chapter 2, then exposing the child to the aversive stimuli related to the abuse so that anxiety can extinguish will be a major component of the individual treatment. Some children may require individual therapy so that they can reexamine and reformulate their attributions and cognitions about the maltreatment. Some children's distress may be a function of their parents' anxiety or the deterioration in parenting skills associated with the discovery of the abuse. In these situations interventions directed at parents may be especially important. Even with children who have been seriously affected by abuse or neglect, individual treatment may not be the treatment of choice. In our experience, many very young children (below 3–4 years of age) do not have the requisite verbal or cognitive skills to benefit from this approach. Second, their psychological well-being is so dependent on their parents and the

TABLE 4.8. Three-Step Treatment Plan Formulation

Step 1: Determine clinical significance of presenting problems.

1. Review findings from the child.
   - Mental status
   - Attachment organization and IWMs/IS
   - Emotional and behavioral self-regulation
     - Externalizing problems
     - Internalizing problems, including dissociation and PTSD
   - Language development
   - Cognitive development and adaptation to school
   - Development of self
   - Peer relationships
   - Coping and defense mechanisms
   - Presence of localized or developmental effects that require attention and intervention

2. Review findings from the family for problems that may require intervention.
   - Family functioning: premaltreatment and postmaltreatment
     - Marital relationship and family functioning
     - Individual functioning of parents
     - Nature of attachment to the child
     - Poverty, stability of supports
     - Single parent
     - Parenting and discipline
     - Accurate perception of the child's needs; appropriate expectations
     - Impulse control
   - Support of child postmaltreatment
     - Acknowledgment of maltreatment
     - Belief in child
     - Emotional support
     - Ability to protect child from further maltreatment
     - Securing appropriate services
     - Provision of adequate parenting postmaltreatment

3. Review environmental problems that may require attention and intervention.
   - Cultural–societal toleration of maltreatment
   - Cultural and religious factors
   - Community reaction to the child and family
   - Supportive milieu for the child and family; provision of appropriate services

Step 2: Develop a conceptualization of the child's problems.

1. Develop a conceptualization about the pathogenic processes and mechanisms contributing to the emergence of clinically significant problems (e.g., internal working models, classical conditioning).

2. Consider moderating variables that compensate (e.g., strengths) or potentiate maltreatment's impact across the child, family, environment, and maltreatment factors.

Step 3: Develop an intervention plan.

1. Examine the EST literature to determine its relevance for the child and family, and how EST interventions may have to be modified to accommodate the child's and family's unique characteristics.

(*continued*)

TABLE 4.8. (*continued*)

2. Consider and set priorities regarding treatment interventions to remediate the impact of maltreatment and prevent further maltreatment. Examples of possible interventions follow:
   - Child domain
     - Need for protection, apprehension
     - Foster home or residential placement
     - Community youth worker involvement
     - Short-term symptom-focused therapy
     - Long-term therapy for developmental impacts
     - Group therapy (e.g., abuse, anger management)
     - Speech therapy, occupational therapy
     - Special school class, tutoring, and the like
     - Day treatment to address school and emotional needs
     - Pediatric consult (e.g., regarding ADHD)
   - Family
     - In-home support (e.g., homemaking, behavioral management training)
     - Parenting training
     - Day care placement and subsidy
     - Low-income housing
     - Public assistance
     - Family therapy
     - Marital therapy
     - Individual therapy
     - Anger management training
     - Drug and alcohol treatment programs
   - Environment
     - Community education
     - Family or individual meetings; communication with extended family
     - Support in further police interviewing
     - Court support to child and family

family environment that intervention should be focused on helping the parents to become the primary agents of change. We have also occasionally encountered children who absolutely refuse to participate in any therapy. Working with parents may be an alternative to help them manage better with their children's behavior.

Although we devote much more attention to ESTs in subsequent chapters, we must note here that familiarity with the scholarly and scientific literature in this area is essential and constitutes an integral component of treatment planning and selection. Most of the empirical research on the effectiveness of psychosocial treatments for childhood disorders has involved the application of treatment packages to children with the same diagnoses, rather than treatments specially tailored for specific pathogenic processes (Shirk & Russell, 1996). Clinicians must review the relevant literature to determine if interventions should be used with a child with the same diagnosis as those of the children in a study *and* with his or her particular constellation of pathogenic processes and moderator variables. The case examples of Geoff and Sam presented at the beginning of Chapter 2 illustrate the need for careful analysis of these processes and variables and their relevance for proper treatment selection.

Although the focus of this book is individual child therapy, we have emphasized throughout that children should never be treated in isolation. Even if they are no longer residing in an abusive or neglectful home and are in an excellent alternate living arrangement, therapists must still engage these latter caregivers in a collaborative alliance and enlist them as allies in the treatment process. Therapists must work with other significant individuals who exert a powerful influence over the children's lives. Similarly, a child participating in individual or family therapy may benefit from group therapy in the course of his or her treatment. Adhering rigidly and solely to one therapeutic modality limits the comprehensiveness of the services that can be offered.

Recommendations about interventions should be built on the child's and family's strengths. For example, children with good verbal skills who, during the assessment, demonstrated a facility in talking about their experiences might benefit from verbally oriented therapy rather than a nonverbal, play therapy approach. Matching the interventions to the needs of the child and the family is crucial; mismatching may lead to the conclusion that the treatment modality was ineffective, that the modality was incorrectly used, or that the child or family undermined treatment, when none of these statements is really the case (Looney, 1984).

Individual psychotherapy may be the principal intervention or one of several components of a treatment plan. Localized effects may require relatively short-term, structured individual child therapy with parental support. Pronounced developmental effects may require the consideration of a wide array of services: long-term individual child therapy; specialized foster home or residential placement; family therapy; and various medical, educational, occupational, and speech therapy interventions. In many cases, the therapist cannot implement such a myriad of interventions simultaneously; they need to be prioritized. Ensuring the children's immediate physical safety is the first priority for those still residing in abusive or neglected homes, followed by the introduction of psychotherapeutic interventions as the child and family can tolerate and respond to them. The transactional model can help in prioritizing interventions and may indicate that some interventions cannot be undertaken until certain factors change. This was the situation in the family described here:

Three children were in the care of George, who was stepfather of two and biological father of one of them. Concerns about multiple types of maltreatment in the family arose shortly after the mother had deserted the children 4 years previously. Various assessments and interventions had been provided to George and the children. George always agreed to such input but seldom actively benefited from in-home support and parent training. He remained passive and noncommittal and was isolated, with no support in the community. When interviewed, the children minimized their concerns and were hesitant to engage with the clinicians or provide information. Child welfare personnel chose not to remove the children from George's care, as they believed they had insufficient evidence. Early assessments indicated that the children were doing poorly in all areas of functioning and suffered from a number of developmental effects. Child welfare personnel exerted increasing pressure on the clinicians to see the children in individual therapy to address these problems. The clinicians took the strong stance, however, that individual therapy would be inappropriate while the children remained in George's care. They reasoned that therapy would be only a small part of their experiences and would do little to change their expectations about others, particularly because George could barely provide basic care for the children. He could not support them in school and peer relationships, let alone give the support they needed to profit from therapy. The clinicians believed that continued maltreatment would likely occur without active intervention from child welfare services and that the children would continue to deny and minimize their experiences. Consequently, the children would have had grave difficulties addressing these issues in therapy.

Despite the children's obvious and increasing needs, the clinicians used the transactional model and also considered the parental and environmental factors in recommending that therapy be initiated only after the children had been removed from George. Eventually George placed the children in care. Once out of the former situation, all three children reported significant emotional, physical, and sexual abuse, as well as neglect. One of the children reported George's maltreatment only after being permanently removed from his care. The boy frankly stated that he had not acknowledged the abuse sooner because he feared more coercion and abuse if he reported the maltreatment and was then returned to George. After being removed, the children engaged in individual long-term therapy and group therapy.

Interventions may be carried out at the level of the child, the family, and the wider community. It is important that any potential treatment plan be formulated in a way that is practical and workable for the child and family. Often, a clinician may formulate a multifaceted and comprehensive treatment plan only to discover that various components are not available, too expensive, or possibly too overwhelming for the family. Clinicians must pay particular attention to developing interventions that are consistent with and respect the family's unique cultural heritage and traditions.

FEEDBACK SESSION WITH PARENTS OR CAREGIVERS

In providing feedback to parents or caregivers, the clinician presents a formulation about the nature of the child's problems and how they might be alleviated to permit healthier development. It is crucial to provide information in a relatively simple and straightforward fashion. The clinician cannot assume that every parent will understand most psychological and developmental terms. Even those parents who have been in therapy or are well educated and articulate may not be familiar with terms used by the clinician. It is often helpful in this presentation to give examples of the child's behavior that illustrate the findings. The therapist should identify strengths in the child's and family's functioning so that therapy can build on these assets while bringing areas of difficulty to the attention of the child and the rest of the family.

Following a review of the child's and family's response to the maltreatment, the clinician describes what interventions will be useful. The treatment plan should follow logically and coherently from the assessment findings so that parents or caregivers can understand why a particular intervention has been recommended. Clinicians should engage parents or other caregivers in an alliance so they can support the child's therapy at both the logistical and the emotional level (Chapter 6 describes strategies for engaging parents); they need to feel they are a necessary part of the child's therapy. Clinicians can achieve this goal by having parents or other caregivers become active participants in setting goals, which should be as specific as possible. The clinician should tell parents what the specific expectations are for their involvement in the child's therapy, what they must do to complement the therapist's work, and should then negotiate a schedule for sessions so that the child can attend therapy reliably.

The clinician may have to provide parents or caregivers with some specific guidance and suggestions during the feedback session that will help them limit or contain particularly troublesome behavior by the child, such as physical aggression or SBPs. For example, restrictions regarding the child's unsupervised contact with other children, substitute activities that may be used to redirect the child's negative behavior, and rewards for appropriate behavior may be essential (Gil & Johnson, 1993). Similarly, caregivers may require immediate specific instructions on how to deal with stealing and hoarding food by a severely neglected child. These plans may need to be written so that parents or caregivers can refer to them daily. Specific plans also decrease the caregiver's, child's, and clinician's anxiety and convey a sense of hope that the negative behavior will diminish and the child will recover.

Clinicians should inform the parents or caregivers of their expectations regarding the child's progress in therapy and explore with parents their own feelings and reactions that may emerge over the course of therapy. The parents or caregivers can have greater trust if clinicians discuss the difficulties and regressions that may be expected, before they occur, during what parents may have expected to be a smooth and easy process. Clinicians also need to clarify the involvement and roles of other professionals, with perhaps a larger case conference being convened to discuss these issues.

Finally, a discussion about the length of therapy and its cost is necessary so that parents or caregivers can give informed consent for the child's participation. The cost includes time commitment and/or monetary investment. The clinician should briefly explain how the end of therapy is determined by referring to its specific goals, so that parents do not feel they are committing to seemingly endless involvement. The therapist should invite questions and comments throughout the feedback session. It is often useful to ask whether the case formulation is congruent with parents' or caregivers' perceptions and expectations. In addition, encouraging feedback about how the treatment plan can be altered or fine-tuned to make the recommendations even more viable can help to engage parents in the treatment process. Even if parents seem to understand clearly all that is said during a feedback session, many are overwhelmed by the content and volume of information they receive. The clinician should not assume that they will retain all this information. Consequently, the clinician may need to review the issues and explanations over the course of therapy. The therapist's willingness to provide even more information as the parent's or caregiver's understanding of the child increases is helpful.

After providing feedback for parents or caregivers, the clinician may also wish to provide the child with formal individual feedback. The amount of detail and the depth of this feedback can vary, depending on the child's developmental status and needs. Again, the clinician should encourage and welcome feedback from the child.

CHAPTER FIVE

Principles and Goals of Treatment

In this chapter we offer a conceptual basis for common treatment goals and strategies for maltreated children. They are derived from our understanding of the sequelae of maltreatment and the mechanisms of impact reviewed in Chapters 1 and 2, as well as from the principles and techniques of assessment described in Chapters 3 and 4. Without an understanding of the theoretical bases for treatment modalities, clinicians may apply indiscriminately the same clinical technique to every maltreated child, regardless of idiosyncratic needs. Although it is important to have a large repertoire of specific strategies and interventions, it is equally important to have a theoretical understanding that guides our choice and application of techniques. Before we discuss the specific goals of treatment and their rationale, we briefly review the basic principles of treatment that guide our work in this area.

BASIC PRINCIPLES OF TREATMENT

Treatment Must Be Comprehensive and Ecologically Based

As already discussed, the clinician must be prepared to address a wide domain of problem behaviors and areas of dysfunction associated with the maltreatment of a child, as well as problems that predated the abuse and/or neglect. Interventions may be necessary in different settings and environments to ensure truly comprehensive and individualized services. Although many maltreated children require direct treatment, intervention must also occur at the family level to maximize the child's recovery and growth. The needs of the families deserve attention; these include "survival needs" (e.g., food, clothing, and shelter); crisis intervention; training in parenting skills; and more traditional individual, marital, or family therapy (Cicchetti & Toth, 1995).

This principle also applies to children who do not live with their families and will have no contact with them. Even in these cases, some adult is assuming responsibility for the child's care, whether it be a foster parent or the staff of a residential treatment facility or group home. Although contact with these adults might be quite different from the interventions directed at biological parents, the clinician must have regular contact with them to facilitate delivery of the most effective and optimal treatment to the child. For example, communication with the staff of a residential facility provides ongoing information about the child's response to treatment and alerts the clinician to any significant developments in the child's life that may have implications for the intervention. It also ensures a coordinated, consistent approach among the important individuals involved in the child's life. The same argument can be made for contact with other collaterals, such as teachers or child welfare workers.

Such contact may yield other benefits. Ongoing communication and consultation with a child welfare worker can help ensure that the broader system meets the child's needs appropriately and sensitively, such as when changes in the child's placement are proposed. Some clinicians resent the time and energy that must be expended on these broad issues of case management or fear that contact with other professionals will somehow contaminate their relationship with the child. However, a failure to play this more active and broader role significantly limits the effectiveness of clinical work with child clients.

Treatment Must Have a Developmental Focus

TREATMENT MUST ADDRESS DEVELOPMENTAL EFFECTS

Abuse or neglect can disrupt a child's ability to negotiate stage-salient developmental tasks and may have a significant effect on the child's ability to handle future developmental tasks successfully. Therefore, clinicians must evaluate and treat, when necessary and appropriate, the developmental effects associated with maltreatment. As well, they must intervene to remedy those localized effects that do not have major developmental ramifications.

TREATMENT MUST BE DEVELOPMENTALLY SEQUENCED

As we have seen, one factor that contributes to the emergence of sequelae associated with maltreatment is the child's developmental level. A child's perception or interpretation of the meaning of the maltreatment may change as a function of progress through different developmental stages. Therefore, therapy must be available to maltreated children at various points in their lives. For example, a child who has undergone serious maltreatment may do some profitable work in therapy at age 8 or 9 years and then again as an adolescent. However, this child may also have to return to therapy as an adult when confronting maltreatment-related issues reelicited by typical adult developmental tasks, such as establishing romantic or sexual relationships with others or parenting one's own offspring.

Another way of thinking about this notion of developmentally sequenced treatment is to conceptualize it as a "family practice" orientation. The therapist functions as a primary care provider, much like the traditional family physician. A clinician offers treatment to clients for different reasons over time in the context of an ongoing relationship. Although the client may not see the family physician for extended periods, he or she regards the practitioner as a resource who can be consulted when difficulties arise. Cummings (1986) suggests that there is no reason why clients cannot interrupt therapy when they are no longer under stress and then return to therapy when they need to. This model of practice speaks to an even larger issue. We need to divest ourselves of the notion that we "cure" people and have only one chance to help a client become problem free for the rest of his or her life, so that if our clients encounter difficulties several years after the termination of therapy, we have in some way failed in our jobs. According to Cummings, this is "absolute sheer nonsense" (p. 429). Returning to psychotherapy is not necessarily a failure either for maltreated children or for the clinicians who treat them. The fact that some ask to return to therapy with the same clinician may speak to a trusting and secure therapeutic alliance. Of course, sometimes clinicians cannot help when clients request future services, inasmuch as they may not have the relevant skills or expertise. Rather than providing direct care, they can serve as a referral source to ensure that former clients receive appropriate help. We would also like to note that this model is not appropriate for all maltreated children, especially those showing more localized effects. Many of these children can be treated quite successfully and usually do not have to have to return for a subsequent course of therapy.

TREATMENT MUST BE DEVELOPMENTALLY SENSITIVE

Like assessment strategies, treatment and intervention must be congruent with the developmental abilities and capacities of the child. For example, a therapeutic approach that places heavy emphasis on verbal exchanges will not be effective with a child with compromised or deficient receptive and expressive language skills. Implementation of such an approach would engender more frustration and a greater sense of failure in a child who is already suffering from a shaky sense of self-esteem. We pay particular attention to this issue in subsequent chapters when we discuss the use of CBT.

Use Directed or Nondirective Therapy with Maltreated Children as Required

There seems to be a common myth that child psychotherapy, especially play therapy, refers solely to a nondirective approach. The best-known proponents of this approach include Allen (1942), who considered certain transactions in the therapist–client relationship to be the crucial elements in successful "relationship therapy." This approach was elaborated and amplified by Axline (1964, 1969). As one of her eight basic principles of nondirective play therapy, Axline (1969) postulated that "the therapist maintains a deep respect for the child's ability to solve his problems if given an opportunity to do so," and "the therapist does not attempt to direct the child's actions or conversations in any manner. The child leads the way; the therapist follows" (p. 73). However, this ability to eventually bring up emotionally sensitive material may not be true of all maltreated children. Contrary to Axline's assertions, some children in therapy may not take the initiative in raising issues related to their victimization.

An exclusive reliance on nondirective play therapy may not be in the best interest of our young clients, although it certainly has a role in the treatment of maltreated children. Clinicians can use it to engage children in a relationship and establish some rapport. Some children do initiate metaphorical play spontaneously as a way of depicting their experiences and feelings regarding their victimization; the therapist needs to do little to help the child begin this process. However, others are so frightened and anxious that they cannot even use the psychological distance inherent in play to express their concerns, and they engage in activities that help them avoid confronting this material. Nondirective therapy may inadvertently strengthen their avoidance. The child must be exposed, either directly or indirectly, to this painful material for anxiety to be extinguished and to begin reformulating the meaning of the abuse or neglect.

Children also may need directed help to develop more adaptive ways of coping with the aftermath of maltreatment. If children engage in highly inappropriate behavior such as physical or sexual aggression, the hope that they will spontaneously or willingly raise these issues is naive. The clinician must be more directive to enable them to confront these often embarrassing patterns that previously brought them much condemnation. Clinicians must possess skills in both nondirective and directed therapy and the flexibility to use different approaches when indicated. Rigidity in both thinking and practice does little to help these children.

Treatment Must Be Culturally Sensitive

As advocated in Chapter 3, clinicians must be sensitive to children's and families' cultural traditions and contexts when conducting assessments and implementing interventions. Cohen and colleagues (2001) summarized the data pertaining to the role of cultural variables in the treatment of abused and neglected children. There are mixed findings regarding the effects of ethnicity on the emergence of childhood psychopathology as a response to maltreatment, although there is considerable evidence that minority children in general, and especially those in foster care (at least in the United States), are less likely to be referred for and receive appropriate mental health treatment than European American children. Cohen and colleagues' review indicated that race is probably not a significant predictor of differential treatment response. However, race as a variable may be too broad and heterogeneous, and clinicians must conduct a more fine-grained analysis of each child's and family's unique cultural and ethnic heritage to identify those specific variables that affect or moderate the child's response to maltreatment. Cohen and colleagues express a similar sentiment:

> Regardless of what the research demonstrates for these children as ethnic groups, cultural issues may be of great importance for certain children and families. It is therefore essential that clinicians treating maltreated children develop cultural competence in discussing and addressing these issues in treatment. (p. 155)

There are a number of cultural variables that influence people's general willingness to seek out, participate in, or benefit from formal mental health care: styles of coping with life events; the cultural meaning of specific symptoms and the stigma attached to behavioral and psychological problems; issues of trust and mistrust, especially vis-à-vis professionals who may be perceived as authoritarian figures; spiritual and religious beliefs; and reliance on formal and informal sources of support and assistance (Saunders et al., 2004). Cultural beliefs, attitudes, and practices also affect the child's and family's response to the maltreatment and their willingness and ability to engage in treatment. These include beliefs about sexuality, nudity, virginity, discipline practices, family boundaries, parent–child relationships, and parental emotional and behavioral reactions to the child's maltreatment (Cohen et al., 2001).

Interventions Should Strive to Use ESTs

ESTs have received a great deal of attention and have generated a fierce debate over the value and imperative of using them (see Wampold & Bhati, 2004, for a comprehensive review of the EST movement). ESTs are considered to be

> those therapies that have shown to be efficacious in treating specific disorders, based on the American Psychiatric Association's (1994) *Diagnostic and Statistical Manual of Mental Disorders* (4th ed.; DSM-IV), in two randomized control trials (RCTs) or in a series of single-case design experiments (Task Force on Promotion and Dissemination of Psychological Procedures, 1995). (Messer, 2004, p. 580)

According to McCabe (2004), "efficacy is a measure of the benefit of an intervention provided for a defined problem under specifically structured conditions of a research investigation" (p. 579). Effectiveness, however, "is a measure of the benefit of an intervention for a given problem provided in a natural clinical setting without concurrent controls (McKibbon, Eady, & Marks, 1999)" (McCabe, 2004, p. 579).

The movement to use ESTs gained powerful momentum in 1995 with the publication of the first of several task force reports by the American Psychological Association (Task Force on Promotion and Dissemination of Psychological Procedures, 1995) and subsequent revisions (Chambless et al., 1998). The task force identified treatments that had been demonstrated through rigorous research to be efficacious for adults and children. ESTs are typically designed for a single DSM-IV Axis I disorder (e.g., PTSD), treatments are manualized and of brief and fixed duration, and patients are selected to maximize homogeneity and minimize comorbid diagnoses. These conditions are imposed to reduce the number of confounding influences that would represent alternative explanations of the results (e.g., differing comorbid diagnoses among patients, varying lengths of treatment, or variations in treatments) (Westen, Novotny, & Thompson-Brenner, 2004).

In subsequent chapters we weave the EST literature for maltreated children into our descriptions of therapeutic strategies. As clinicians, we have a responsibility to be aware of this body of knowledge and to strive to use ESTs when appropriate. The Chadwick Center for Children and Families (2004) and Saunders and colleagues (2004) both conducted comprehensive reviews of empirical research supporting the efficacy of certain treatment protocols with maltreated children. Although we frequently reference the literature throughout this book, we strongly recommend that clinicians review these two excellent sources. Despite the importance of evidence-based practice, however, there are four caveats that temper a wholesale, indiscriminate application of ESTs to adults' and childrens' psychological problems.

First, the EST research methodology attempts to include patients with a single disorder, or "pure" cases, to avoid the confounds that would arise if they had comorbid or cooccurring conditions or problems. Westen and colleagues (2004) and Messer (2004) point out that most patients seen in clinical practice are polysymptomatic, with most adult studies consistently finding that most Axis I conditions are comorbid with other Axis I or Axis II disorders in the range of 50–90%. Children also exhibit high rates of comorbid conditions, including some of the more frequent symptoms presented by maltreated children. If EST research excludes these patients, who seem to be the majority of children we see, we cannot assume that the results of the intervention study are necessarily generalizable to these patients. As asked by Westen and colleagues, are interventions developed in the laboratory transportable to everyday clinical practice?

Second, as we argued in Chapter 2, formal diagnostic labels may not reflect differences between patients in a given diagnostic category. There may be varying pathogenic processes underlying behaviors that look the same but which may require different interventions. Selecting an intervention or treatment package solely on the basis of research that demonstrated that other patients with the same diagnosis showed, as group, significant improvement, is unwarranted and must be accompanied by a consideration of pathogenic processes and other variables (e.g., child's developmental level, ability of the family to support the intervention).

Third, EST research usually employs manuals to standardize interventions and to minimize within-group variability; that is, subjects in a specific treatment condition all receive the same ingredients, for the same amount of time, and at the same time. The more a manual and the clinician deviate from this standardized practice, the more difficult it is to draw conclusions about precisely what caused the experimental effects. If clinicians are to use ESTs in their daily practice, then the most empirically defensible way to do so is to adhere closely to the manual. However, manualization may come with a real cost. As articulated by Westen and colleagues (2004):

> A good clinician in an efficacy study (and, by extension, in clinical practice, if practitioners are to implement treatment manuals in the ways that have received empirical support) is one who adheres closely to the manual, does not get sidetracked by material the patient introduces that diverges from the agenda set forth in the manual, and does not succumb to the seductive siren of clinical experience. The more researchers succeed in the scientifically essential task of reducing the clinician to a research assistant who can "run subjects" in a relatively uniform (standardized) way, the more they are likely to view psychotherapy as the job of paraprofessionals who cannot—and should not—exercise clinical judgment in selecting interventions or interpreting the data of clinical observations. (pp. 638–639)

Strict adherence to a manual and a corresponding erosion of the role of clinical judgment can sometimes have adverse effects on patient care, such as the development of a poor therapeutic alliance (Goldfried & Eubanks-Carter, 2004; Wampold, 2001). Consider an 8-year-old girl who is being treated for PTSD after witnessing multiple episodes of domestic violence. In one session the child quickly divulges that her pet dog died the previous day. A clinician who follows the manual and proceeds to the next step in an anxiety management protocol without addressing the child's level of distress and helping her to process this loss is showing a significant failure in clinical judgment. Dismissing or ignoring the child's concerns will probably have a detrimental effect on the therapeutic relationship and inhibit the girl from disclosing other relevant information. Why would she talk about other relevant issues with an insensitive individual who ignores what is really important to her? Furthermore, the clinician may have missed a wonderful opportunity to address issues possibly linked to the maltreatment. Exploration of the girl's reactions to her pet's death may have revealed feelings of abandonment by parents who were so involved in their own conflictual relationship that they had little time left for their daughter; the dog may have represented the only figure who unconditionally accepted this child. Although this is a hypothetical example, the point is that a failure to at least explore the child's feelings and thoughts around this event may have left a lot of rich clinical material untouched. Strict, unthinking adherence to a manual reflects a broader philosophical stance: Therapy is something that is done to a client by a clinician who has control over the sessions, "rather than a transactional process in which the patient and therapist collaborate" (Westen et al., 2004, p. 639). Without such control, standardization suffers and within-group variance attributable to other sources increases, but skilled therapists realize that clients, including children, often bring their own agendas to sessions and they "are always coauthors and coconstructors of the treatment process" (Ablon & Marci, 2004, p. 666).

Fourth, a substantial proportion of the EST literature focuses on treatment packages, including much of the research on the efficacy of interventions for maltreated children. Although this is undeniably helpful, we still have little data identifying the specific, active ingredients of these packages, especially for complex children who have not only been maltreated but present with several other comorbid conditions and who reside in dysfunctional families. As recommended by Westen and colleagues (2004) and Ablon and Marci (2004), we need to isolate specific intervention strategies that clinicians can integrate into their practices. The following statement by Westen and colleagues summarizes our position regarding ESTs:

> We might do well to realign our goals, from trying to provide clinicians with step-by-step instructions for treating decontextualized symptoms or syndromes to offering them empirically tested interventions and empirically supported theories of change that they can integrate into *empirically informed treatments*. . . . Perhaps most important, it would require the assumption of clinically competent decision makers (rather than professionals trained to stay faithful to a validated manual) who have the competence to read and understand relevant *and* basic research, as well as the competence to read people—competencies we suspect are not highly correlated. (p. 658)

COMMON GOALS OF THERAPY

The basic principles discussed above provide us with a general orientation to psychotherapy with maltreated children. We now discuss some common goals of therapy, with particular attention to their rationale and implications for clinical intervention. We wish to make it clear, however, that this discussion can serve only to provide the clinician with general direction in choosing possible treatment goals and interventions. Although the goals described here are clearly not applicable to every maltreated child, they are derived from our previous discussion of maltreatment's impact and possible mechanisms that may be responsible for outcome. Each child requires an individualized treatment plan that identifies specific goals and interventions.

Acknowledging the Maltreatment and Expressing the Associated Feelings and Cognitions

The overarching goal of psychotherapy with maltreated children is to help them develop more adaptive ways of coping with the impact of the maltreatment to ensure a healthy developmental trajectory. Attainment of this goal is associated with a decrease in clinically significant behavioral and emotional difficulties and a resumption of the child's healthy developmental trajectory. However, for a child to attain these goals, the youngster must first acknowledge (either directly or indirectly) that the maltreatment did indeed happen and then begin identifying and expressing the feelings and cognitions (e.g., attributions regarding responsibility) linked to such experiences. Doing so is the first step in the change process, and articulating details of the maltreatment and the associated feelings and cognitions is a means to an end. For example, the clinician can help the child to modify cognitive distortions and misattributions only after the child has identified them.

Talking about the maltreatment may also have direct therapeutic effects. Exposing children to stimuli (e.g., memories, feelings, cognitions) related to their maltreatment is an important component of anxiety reduction interventions. As we saw in our discussion of conditioning theories in Chapter 2, many maltreated children develop anxiety-related symptoms, including PTSD, owing to the pairing of previously neutral stimuli with stimuli associated with the maltreatment. These neutral stimuli then acquire aversive properties such that their presence elicits anxiety and the child learns to avoid stimuli associated with the maltreatment, including thoughts or feelings. Thus, if a child avoids thinking about the maltreatment, his or her discomfort is minimized. However, this strategy is maladaptive in the long term. By not examining or talking about the maltreatment, the child eliminates the possibility of exposure to cues and affects. Therefore, the anxiety does not extinguish and symptoms continue. Furthermore, avoidance of thoughts or discussion about the maltreatment is reinforced and the child never learns at what point, if any, the fears are no longer justified or adaptive. We can derive a principal method of intervention from this conceptualization of anxiety and the associated pathogenic processes: the child must be exposed to the feelings, cognitions, and memories associated with the maltreatment so that his or her anxiety can be extinguished. Forms of exposure range from more direct modes in which the child talks directly about the maltreatment, to more indirect methods such as exposure to these themes via metaphorical play. In subsequent chapters we describe specific cognitive-behavioral techniques (e.g., gradual exposure, relaxation training, thought stopping) and other strategies that are useful in reducing a child's anxiety.

Developing More Adaptive Behavioral and Emotional Self-Regulation

Rather than immediately expressing feelings through overt behavioral displays, a child can use words to represent these affective states symbolically. The child's growing ability to use language to label and communicate emotions contributes significantly to self-control and self-regulation. In Chapters 1 and 2 we reviewed how the ability to regulate feelings and behavior is often disrupted in maltreated children. For example, they display compromised internal state language.

A good example of an approach based on this conceptualization of pathogenic processes is helping children learn more appropriate ways of expressing their anger. The maltreated child may experience strong feelings of rage but may not have the ability to put these feelings into words; instead, the child expresses this anger through overt, behavioral displays, such as physical aggression. These displays not only hurt others but also invite retribution and rejection, which in turn exacerbate the child's negative self-esteem, feelings of isolation, and negative IWM/IS. Helping the child express this anger in more appropriate ways, such as through words, may lead to better emotional and behavioral self-regulation.

Reformulating the Meaning of the Maltreatment

Uncovering the maltreatment provides an opportunity for a child to explore and possibly reformulate the meaning and implications of his or her maltreatment. Chapter 2 included an extensive discussion of the meaning (different types of attributions) the child may impute to the maltreatment and the role these attributions play in the child's subsequent adaptation to the trauma. Besides being exposed to the aversive stimuli, the youngster must have an opportunity to cognitively restructure the traumatic events, that is, examine and revise their meaning. In his discussion of psychotherapy with sexually abused children, Friedrich (1990) argues that uncovering the abuse provides the child with an opportunity to understand the experience. Maltreated children may well have to address important attributions and appraisals: "What actually happened to me?" "Why did the perpetrator hurt me?" "Was it my fault?" "How did I react to the maltreatment, and why did I react that way?" "Does the fact that I was hurt mean that I can't trust anyone, or was this just an isolated experience?" "Will I be powerless in the future to prevent other assaults, or is there something I can do to protect myself?" It is essential that maltreated children have the opportunity to explore these questions. Examining the meanings and implications of maltreatment may become a central task of therapy, especially for those children who have undergone chronic and repeated episodes of abuse and neglect. The therapist must help correct cognitive distortions, such as the belief that the child was responsible for the abuse. Children exposed to more isolated episodes of abuse, and who now display localized effects, also require an opportunity to explore these issues. Bringing the maltreatment into the open is a prerequisite for the discussions, explorations, and critical appraisals that integrate these experiences into the child's life.

Modifying IWMs and IS

The notion that earlier relationships influence later ones has been a basic tenet of attachment theory, and subsequent work on IS and models of social information processing has further extended this concept beyond the caregiving relationship to other social relationships. Many children who have experienced chronic maltreatment from an early age expect the same or similar maltreatment in new relationships, and they may adopt some of the same coping strategies learned when they were much younger. These new figures on whom maltreated children impose their IWMs/IS include a variety of people: teachers, foster parents, peers (e.g., in friendships, subsequent romantic/marital relationships), and therapists. These are not new concepts and are consistent with Freud's conceptualization of transference (Bowlby, 1988b). Working from a traditional psychoanalytic perspective, Littner (1960) argued that maltreated foster children bring expectations and beliefs to new relationships. They often interpret the actions of new figures as hostile and negative and then behave in ways to provoke these individuals into rejecting or abusing them. Shirk and Saiz (1992) label this difficulty in experiencing others as positive and benevolent and in forming a positive working relationship with a therapist as an "attachment casualty": "In brief, children who are difficult to engage in therapy, whose affective orientation to the therapeutic relationship is negative, are hypothesized to have experienced unreliable, ambivalent, or hurtful early caregiving relationships" (Shirk & Saiz, 1992, p. 721). Consistent with this perspective, adolescents with relationship problems and more negative IS had greater difficulty with establishing an alliance than comparable youngsters without such problems and expectations, However, alliance formation was strongly predictive of outcome for the clinical group (Eltz, Shirk, & Sarlin, 1995).

A child may react to the therapist in ways characteristic of the earlier attachment patterns described in preceding chapters. The child with an avoidant attachment history may withdraw from the therapist, ignore overtures for interpersonal contact, and display little or no affect. By doing so, the child attempts to avoid the rejection, abuse, and hostility expected from the therapist, as well as the distress engendered when needs for security and comfort go unmet. Other children exposed to early inconsistent and neglectful parenting may react to a therapist in the angry, aggressive, but dependent and clingy fashion characteristic of ambivalent–resistant attachments.

There is continuity in development when interpersonal and other environmental experiences maintain already established developmental pathways or trajectories. In particular, continuity occurs when experiences are consistent with the individual's IWM/IS. For example, further abuse will reinforce the child's negative beliefs and expectations about relationships initially generated by earlier and repeated incidents of maltreatment. Conversely, positive experiences with others may engender some positive change or accommodation in the child's negative IWM/IS. For children whose experiences have been consistently unfavorable, introducing an element of discontinuity into their lives through favorable, positive experiences is critical. It increases the chances that deviations in developmental pathway will diminish as new perceptions and interpretations of others and self emerge and lead to more adaptive functioning. Thus, besides being mechanisms for continuity, IWMs/IS have the potential to be mechanisms for change.

Although the clinician, from his or her perspective, relates in a nonabusive and caring manner, the child may not initially perceive it as such and interpret it according to his or her own representational model. The degree to which social supports and caring interactions will be perceived positively may depend partially on models of relationships derived from earlier years (Flaherty & Richman, 1986; Littner, 1960; Parker et al., 1992). We cannot assume that a maltreated child's psychological functioning will automatically improve if he or she is removed from an abusive or neglectful environment and then provided with what we regard as supportive and positive caretaking. As we described in Chapter 2, children are strongly predisposed to interpret social interactions in ways consistent with their IWMs/IS and will not necessarily change their models or expectations as a function of these new social experiences. Although removing children from substandard and maltreating environments is necessary for their enhanced functioning, it may not be sufficient. They may require much more active and intensive guidance and assistance to accurately perceive and interpret others' behavior as supportive and helpful. These interactions include the relationship with the therapist, who helps the child to identify the archaic models and expectations underlying his or her distorted reactions and encourages and facilitates a reevaluation and modification of the IWM/IS. Uncovering these experiences and the attendant feelings and cognitions, revising distorted beliefs, and developing adaptive strategy mechanisms to better cope with negative IWMs/IS allow children to process information without distorting or excluding it. In turn, they are more open in the future to new information and more willing to experiment with alternate responses and interpretations of their experiences. "Resolving" histories of abuse or neglect does not mean forgetting them. Rather than being disavowed, denied, or dissociated, abusive, neglectful, or frightening episodes remain in children's memory but lose their power to significantly disrupt their current functioning or developmental course. Episodes of abuse or neglect are integrated into their lives in the proper perspective.

Psychotherapy, especially the relationship between the child and therapist, can be one opportunity to modify the skewed and biased IWM/IS by introducing some discontinuity into the child's life. The psychotherapeutic relationship, often so different from earlier ones marked by maltreatment and rejection, can counter the child's pessimistic and negative beliefs and expectations of others and self. In this way, *the therapeutic relationship is a medium far change.*

This perspective on the therapeutic relationship has formed the basis of various approaches to psychotherapy with adults and children. In an early work, Alexander and French (1946) describe this warm, positive relationship with the therapist as a corrective emotional experience that instills hope of something better in the client.

The second major perspective on the relationship in child psychotherapy regards the interactions between the child and therapist as serving a different function (for a cogent review of these two perspectives, see Shirk & Karver, 2003). Rather than being the principal curative agent, Shirk and Saiz (1992) indicated that the relationship or treatment alliance referred to

> positive feelings the child had for the therapist that enabled the child to accept the therapist as an aid in overcoming emotional or interpersonal problems. In essence, the alliance was a means to an end. It referred to the affective quality of the relationship between child and therapist that enabled the child to work purposefully on resolving problems. (p. 715)

From this perspective, it is assumed that there are specific therapeutic tasks or interventions the child must experience for change to occur. The therapeutic relationship serves to facilitate and encourage the child's participation in this treatment regimen and has been given more prominence in therapies that traditionally have not emphasized its importance. For example, Kendall (Kendall, 1991; Southam-Gerow & Kendall, 1996) reported that a positive therapeutic relationship is essential for CBT and that children who have completed a course of CBT viewed the relationship with the therapist as highly important.

What does the empirical research tell us about the importance of the therapeutic relationship? In a meta-analytic examination of 23 studies investigating the association between therapeutic relationship variables and treatment outcome in child and adolescent therapy, Shirk and Karver (2003) found a modest association between the therapeutic relationship and outcome, which was consistent with the correlation between therapeutic relationship and outcome for adults. Type, mode, structure, and content of treatment did not moderate the association between the therapeutic relationship and treatment outcome, although studies showed a stronger association for children with externalizing diagnoses than for those with internalizing problems. As in the results presented by Eltz and colleagues (1995), establishing a therapeutic relationship with them may be more challenging, yet more important for outcome, for externalizing children than for internalizing youngsters.

The studies in Shirk and Karver's (2003) meta-analysis used numerous alliance/therapeutic scales, and no measure was commonly employed in most of the studies. Consequently, it is difficult to specifically define the components that constituted the term "therapeutic relationship," and to identify, in a more fine-grained manner, the specific ingredients or interpersonal processes that contributed to the association in Shirk and Karver's meta-analysis. However, the adult literature provides more data regarding specifically the importance of therapist and therapist–client variables, sometimes referred to as "common factors." According to Messer and Wampold (2002):

> Common factors and therapist variability far outweigh specific ingredients in accounting for the benefits of psychotherapy. The proportion of variance contributed by common factors such as placebo effects, working alliance, therapist allegiance and competence are much greater that the variance stemming from specific ingredients of effects. (p. 23)

Therapist empathy, agreement and collaboration around goals, and the quality of the therapeutic alliance correlate with therapy outcome (Messer, 2004). But how do we establish a therapeutic alliance? The adult literature offers some direction. Ackerman and Hilsenroth (2003) reported that the following personal attributes of the therapist enhanced the therapeutic alliance: flexibility, honesty, trustworthiness, confidence, warmth, and being interested and open. These personal qualities are not the only factors. The following techniques also contributed to the alliance: exploration, reflection, identifying past therapy success, accurate interpretations, facilitating the expression of affects, and attending to the patient's experience (Ackerman & Hilsenroth, 2003).

We maintain that therapists should not assume a rigid and doctrinaire position that excludes either of these two perspectives, as they are not mutually exclusive. Therapists must have sufficient flexibility to develop and implement treatment programs that incorporate strategies designed to establish a therapeutic alliance with children and to strategically use the therapeutic relationship as a major agent of change, at least with some maltreated youngsters who evidence, for example, social information-processing deficits or biases. We describe these techniques in Chapter 7.

There are other conditions that maximize the benefits of the therapeutic relationship as a medium for change. A greater probability of changing maladaptive IWMs/IS exists when children have multiple experiences or relationships that consistently counter these negative beliefs and expectations. The direct psychological treatment of maltreated children is just one component in an overall strategy to help reestablish progress along an adaptive developmental trajectory. We agree with Graziano and Wells (1992) that, although we must approach maltreated children's problems directly, develop effective treatment strategies, and evaluate them rigorously, psychological treatment constitutes only a "partial solution" to the problem of child abuse and neglect, albeit an important and significant one. An exclusive reliance on psychotherapy with maltreated children, whether based on attachment theory or other theoretical orientations, is usually insufficient to fully ameliorate significant difficulties. Psychotherapy is not a panacea; it is one part of a comprehensive, ecologically based treatment plan in which interventions are directed at the level of the child, family, and factors in the broader environment. The failure to change or modify those aspects of a child's life that maintain or reinforce negative beliefs and expectations (e.g., a child who continues to be maltreated while receiving therapy) will attenuate or even obviate any positive outcomes of direct therapeutic involvement. Similarly, caregivers can do much to help children develop more adaptive coping mechanisms to decrease or eliminate symptoms. As we have stressed throughout this book, the therapist must intervene directly with these other individuals and conditions to maximize therapy's benefits.

Some maltreated children do not exhibit impaired attachment patterns or negative IWMs/IS. For example, a child who has always received consistent and appropriate care and is then sexually assaulted once by an adolescent babysitter may not manifest these developmental effects. This child may require therapy to address symptoms of PTSD, but the focus will not be on the therapeutic relationship as the principal means of resolving this particular problem, although a positive therapeutic alliance is necessary for the child's active collaboration and cooperation with the treatment plan. Other youngsters may present with both developmental and localized effects and may require a wider array of interventions. The clinician can use the therapeutic relationship to change IWMs/IS as well as specific anxiety-reduction strategies for PTSD symptoms. Developing a therapeutic relationship, although a potent strategy, is usually not sufficient by itself to counteract all the diverse emotional and psychological damage associated with abuse or neglect. The therapist must be well versed in other techniques, especially ESTs, for treating a wide range of psychological and behavioral difficulties in children and be able to implement them. Consistent with the transactional model, ameliorating these localized effects may generate more positive expectations of others (via the perception that others are sensitive to one's distress and willing to help) and of the self (via the perception that one can change and overcome one's difficulties).

Modifying Self-Perceptions

A common theme in the treatment of maltreated children is helping them change their perceptions of themselves and develop greater feelings of mastery and self-efficacy. Internal attributions, such as "It was my fault that I was abused," contribute to the psychological distress of victims of interpersonal violence. Some children need to achieve a sense of mastery over their maltreatment to reduce feelings of fear, powerlessness, helplessness, and low self-esteem. For example, a child has to review what he or she could have done or could do in the future to protect him- or herself from further maltreatment. Chapter 10 describes specific techniques that help children transform feelings of passivity and impotence into those of activity and power. Furthermore, clinicians may have to help children address more general issues of low self-esteem or an unintegrated sense of self associated with the operation of defense mechanisms such as splitting and dissociation. These mechanisms are particularly evident in children who have experienced chronic maltreatment.

These are some of the broad themes that confront clinicians who work with maltreated children. At this point, we need to reiterate one of our central guidelines: The clinician must conduct a comprehensive assessment of the child and family in order to identify specific treatment goals and plans. Although these broad themes provide some direction about possible intervention targets and the mechanisms of change, a treatment plan must be individually tailored to meet the child's and family's unique needs.

CHAPTER SIX

Working with Parents and Caregivers

We have stressed throughout this book that the child's adaptation to maltreatment is influenced by multiple variables. One of the most important is the risk of further maltreatment. Clearly, if a child is currently being abused or neglected or is at significant risk for further maltreatment, immediate and intensive intervention is required to ensure the child's safety. Working with abusive or neglectful parents to change these maladaptive patterns is a critical topic but one so vast that it exceeds the scope of this book. Rather, this chapter focuses on interventions with nonoffending parents and caregivers to support the child's recovery and maximize the benefits derived from individual psychotherapy. First, we discuss some reasons for contact between a therapist and parents or caregivers. Second, we present concrete strategies therapists can use to help parents support their children after the maltreatment has been disclosed or discovered. Third, we discuss more long-term interventions with parents, alternate caregivers, and other important adults in the child's life to remediate some of the developmental effects associated with maltreatment. Subsequent chapters, although focused on individual therapy with the child, include other suggestions for intervening with parents that support and amplify the therapist's efforts.

REASONS FOR CONTACT BETWEEN THERAPISTS AND PARENTS/CAREGIVERS

Establish a Collaborative Alliance

As discussed in Chapter 3, psychotherapy with children whose parents do not support their participation is likely to result in premature termination. A lack of support is reflected in responses that range from active refusal to bring the child to therapy sessions to more covert sabotage, exemplified by parental remarks to the child such as "therapy isn't all that important." These ambivalent and hostile attitudes erode children's trust in the therapist and the psychotherapeutic process and detrimentally affect their engagement and participation in therapy. Furthermore, premature termination means that the child has had another unrewarding experience with adults who have been unable to meet his or her needs for support and assistance. To establish and maintain a collaborative alliance, the therapist must have regular contact with parents or alternate caregivers. In this chapter we describe a number of ways to establish and maintain this alliance.

Ensure the Child Is Exposed to Multiple Experiences That Promote Adaptive Functioning

We have stressed this point throughout the book: Psychotherapy is not a panacea for maltreated children, but rather one component of a comprehensive treatment package. The failure to intervene at a broad level attenuates the chances of helping children recover. Chapter 3 reviewed the empirical data linking children's outcome to parental and family variables. Contact with parents or caregivers is an opportunity to offer helpful suggestions about managing children's problematic behavior, guidance on how to support their children, and suggestions on coping with their own reactions to their children's victimization. These and other interventions increase the chances that children will be exposed to multiple experiences and interventions that counteract their maladaptive behavior patterns.

Parents and Caregivers Are Sources of Important Information about the Child's Functioning and the Outcome of Therapeutic Interventions

It is vital that therapists gather ongoing information about the child's functioning, particularly in relation to their interventions. For example, they may expose the child to stimuli related to the maltreatment too quickly, which overwhelms the child's defenses and results in significant behavioral deterioration. Feedback from others, including parents or teachers, is essential to evaluate the outcome of interventions and make appropriate adjustments. As well, contact with parents or caregivers provides information about significant events in the child's life that have implications for therapy (e.g., death of an extended family member or changes in criminal proceedings related to the maltreatment, such as an adjournment of a case in which the child was scheduled to testify). This information allows the therapist to plan appropriate interventions, such as being sure to raise these issues in therapy. We now turn to a discussion of concrete and practical strategies therapists may use in working with these significant caregivers.

SUPPORTING PARENTS OR CAREGIVERS IN THE POSTDISCLOSURE PERIOD

Chapter 3 identified family support as an important moderator of the effects of child sexual abuse in empirical studies that have examined this variable. Family support includes the family's belief in the child, emotional support (e.g., the parent does not blame the child), instrumental support (e.g., the parent ensures that the child receives appropriate medical or psychosocial interventions and responds to the child's symptoms or behavior in ways to promote more adaptive functioning), and appropriate actions toward the perpetrator (e.g., notifying the police and protective services). In this section of the chapter we review interventions and strategies therapists can implement with parents or caregivers in the postdisclosure period. But before we describe these in detail, we briefly review EST outcome studies that have incorporated parental involvement as a significant component in the treatment of abused children. The research provides us with some directions to pursue in our clinical work with maltreated youngsters and their families, although comprehensive evaluations are necessary to identify the unique strengths and weaknesses of a family's ability to support the child in the postdisclosure period.

There is considerable similarity in the actual components of parental interventions investigated across empirical studies. Cohen and her colleagues (Cohen, Deblinger, Mannarino, & Steer, 2004; Cohen & Mannarino, 1996a, 1996b, 1997, 1998a, 1998b, 2000; Cohen, Mannarino, & Knudsen, 2005) examined the importance of parental variables in the treatment of sexually abused children and developed treatment packages to address three broad areas when working with parents: decreasing parents' emotional distress (e.g., distorted attributions about the abuse; parental feelings about the perpetrator; parental feelings of stigmatization; parental history of sexual abuse if applicable; increasing support for the parent; parental anxiety and anger management skills); enhancing parental support for the child (e.g., belief in the child's disclosure; appropriate supportive management of the child's distress symptoms; appropriate limit setting); and management of child behavior difficulties related to the abuse (e.g., recognition of, and interventions for inappropriate behaviors; problem-solving skills). Deblinger and colleagues (Deblinger, Lippmann, & Steer, 1996; Deblinger, McLeer, & Henry, 1990; Deblinger, Stauffer, & Steer, 2001; Deblinger, Steer, & Lippmann, 1999; Stauffer & Deblinger, 1996) also examined the association between parental response and treatment outcome and incorporated similar ingredients in interventions they directed to parents: educational information to address and modify parents' emotional responses and distress; communication, modeling, and gradual exposure; and child behavior management skills. The gradual exposure component deserves more comment, given its central prominence in many treatment programs for sexually abused children. Therapists provided parents with guidelines for effective parent–child communication and specifically focused on helping them talk to their children about the sexual abuse. The goal was to have parents expose the youngsters to the cues and stimuli associated with the abuse via these discussions so that the children's anxiety would extinguish and they could begin reprocessing these experiences, a process similar to that followed by professional therapists.

Cohen found a strong correlation between parents' emotional distress related to their preschool children's sexual abuse and the children's outcome at posttreatment. Cohen and Mannarino (1996b) speculate that this association may be mediated by modeling in cases in which the child is exposed to fewer adaptive coping skills by a highly distressed parent, or in which a distressed parent is less emotionally and/or physically available to provide the child with support. Interestingly, although parental distress was the strongest predictor of children's difficulties at posttreatment, parental support for the child was the overall strongest predictor of preschoolers' outcome at the 6- and 12-month follow-ups. Emotional distress may diminish over time, and parental support may become more important in facilitating symptomatic improvement in young children who are particularly dependent on parents for the fulfillment of their physical and emotional needs. Consistent with this notion, poorer child outcome was associated with a higher level of parental tolerance for negative or inappropriate behaviors and more lax routines and structure.

Cohen and colleagues also studied sexually abused school-age children and found the same significant association between parental support and treatment outcome, but there was no association between parents' emotional distress and child outcome (Cohen & Mannarino, 1998b). They argue that children's response to treatment was more dependent on their abuse-related attributions and family predictability and structure; again, lax limits were associated with worse outcome. A multisite, randomized control trial for sexually abused 8- to 14-year-old children with PTSD demonstrated that parents assigned to trauma-focused CBT (TF-CBT) that addressed the three themes described above (i.e., decreasing parents' distress, enhancing parental support for the child, management of abuse-related child behavior problems) reported lower levels of depression and abuse-specific distress, and greater support of the child and more effective parenting practices, than parents assigned to a nonspecific, supportive therapy program (Cohen et al., 2004). The children of the first group showed greater improvement with regard to PTSD, behavior problems, shame, and abuse-related attributions.

An initial study by Deblinger and colleagues (1996) found that mothers who participated in a CBT program that addressed their emotional reactions, communication patterns with their children, and child behavior management skills reported significant reductions in their children's externalizing behaviors and increases in their use of effective parenting practices. Their children were less depressed than those whose mothers were assigned to a community support program. The CBT interventions with the mothers were aimed to increase their level of confidence and efficacy and encouraged them to model appropriate coping strategies for handling their feelings, thereby contributing to the reduction in their children's self-reports of depression (Deblinger et al., 1996). Children treated by professional therapists showed a greater reduction in PTSD than children not seen by professionals but whose mothers implemented gradual exposure techniques with them. Deblinger and colleagues suggest that these mothers may have been less successful than professional therapists because of their emotional involvement.

Stauffer and Deblinger (1996) enrolled nonoffending mothers in an 11-week CBT group that addressed the same areas of parental functioning incorporated in the Deblinger and colleagues (1996) study just described. Parents reported lower levels of general distress, less avoidance of abuse-related thoughts and feelings, and more appropriate responses to their 2- to 6-year-old children's abuse-related behavior after participation in the group. The children, treated in a concurrent CBT group, showed a decrease in sexualized behaviors. Stauffer and Deblinger posit that a diminution of the mothers' distress enabled them to respond more appropriately to their children, especially if they were less avoidant of sexual abuse themes and had improved their parenting practices. A subsequent study (Deblinger et al., 2001) compared mothers participating in a similar CBT group to those in a nonspecific support therapy group. The CBT mothers reported greater reductions at posttreatment in their intrusive thoughts and their negative emotional reactions to the sexual abuse.

These studies have several limitations. They included only sexually abused children and nonoffending mothers, making it difficult to draw conclusions about the influence of parental support for children exposed to other forms of maltreatment or the role fathers may play. Parental support included several different components, and no dismantling studies have yet been conducted that identify the specific interventions that predict outcome. Likewise, the Cohen and Deblinger studies usually included interventions directed to children as well as those involving parents. Consequently, it is difficult to make any firm statements about the differential effects of treating children versus treating nonoffending mothers. Despite these limitations, the data do point to the importance of involving parents in treatment programs for maltreated children. We now describe a number of interventions in some detail.

Educational Interventions

Using a psychoeducational approach, the therapist can give parents and caregivers considerable information to attenuate their anxiety and to encourage more adaptive responses to their children's distress. Parents are often shocked or dismayed at the symptoms or problem behaviors children display in reaction to maltreatment. Informing parents that other maltreated children show similar behavior and providing them with an explanation of the possible mechanisms leading to these problems can decrease their anxiety. Clinicians can make other inexplicable behavior, such as a child's tendency to recant the initial disclosure, more understandable by discussing some of the short-term adaptive functions of such responses (e.g., avoiding the consequences threatened by the perpetrator). The explanation may also prevent adults from personalizing the behavior or attributing the recantation to their being bad parents. Education about the widespread prevalence of maltreatment such as sexual abuse may counter parental feelings of isolation and inadequacy.

Education about other aspects of the maltreatment can be of real benefit to parents. They need clear statements about the critical role they play in the child's recovery and the importance of family support for a positive outcome. Some parents believe that their children will be irreparably scarred for life. The therapist can instill some hope by citing the evidence that such damage is not inevitable and that the parents can do much to facilitate a positive outcome. However, psychotherapy with many maltreated children, especially those exposed to years of abuse and neglect, is often difficult and arduous. Many do not show immediate improvement, and their behavior deteriorates during therapy as memories and feelings about their experiences emerge. Parents or caregivers with unrealistic expectations about the immediate benefits and improvements associated with therapy are quickly disappointed. They begin to wonder about the usefulness of therapy, particularly when faced with children who now present even more challenging behavior. Therapists must educate them about the process of therapy and the sometimes slow pace of change.

As professionals, we sometimes assume that everyone has our specialized knowledge about maltreatment, its sequelae, and the mechanisms associated with it, and the response of legal, child welfare, and medical/psychosocial systems to such cases. Becoming involved with these larger systems is often a confusing and perplexing experience for many parents or caregivers, which exacerbates their anxiety and distress. Therapists can help these families by explaining the roles of various professionals who are or will become involved with them or their children. Sometimes parents assume that the involvement of child welfare authorities automatically results in the removal of their children. Although professionals must guard against giving false assurances, they should present the range of possible responses from agencies in order to significantly reduce parents' anxiety and thereby allow them to more adequately support their children.

Helping Parents Cope with Their Own Reactions and Feelings

The therapist's task in helping parents is twofold. While validating and normalizing their feelings or reactions, the therapist must also help parents or caregivers learn healthy ways to express these feelings in a manner that supports children's recovery. As we have seen, alleviating parents' distress may be especially important for the treatment outcome of young children. Clinicians must directly tell parents that children are strongly influenced by parental attitudes and reactions to the victimization and that catastrophic displays of emotion will just heighten a child's distress. In other words, although parents may have many strong and understandable feelings about their child's experiences, they must learn how to contain and express these feelings appropriately. What follows is a discussion of common reactions of parents or caregivers and interventions that may ameliorate their distress.

GUILT

Parents or caregivers sometimes feel extremely guilty about their child's victimization, especially if they themselves have a history of maltreatment. When their children were younger, or even not yet born, these parents may have promised themselves that they would never allow their children to be similarly maltreated. When the unthinkable happens, they are consumed with guilt and feelings of inadequacy, which in turn may influence their parenting practices. As mentioned in Chapter 3, guilt feelings may contribute to the difficulty some parents have in placing firm and consistent limits on their children's behavior. The empirical research we reviewed suggests that lax limits are associated with poorer child outcome (Cohen & Mannarino, 1996a, 1996b). Strong feelings of guilt may also provoke parents to prematurely terminate therapy, because the child's participation is a powerful reminder of the child's abuse. Other parents, out of a desire to protect their child from any future victimization, become extremely overprotective and severely restrict the child's activities. Unfortunately, such children then begin to regard themselves as even more powerless and inadequate and less able to protect themselves from future dangers. Parents may even feel guilty about pressing charges against the perpetrator, especially if that individual is a family member. The child may interpret the ensuing reluctance as a reflection of parental skepticism about the disclosure or a wavering commitment to protect the child from further assaults.

What can therapists do to help these parents who feel so guilty? Some parents truly knew nothing about their child's victimization, yet still feel guilty because they failed to identify the child's behavioral cues as indicators of maltreatment. However, these behaviors may have been so subtle that they would have escaped the notice of the most sensitive and astute observer. Some children are asymptomatic and show no signs of distress. Clinicians can explain to parents that their guilt is unjustified, although some will probably still feel guilty. In these situations, therapists can tell them that even though they still experience guilt, they can do much to expedite their child's recovery, such as by cooperating in treatment. Other parents have actively contributed to their child's maltreatment or have not adequately protected their youngster. Rather than trying to automatically absolve their guilt, therapists should affirm their feelings of remorse and contrition. Therapists should also inform them that their guilt and ability to acknowledge their inadequacies as parents, as opposed to an outright and rigid denial of their responsibility, may reflect an authentic sense of commitment to the child and a solid base on which to build. Rather than focusing exclusively on guilt, therapists should assist the parents in identifying and implementing more appropriate parenting strategies (e.g., alternate child care arrangements, or a better choice of partners) to decrease the probability of future occurrences of maltreatment and strengthen the parent–child relationship. Within limits, guilt can be a potent motivator that helps parents to make healthy changes in their relationships with their children. However, therapists must not allow parents who feel extremely guilty to become immobilized in their efforts to set firm and consistent limits. Children who act out as a result of their maltreatment do not need parents or caregivers to ignore or excuse inappropriate behavior. Instead, at this time of crisis, they need parents who, although sensitive and empathic to their underlying affects and dynamics, help them contain this behavior and develop healthier ways of functioning.

ANGER

Parents whose children have been maltreated are understandably angry and outraged. In fact, sometimes the absence of anger is a worrisome sign: one might begin to question the parents' commitment to the child or their ability to empathize with the child's experience. Chapter 3 described how parents' unmodulated and extreme displays of anger may invalidate children's feelings of ambivalence toward the perpetrator. Children also become anxious, fearing that their parents cannot control this rage, to the point that these caregivers might take action that could well lead to their incarceration. Given these fears, children's reluctance to talk about their maltreatment is understandable. Parents benefit from an opportunity to ventilate their unmodulated anger when the child is not present. Therapists can encourage them to identify individuals in their natural environments with whom they can talk about their anger. Although empathic with parents' feelings, therapists must educate them about the detrimental effects on children who are exposed to dysregulated displays of rage and help them develop healthier ways to express the anger and fulfill their desire for retribution, such as by cooperating with criminal investigation personnel and pressing charges against the perpetrator. After a parent has learned to control and express this anger more adaptively, joint sessions with the child and family may be particularly useful. The child may benefit from learning directly that the parent too is angry with the perpetrator, thereby validating the child's affects and experiences. We have used these sessions to encourage the family to develop healthy ways to express this anger together. One creative mother proposed to her 8-year-old daughter that they jointly draw some pictures that depicted their anger. Many parents, especially in intrafamilial cases of physical and sexual abuse, are similarly ambivalent about the perpetrator and they, too, require assistance to express these feelings.

Parents may also feel some anger toward the child. Perhaps they expected the child to protect him- or herself from the perpetrator or to have disclosed the maltreatment sooner. Again, they can probably benefit from information about the typical reasons why children cannot stop the abuse or readily disclose it. Therapists can identify the normalcy of feelings of powerlessness and helplessness children typically experience in these situations, even without being exposed to overt threats or force. The parent may be angry about the involvement of child welfare agencies with the family, especially if they previously had conflictual or negative experiences with such agencies. Educational efforts directed toward clarifying the possible (and potentially positive) role of child welfare services and an opportunity to ventilate this anger may attenuate some of the parents' hostility.

ANXIETY

Besides feeling guilt and anger, parents or caregivers usually experience considerable anxiety. They worry about the child's physical health. A child who has been physically abused may have serious medical problems. Parents require clear and direct information about the child's medical status, most likely prognosis, and what they can do to help. Given the prevalence of problems such as HIV/AIDS and sexually transmitted diseases, parents of sexually abused children may share similar concerns and require information and guidance about these diseases.

Parents also worry about their child's current and future emotional and psychological well-being. Parents of sexually abused children may feel that their child is tainted because of exposure to sexual activity and is now "spoiled goods." They wonder whether the child consented to the sexual activity, enjoyed it, or in some way initiated the sexual interaction with the perpetrator. Regehr (1990) postulates that parents may project their own issues about sexuality onto the child and require assistance to express these feelings and issues. For example, a father may worry about a young son who did not immediately disclose sexual abuse by an adult male who was a family acquaintance. The father fears his son is gay, rather than realizing that there were probably many factors, including coercion or threats, that inhibited the child from disclosing sooner. The opportunity to discuss such issues and receive feedback or information from the therapist counteracts parents' fantasies or distortions. Family sessions during which children have an opportunity to explain the reasons for their delayed disclosure help parents gain a more accurate understanding of the issues. Prior to these joint sessions, both children and parents may require some individual work. Children will need assistance to identify their reasons for the delayed disclosure, and clinicians can encourage parents to begin thinking about how to respond to the children's statements in a constructive and supportive fashion, such as by empathizing with their fear. Role play can also be useful in coaching parents to respond sensitively and constructively.

Parents also become anxious at the thought of the involvement of larger systems in their lives. Their child may have to testify in court, or child welfare agencies may take a more active role in the family. Parents' anxiety may decrease if they have more information about these agencies and the possible consequences for the child and themselves.

DENIAL

Some parents deny that the maltreatment ever happened in order to ward off their own feelings (e.g., guilt, anxiety, anger). Others deny the child's victimization because the perpetrator is someone they love, trust, or depend on to meet their psychological and physical needs. In cases in which the perpetrator is a family member, other family members or relatives can pressure parents to refute the child's disclosure and take no further action.

One of the most important things the therapist can do when confronted with this reaction is to openly and directly acknowledge the parents' distress over these divided loyalties. The therapist should explore the possible consequences that might accrue if the parent acknowledged the maltreatment. The perpetrator might be incarcerated and the family might go on public assistance, or there might be an emotional loss for a nonoffending parent. Some parents feel extremely guilty about not protecting the child. Denying the maltreatment is another way to protect themselves from the ensuing remorse, guilt, and feelings of inadequacy. A clear statement regarding where the responsibility for the maltreatment lies, that is, with the perpetrator, may alleviate some parental guilt and denial. Others deny their children's victimization as a way to deny personal histories of abuse and the attendant feelings. Again, the therapist should inquire about the existence of these factors, empathize with the parents' distress, and clearly describe the dangers associated with denying the child's experiences, while simultaneously reinforcing the parents' critical role in the child's recovery. By quickly acknowledging any strengths the parent may have, particularly as they pertain to allying with and supporting the child, the therapist may further decrease the parents' reliance on denial.

Counteracting parents' or families' denial of maltreatment probably deserves its own chapter, but a more detailed discussion is beyond the scope of this book. We refer the interested reader to Friedrich's (1990) book on the psychotherapy of sexually abused children and their families. It contains an excellent chapter on treating the family, including useful strategies and interventions for establishing a therapeutic relationship and countering the family's reluctance to acknowledge the abuse. Although that chapter focuses specifically on sexual abuse, therapists can apply many of Friedrich's ideas and suggestions to other types of maltreatment.

PARENTS' ISSUES AND REACTIONS BASED ON THEIR OWN HISTORY OF MALTREATMENT

Chapter 3 contains a review of reactions of parents with personal histories of maltreatment. They deny and minimize the child's experience, deal with it intellectually, or become so preoccupied with their own issues that they are physically and psychologically unavailable for their children. The last situation leads to a deterioration in such parenting skills as monitoring the child's behavior, supervision, limit setting, and providing emotional support. Parents' maladaptive reactions, such as substance abuse, further compromise their ability to provide emotional and behavioral support.

What can the therapist do to help these parents at this time of crisis? The goal in this phase is to quickly provide sufficient support and guidance so that parents can then adequately support their child. It is clearly unrealistic to expect them to now fully resolve personal and sometimes longstanding issues related to their own maltreatment. However, the crisis is also a window of opportunity for the initiation of more long-term interventions.

First, the therapist should empathize with the intense affects elicited by the child's victimization and reassure parents that they are not crazy for experiencing powerful and sudden reactions. Individuals who experience symptoms such as intrusive memories are often uncertain about the reasons for their distress, and their perceived lack of control over their symptoms compounds their anxiety. The therapist can help by providing an explanation of the processes and mechanisms that lead to these reactions (i.e., by referring to conditioning and attribution theories in the PTSD formulation described in Chapter 2). This knowledge may lead them to realize that they are not crazy and that others have gone through similar experiences.

Although parents or caregivers may be experiencing significant distress, they must still be available to support their children. Therapists can facilitate supportive and appropriate parental responses by again explaining that their reactions will be a significant determinant of their child's adaptation to the maltreatment. Parents should be told they must contain some of their own anxiety, anger, and sadness while in the child's presence and that prolonged and intensive affective displays will just overwhelm the youngster. Parents may need their own therapy to more fully explore and process some of these feelings and develop effective coping mechanisms (e.g., relaxation training). Unfortunately, waiting lists are ubiquitous, and they may wait for lengthy periods before beginning their own counseling. The therapist can encourage parents to find alternate supports, such as good friends, clergy, and family physicians. If none are available, the therapist may have to continue providing this support on an interim basis. However, therapists must be cautious about exploring a parent's own history of maltreatment and associated issues too deeply, especially if an assessment has not been conducted that evaluates the parent's ability to cope with powerful feelings. Rather, the principal goal is to offer the adult opportunities to express and cope with some of these feelings while concurrently promoting the parent's adaptive response to the child.

Highly distressed parents probably need guidance and suggestions about how they can best help their child. The therapist and parent should develop *specific* statements or phrases the adult might use with the child that convey the adult's belief in the disclosure, acceptance of the child, ongoing willingness to protect the child from further maltreatment, and support for the child's recovery. Similarly, they should develop and rehearse specific child management strategies (discussed in more detail below). For example, if a sexually abused child begins involving other children in inappropriate sexual activity, the parent or caregiver needs concrete strategies to quickly deal with this situation.

We cannot emphasize enough the importance of parents having a repertoire of child management strategies and responses. Although they may not always be effective in quickly calming a highly distraught or acting-out child, the use of such strategies may attenuate parents' feelings of powerlessness and lack of control. The therapist should encourage a parent to anticipate difficult situations that arise by asking, "What's the worst thing the child could say or ask you about the abuse?" or, "What would be the most upsetting thing your child could do?"

Parents or caregivers with a history of maltreatment may also harbor negative feelings about their children's participation in therapy. Some parents become jealous of the attention their child receives from the therapist, especially if they are emotionally needy, dependent adults who were never adequately parented. Their jealousy may be so strong that they terminate their child's participation in therapy, as it is a too potent reminder of the attention and nurturance they missed receiving. Others are dependent on their child to meet their emotional needs and regard the child's close involvement with a therapist as a real threat, then ending therapy prematurely to preserve their exclusive relationship with the child. The child becomes aware of the parents' reaction and subsequently feels torn between feelings of loyalty to the parents and a growing connection to the therapist. Regularly scheduled contact between parents and the therapist, or the parents' involvement with their own therapist, may diminish this jealousy. Furthermore, the therapist can suggest ways to strengthen the relationship between parents and child (discussed in a later section of this chapter). By so doing, the therapist makes it clear that he or she has no intention of usurping a parent's role in the child's life.

Helping Parents Support Their Children Directly

Besides managing their own feelings appropriately to help their child, parents and caregivers can provide the child with more direct support on two levels. First, the parent's direct interaction with the child, such as talking with the child about the maltreatment and managing problematic child behavior, contributes to the child's healthy adaptation. Second, clinicians sometimes have to address parents' ability to support the child via other agencies and systems.

TALKING WITH CHILDREN ABOUT THE MALTREATMENT

Parents must be able to respond to their child's initial disclosure of maltreatment in a way that conveys belief of the allegation. Parental skepticism about its validity, or outright statements of disbelief, may well result in the child's recanting the disclosure, thereby placing the child at even higher risk for abuse. Such parental reactions increase the child's level of guilt and reinforce feelings of stigmatization and low self-esteem. Therapists must coach parents to empathize with the difficulty children encounter when they disclose episodes of abuse or neglect. Statements such as "We know how hard it must have been for you to tell us, especially when he told you he'd beat you up if you ever said anything about this" may be very reassuring. Again, family sessions wherein these issues are discussed with the therapist's guidance afford parents an opportunity to convey these messages.

Parents must be able to empathize with the ambivalence many children feel about the perpetrator. As we have seen, this empathic appreciation of such mixed feelings is often difficult for parents consumed with rage. However, they must be attuned to the possibility that their child may experience a real sense of sadness about losing the relationship with the person who hurt him or her. Parents must give the child an opportunity to express these feelings and to normalize and validate them. Many parents themselves harbor similar feelings of ambivalence and sadness about the perpetrator. Sharing feelings again validates the child's feelings and creates, in our experience, a closer relationship between child and parent. Therapists may also help parents respond to children's misattributions, such as blaming themselves for the abuse. Simple statements like "He was the adult and shouldn't have done those things to you" can be helpful.

Therapists should also warn parents or caregivers about providing children with a blanket reassurance that "everything is going to be OK now that you've told." For many children, disclosures are followed by even more stress and disruption. In response to children's inquiries about what will happen next, parents should tell them about the most probable outcome, such as having to talk with police or child welfare authorities. Although there are no definitive answers about the consequences of this involvement, a parent should reassure the child that he or she will do everything possible to support the child throughout this process. Some children may undergo medical examinations because of physical or sexual assaults, and they require appropriate preparation for these procedures. Clearly, the parent or caregiver must use vocabulary and language appropriate to the child's developmental age and convey sufficient information that the child can understand. Giving too much information, as in describing all the details of a gynecological examination, will just overwhelm a young school-age child with anxiety. Parents must consider the child's developmental age when making a decision about the timing of this preparation. Telling a young child weeks in advance about an intrusive medical examination exacerbates anxiety and confusion. Moreover, the parent or caregiver must provide an opportunity for the child to express anxieties or concerns after completion of a medical examination or legal/forensic interview. The child should not undergo a severe interrogation but should be gently asked about any worries or concerns. Likewise, parents or caregivers may be highly distressed when their child undergoes this type of investigation, and they should have an opportunity to vent their feelings to other adults and seek clarification about the proceedings and subsequent findings.

There are other things parents or caregivers can do to help their children. Sometimes maltreated children worry that others, including peers, will find out about what happened and ask for information. Classmates may ask why a child leaves school early to attend therapy sessions, missing the last 2 hours of school every Tuesday afternoon. The parent or caregiver can make some direct suggestions about what to say, informing the child of a right to privacy and suggesting a vague answer about ongoing appointments. Classmates may also ask for details of the abuse or neglect if they are aware of what has happened. The child might politely respond with "I'd rather not talk about it." Of course, if people who have regular contact with the child continue to press for more details, a parent or caregiver will need to intervene and tell them to stop that line of questioning. Parents should understand they do not owe these other individuals an explanation and that they have the right to privacy.

Some maltreated children, especially younger ones, talk indiscriminately about their experiences to anyone who will listen. Unfortunately, other people may then use this information to tease or taunt the child. It may also be a way for the child to obtain attention from others. Parents can help the child discriminate among people who should have this information and the conditions in which he or she should divulge it. Parents should avoid using terms like "It's our secret," which reinforce the perpetrator's original instructions; rather, parents or caregivers should teach the child that it is important and healthy to discuss the maltreatment openly with certain people and in particular contexts.

Parents can also assume that the child has resolved all the feelings and issues associated with the maltreatment if the child no longer discusses these events. The child may have stopped talking about it to spare a parent or the family further distress or because he or she has remembered more incidents that are particularly anxiety provoking. Rather than ignoring the issue, a parent should provide opportunities for the child to talk about the maltreatment if the child so chooses. For example, when alone with the child at home, the parent can broach this issue with the following statement: "You and I haven't talked for a while about what your uncle did to you. I was wondering if you want to talk any more about it." The parent must inform the child quite regularly that he or she is willing and able to talk about what happened. By talking with a supportive adult, the child typically feels accepted, understood, and validated. Conversely, incessantly badgering the child to talk can be another coercive experience, leading to greater resistance to discussion of these matters. Discussions also constitute opportunities for gradually exposing the child to the abuse-related material so that anxiety extinguishes and to clarify any of the child's misconceptions.

PARENTAL MANAGEMENT OF A CHILD'S PROBLEM BEHAVIOR

One of the most important ways parents and caregivers can help maltreated children in the immediate postdisdosure period is through active management of their problem behavior. Although some maltreated children may be asymptomatic, others show a diversity of behavioral symptoms, ranging from those based on anxiety (e.g., nightmares, somatic complaints) to more externalizing behaviors (e.g., sexually inappropriate behavior, physical aggression). As well as explaining the emergence of these symptoms, the therapist must help parents develop some management strategies to alleviate a child's distress and acting out and to promote a child's behavioral and emotional self-regulation.

Externalizing Behaviors: Sexual Behavior Problems and Physical Aggression. Externalizing behavior often poses the greatest problem for parents, especially if it is generalized to other environments, such as school or the neighborhood, and if other people begin to complain to parents or demand they do something to control the child. Sexualized behavior is one of the more common sequelae associated with childhood sexual abuse. This pattern frequently merits the child's direct involvement with a therapist. Chapter 9 describes an intervention approach with children based on cognitive-behavioral principles. However, parents and other significant adults must receive immediate guidance and assistance regarding the management of the sexualized behavior. In the following discussion, we review in some detail our approach to working with parents and families on this issue and draw upon some of the treatment components identified by Gil and Johnson (1993). Many, if not most, of these principles and techniques can be applied to cases of physical aggression.

First, parents must be able to talk with the child about sexuality in general. If they cannot, their ability to communicate about inappropriate sexual behavior is severely compromised. There are several things the therapist can do to facilitate this process. Inquiring about the basis of the parent's discomfort may reveal a personal history of sexual abuse, in which case discussions about sex arouse considerable parental anxiety. The parent may benefit from therapy geared to addressing these issues. Alternatively, the parent may have been raised in a family in which no one talked about sex. We have found that family sessions in which parents read sex education books to their children are particularly useful. The parents' anxiety decreases because of the structured format in which to talk about sex. With some extremely anxious parents, we begin to read such material to the child in the parent's presence to desensitize both child and adult; they must only sit and listen. When parents feel more comfortable, the clinician may ask them to start reading. The therapist may prompt the parent to encourage the child to ask any questions about the material and to respond appropriately.

After parents have attained this level of comfort, they may be more ready to talk with their child about the child's sexual behavior, particularly about their expectations for healthy and appropriate behavior, in a manner much as they would talk about their expectations regarding nonaggressive ways of solving interpersonal disputes. In our experience, many parents have never considered what sexual values and mores they want to impart to their children. Consequently, the therapist must encourage parents to reflect on this issue and make some decisions about what constitutes healthy or appropriate sexuality for their children. Cultural values often play an enormous role in parental conceptualizations of sexuality, and the clinician must remain sensitive to them. In a two-parent family, partners must reach a consensus about acceptable sexual behavior. We have asked couples to discuss this issue at home and report on their success in the next session. Were they even able to talk about the subject? If they did talk, were they successful in reaching an agreement? The therapist must facilitate discussion and assist them in achieving a consensus if they did not reach an agreement. Parental consensus is critical before children are included in these discussions, as they need to know that their parents are united on this issue and both will consistently enforce limits and expectations. In subsequent sessions, parents can inform the child of their values and expectations about sexuality. First, the therapist and parent may have to rehearse what the parent will say, especially what words will be used to refer to sexual behavior such as masturbation. As well as identifying unacceptable sexual behavior and providing an explanation geared to the child's developmental level, parents should identify what they consider appropriate behavior. For example, we have seen many parents who have told their children that masturbating in private is acceptable.

If other children live in the home, they too should be included in these family sessions, especially if they are at risk for being victimized by the youngster who is demonstrating coercive, compulsive behavior that has been refractory to normal limit setting and prohibitions. Family sessions are an opportunity for parents to articulate clear expectations and limits for all their children. Parents should give other children in the family explicit permission (including the actual words they may use) to inform parents if the child who has been maltreated attempts to engage them in sexual behavior or resorts to physical aggression. The danger of avoiding these explicit discussions is that by doing so the family is, in effect, colluding with the often furtive nature of the child's sexual behavior, thereby placing other family members at risk of being abused.

The family will also benefit from open discussion about personal boundaries and privacy in the home, such as ensuring that bedroom doors are closed when family members are changing clothes. They may require clear limitations on the type of sexually explicit material that can be brought into the home. A number of sexualized children we have treated found such material to be very arousing and subsequently reported that this arousal preceded their coercive sexualized advances to others. Sometimes therapists must engage in intensive dialogues with parents who allow or themselves bring this material into the home, alerting them to the role it may play in the genesis and maintenance their child's sexualized behavior, and suggesting they keep it securely out of reach if they refuse to dispose of it. However, the therapist should not assume that parents have complied even if they say they have. One father seemed genuinely surprised when he found that his 11-year-old son continued to watch the father's pornographic movies. He explained that he had "hidden" the videotapes on the top shelf of his bedroom closet. When his resourceful son discovered that the tapes were no longer in the living room bookcase, he systematically searched the house and quickly found them. Although the father refused to part with the tapes, he agreed to keep them in a locked toolbox and always carry the key with him.

Family sessions can teach and even model nonsexual expressions of affection. Some sexualized children invade others' body spaces, for example, by pressing themselves, including their genitalia, against others. With the therapist's help, parents can propose alternate ways of giving and receiving physical affection, such as sitting closely beside each other or hugging without this kind of body contact. Therapists can teach and coach parents to positively reinforce these healthier responses, just as parents would reinforce the prosocial, nonaggressive interactions of children who had been referred for problems of physical aggression.

Children with significant SBPs often require stringent external controls on their behavior. There are two major components to this control: supervision and limit setting. A continuation of the sexual behavior places other children at risk and provides even more reinforcement to the child (via physiological arousal or gratification of psychological needs, such as a need to dominate others), while exposing the child to further rejection and censure from others. Some require maximum supervision, even to the extent of never being left unsupervised with other children. Although this seems drastic, parents can be told of its necessity to prevent the child from doing something that would get him or her in trouble. The therapist and parents should develop a specific supervision plan and share it with all family members. Typical components of a supervision plan for children with SBPs address the following issues: Can the child ever be left alone with other children? If not, who will supervise and how (e.g., the child always being within eyesight of the supervising adult)? Does the child share a bedroom or a bed with siblings? Who will supervise in other environments, such as at school or in recreation activities? What information should be conveyed to responsible adults in these other environments? The parents might tell the child that they are instituting this measure because they care about the child and want to ensure that he or she does not display such behavior again. We have found that such firm statements, accompanied by consistent monitoring, often attenuate children's anxiety about repeating harmful behavior and convey the parents' authentic commitment to their welfare. Parents can taper the level of supervision as the child demonstrates increasing ability to control the sexualized behavior. They should clearly identify the specific behaviors they will use to make this determination. The therapist may initiate this process by asking the family, "How will you know when [the child] is doing better?" It is better to set small and attainable goals (e.g., the child can spend 5 minutes in the home with another child with an adult present but not directly observing the interaction, and without sexual behavior occurring). It is often useful for the parents, child, and therapist to review and renegotiate these goals weekly. Children and parents need concrete evidence of their progress at regular intervals to maintain the hard work of therapy, along with positive reinforcement for attaining these goals.

Therapists can help parents set appropriate limits when children behave in sexually inappropriate ways. This is often a major task of therapy, especially when parents have had long-standing problems in setting consistent limits on other undesirable behaviors. Therapists can help parents identify the consequences of children's sexualized behavior and learn how to deliver limits in a clear, no-nonsense tone of voice. Clinicians should caution parents against appearing repulsed by their youngster's behavior, inducing shame or guilt, or devoting excess attention to the issue—for example, haranguing the child for hours and inadvertently supplying even more reinforcement and attention. Instead, therapists can teach parents to reinforce the child's interactions with others that do not include unhealthy expressions of sexuality. Parents often require much reinforcement and encouragement, as well as practical guidance and concrete suggestions regarding behavior management, to become firmer and more consistent with their children. In-home teaching services, if available, are often valuable in helping parents improve these basic parenting skills.

This is but one area in which the therapist can provide assistance to parents or caregivers so that they can learn effective ways of managing children's externalizing behaviors. Therapists can help parents to devise a similar plan to manage other types of externalizing problems, such as physical aggression. Parents learn to convey their expectations concerning this behavior directly to family members and to develop a plan that ensures the safety of other children in the home. Consistent monitoring and supervision, limit setting, and reinforcement of prosocial, nonaggressive behavior complete the process. Patterson, Redi, Jones, and Conger (1975), Patterson (1980), and Alexander and Parsons (1982) incorporate social learning theory in the treatment of aggressive and coercive children by their parents, and readers may want to refer to these works.

More germane to the topic of parents assisting maltreated children to reduce externalizing behaviors, Jouriles and colleagues (2001) evaluated the effectiveness of interventions in reducing conduct problems among 4- to 9-year-old children of battered women. The interventions consisted of two components: providing mothers with instrumental and emotional support, and teaching child management skills. Consistent with social learning approaches, the latter included contingent praise and positive attention, appropriate instructions and commands, and contingent consequences for noncompliance and aggressive behavior. Children in this intervention group improved at a faster rate, the proportion of children displaying high levels of conduct disorders greatly diminished, and mothers exhibited greater improvements in child management skills as compared with an existing services condition. Jouriles and colleagues noted that an instrumental and emotional support component was also essential in the recruitment and retention of these families in treatment. This included emotional support during their transition from a shelter to help mothers obtain physical resources and social support central to their efforts to become self-supporting. These data again speak to the necessity of providing comprehensive services to maltreated children and their families.

Internalizing Behaviors: PTSD and Anxiety-Related Symptoms. One of the simplest things parents can do to help manage their children's anxiety is to learn to talk with them about their fears and worries. We present a short review of some helpful things parents might say. Parents can empathize with their child's anxiety, reassure the child that he or she is not crazy, and that the parents will do everything to ensure the child's safety. However, as we described earlier, parents must be warned against giving glib reassurances, such as telling the child that "everything is going to be fine," when in reality the future is uncertain. They must sensitively and realistically acknowledge these challenges rather than denying them or reacting catastrophically, either of which will exacerbate the child's anxiety. Parents should monitor their child's emotional state more closely and identify changes in the child's presentation that reflect escalating anxiety. Parents might then offer the youngster an opportunity to talk about worries or even engage in breathing and relaxation exercises together. These discussions gradually expose the child to the stimuli and the cues to extinguish the anxiety.

Therapists can teach children to identify the signs and signals that indicate their anxiety is rising, such as somatic complaints like abdominal pain, and then to request their parents' assistance. They can graphically depict these reactions and feelings on an outline of the child's body to make them more observable and concrete. The therapist encourages the child to identify the adults he or she could approach for help and what the child would say (e.g., "I feel really worried right now, and I'd like to talk to you") to gain their assistance. It is important to inform adults that the child may approach them, and ask them to think of ways to best respond to the child's expressions of anxiety. Sessions with the parent and child in which they reach an agreement about when and how the child will approach a particular adult for help are especially useful. A child who has difficulty sleeping may benefit from certain measures, such as having a nightlight and a well-defined bedtime routine.

Parents can provide practical and logistical assistance using child-focused techniques (e.g., helping the child "freeze" the perpetrator or assisting the child in tacking a positive dream picture on a wall). Chapter 9 describes these techniques and the caregiver's important role in helping children implement them in natural environments.

Helping Parents Cooperate with Other Agencies

Parents' effectiveness as advocates for their children may be compromised by having few practical skills and little knowledge necessary to secure outside services. As mentioned earlier, the therapist can educate parents about the role of various professionals and agencies in helping their child recover and by identifying the possible range of outcomes. Parents, especially those responsible for their child's abuse and neglect, may feel especially threatened and frightened at the prospect of dealing with other agencies. The therapist should empathize strongly with parents' underlying fear and anxiety while coaching them in how to be effective advocates for their children. The therapist and parents can "brainstorm" all the questions the parents have for physicians or child welfare staff and then rehearse by asking these in an assertive but nonaggressive manner.

SERVICE DELIVERY

Clinical services for parents in the immediate postdisclosure period may be implemented in several ways. The therapist might work individually with parents or in a group format. The advantages of a group format include the greater number of parents who can be accommodated and that participants may benefit significantly from talking with others who are undergoing similar experiences, thereby reducing their sense of isolation and stigmatization. We have already reviewed the empirical evidence regarding the effectiveness of CBT groups for parents in reducing their distress associated with their children's sexual abuse (Stauffer & Deblinger, 1996). Some parents also benefit from reading books or other materials that describe common reactions of abused children and parents and the ways parents can help and support their offspring (e.g., Hagans & Case, 1988).

Possibly more important than the type of modality in which information and assistance are delivered is the timing of the intervention. Services delivered as quickly as possible after the child's disclosure may have greater impact because parents are more open to change at that time. The Child Abuse Service at Alberta Children's Hospital, Calgary, operates a Fast Track Program in which parents are seen within 72 hours after contacting personnel about their physically or sexually abused child. Although hospital based, this program has an open referral system whereby parents can directly contact the intake worker and refer themselves and their children without a physician's referral. The program offers parents many of the services described above: education about typical responses of maltreated children, information about the roles of various professionals and agencies, the typical course of investigations, an opportunity to express their own feelings about and reactions to the child's victimization, and concrete suggestions and guidance on how to deal with the child's behavior. Longer-term clinical services are subsequently provided to those children and families that require them. The following is a typical case handled in this program.

Janet, the 37-year-old single mother of 14-year-old Brad and 9-year-old Cheryl, called the Child Abuse Service after Cheryl disclosed to her the night before that Brad had been sexually abusing her for the past 2 years. Janet was highly distraught during her phone conversation with the intake worker and asked for help in managing this situation. The intake worker informed her that child welfare authorities would have to be notified immediately. Although reluctant, Janet agreed to do this herself, and the case was assigned to a child welfare worker for investigation. The police also planned to investigate this matter. Given her level of distress, Janet was accepted for the Fast Track Program and was seen 2 days after she called.

Janet was seen for two sessions that had a crisis intervention orientation. The therapist explained that her involvement was short term; she would focus on helping Janet and the family cope with the immediate stressors and demands of the postdisclosure period, and another therapist would be assigned as soon as one was available if ongoing therapy was necessary. After Janet agreed to this plan, the therapist invited her to identify the concerns she wanted to address. She said the child welfare agency's involvement with her family was especially troublesome (at the time of this first appointment, this agency's investigation had not yet been initiated). Janet had had no previous contact with child welfare services but was worried that her children would be removed from her care because she had read some sensationalized reports in the press about the child welfare agency "snatching kids." The therapist explained the mandatory reporting laws, the need to ensure the safety of children, and that Brad's removal from the family would depend on the risk he posed to Cheryl. The therapist also explained that the child welfare authorities would be able to provide useful services to the family, such as referring Brad to a treatment program for adolescent sex offenders sponsored by the child welfare agency. This information alleviated some of Janet's anxiety, although she remained dissatisfied with the investigation's slow pace. No one had yet interviewed Cheryl, which just escalated the mother's and daughter's anxiety. Janet and the therapist discussed various ways to approach child welfare staff with these concerns. She subsequently contacted the assigned worker and expressed her concerns in an assertive but measured way. Fortunately, the worker responded and agreed to see the family sooner.

In the first session, the therapist raised the issue of Cheryl's safety, as Brad still resided in the home. Janet was concerned about protecting her daughter, particularly because Cheryl had told her mother that the assaults always happened after school but before Janet returned home from work. With the therapist's guidance, Janet arranged for alternate child care for Cheryl after school at the home of a neighbor who was Janet's close friend and knew about Cheryl's disclosure. Janet and the therapist discussed other ways of ensuring Cheryl's safety, such as closely supervising and monitoring the two children.

Janet was extremely angry with Brad. Although she had not yet confronted him with his sister's allegations, Janet believed she must do this quickly. While normalizing and empathizing with Janet's anger, the therapist pointed out some drawbacks to confronting Brad at this time, such as the possibility of contaminating the criminal investigation and giving Brad an opportunity to force his sister not to talk with the authorities. Janet agreed to let the authorities confront her son, but she was finding it harder to contain her anger. She and the therapist identified several individuals with whom she felt she could talk when she felt especially angry. These people included some good friends whom she trusted. Janet discussed how she would approach her friends and how she would tell them about Cheryl's disclosure.

Cheryl had been having nightmares for the past several months, which had increased in frequency after her disclosure to her mother. Cheryl revealed to her mother that Brad had threatened to beat her up if she ever disclosed the abuse. The therapist incorporated this information in her explanation of why Cheryl's nightmares worsened after disclosing the abuse. She and Janet developed ways to help Cheryl with this problem. Janet kept reassuring her daughter that she had done the right thing in disclosing, and that she would do everything possible to ensure her safety, especially in the light of Brad's threats. The therapist encouraged Janet to institute a more regular bedtime routine for Cheryl, to buy a nightlight for her room, and to ask Cheryl regularly if she wanted to talk about her fears. Cheryl was responsive to her mother's invitations to talk and found Janet's reassurances comforting.

After two crisis intervention sessions, another therapist became available who assumed responsibility for the case. Cheryl began her own therapy to deal with a number of issues engendered by her brother's assaults, including PTSD symptoms, feelings of powerlessness and stigmatization, and guilt about her brother's subsequent removal from the home and placement in a residential treatment program for adolescent offenders. Janet actively collaborated in her daughter's treatment and attended some individual sessions to deal with her own feelings of guilt about having been unaware of what was happening to Cheryl.

A family therapist subsequently initiated joint sessions for Janet and Cheryl to discuss Cheryl's anger about her mother's lack of awareness of her victimization. She felt that her mother "should have known" what was happening, and Janet felt very guilty. Family sessions brought these feelings into a forum wherein they were directly addressed. Brad eventually joined the sessions after his own individual therapy enabled him to accept responsibility for his behavior. He had gained a better understanding of the basis and precipitants of his sexual assaults on his sister.

Although the two crisis intervention sessions did not address or resolve many of the significant or long-standing issues in this family, they provided Janet with the support and guidance she needed to make and implement decisions that supported her daughter at this crucial time. For example, Janet fought for a quicker response by child welfare authorities, supported involvement of child welfare authorities and police with her son, and instituted alternate child care arrangements to ensure Cheryl's safety. Although still terribly upset by her daughter's victimization, Janet felt some relief from her anxiety as she began expressing these feelings and discovered that they were normal and expected reactions. Cheryl found her mother's greater psychological availability to be a real help, which in turn augmented Janet's sense of efficacy and attenuated her feelings of guilt.

INTERVENTIONS FOR PARENTS FOR DEVELOPMENTAL EFFECTS OF MALTREATMENT

Parents and caregivers of maltreated children may require interventions after the immediate postdisclosure period, particularly if the children have been exposed to severe and chronic abuse and neglect and now display some of the serious developmental effects described in Chapter 1. These children frequently present formidable challenges to even the most skilled parents. A regimen of 1 or 2 hours of psychotherapy per week, although useful, is often insufficient to remedy pervasive and profound developmental effects. Maltreated children require multiple and repeated experiences throughout their daily lives, that is, a therapeutic milieu, in order to have any significant chance of recovery. Involving parents or alternate caretakers (e.g., foster parents) and other adults who have significant contact with the child (e.g., teachers) and ensuring their collaboration and cooperation in a comprehensive treatment program are essential. Just as the therapist functions like a family physician to the child, the same kind of orientation to parents or caregivers may be necessary. There are some adults who require consultations from a therapist at different periods while caring for a maltreated child. For example, the child's entry into adolescence may pose particular difficulties for parents or caregivers. The therapist's reinvolvement is expedited for everyone if the therapist, parent, and child already have established a relationship characterized by trust and respect. Although some parents may become overdependent, the therapist should not automatically dismiss their requests for reinvolvement. Their need to return to therapy is not necessarily pathological or indicative of a failure in helping the child or family when therapy first began. We must never forget that raising these children is often hard work with few rewards; adults who assume these responsibilities require and deserve generous and competent support and assistance.

This section of the chapter reviews some selected interventions for use with parents who care for these children, rather than interventions designed to change abusive or neglectful parental behavior. We describe strategies that enable parents and caregivers to complement and support the therapist's work. The last section of the chapter discusses consultation to school staff and representatives of the child welfare and legal systems.

Because a principal focus of this book is the relevance of attachment theory and research for treating school-age maltreated children, we now review strategies to enhance the attachment relationship between parents or caregivers and children. As abused and neglected children are at significantly higher risk for forming insecure attachments, a major goal of psychotherapy is the remediation of insecure attachment patterns and associated pathogenic processes. However, because parents or caregivers have much more extensive contact with the child and more opportunities to intervene with this problem than the therapist, they must be enlisted as integral and crucial allies in the treatment process.

Promoting Trust in Availability

Through small, repeated demonstrations of the parent's physical and psychological availability, the child's IWM/IS may begin to change. This availability constitutes evidence that disconfirms the child's skewed IWM/IS. The child may well have to undergo a great many of these experiences before actually beginning to trust the authenticity of the parent's positive intent. The therapist can help the parent or caregiver to identify opportunities to prove this commitment and to formulate concrete ways to show this caring attitude. For example, caregivers can ask children who appear ill or tired how they are feeling, commenting, "You look like you're not feeling very well right now. What can I do to help you?" and then quickly follow through with any appropriate requests. Children with an avoidant attachment organization may deny distress or that they need anything, and the caregiver can encourage expression of the simplest of needs (e.g., "If you need a drink of water, just ask me: say, 'I'm thirsty, I need a drink,' and I'll get you one"). Parents or caregivers should follow through with any promises made, or appropriately accommodate special requests or needs, such as preparing a child's favorite meal. These gestures serve as concrete reminders of the caregivers' commitment and availability, and that they are thinking of the child—that is, they are holding the child in their minds (Schofield & Beek, 2005). In addition, the therapist can help caregivers become more attuned to the feelings and conflicts underlying the child's sometimes provocative and perplexing behavior (described below). Exposure to sensitive adults who articulate empathy is a novel experience for many children and starts a reparative process that restores their trust in others.

James (1994) also recommends that maltreated children need "positive, intimate, physical touch" (p. 76). To prevent an escalation in the child's anxiety, James advises caregivers to explain the touching behavior to the child. She suggests that they begin with grooming behavior, such as shampooing and styling the child's hair. We also believe it is critical for the parent or caregiver to proceed slowly and gradually in this area. Physically or sexually abused children may associate touching that seems innocuous to most people with some frightening and painful experiences. For instance, an adult who sexually abused a child may have initiated the assaults by giving a back rub before progressing to sexually intrusive behavior. Other sexually abused children might find this touching to be sexually exciting, thereby eliciting significant anxiety. Parents or caregivers should proceed gradually and take their cues from the child's ability to tolerate touching. Parents must also explain the distinction between the current touching and that associated with the maltreatment (e.g., "When I hug you like this, it means that I like you and care about you. It does not mean that I am going to touch your private parts").

Promoting Reflective Thinking

If parents successfully demonstrate their availability, children start to feel a greater connection to their caregivers. However, forming intimate relationships with others is often a threatening experience for many maltreated children. When they become closer, they feel more vulnerable. They equate intimacy with harm, threat, and betrayal and therefore try to put some much-needed distance into the relationship, sometimes via oppositional, defiant, or rejecting behavior. This behavior allows a sense of control over the rejection they believe is inevitable. A child may derive some measure of security and control by provoking rejection rather than passively waiting for it to happen.

There are other reasons that inhibit maltreated children from establishing close relationships. They may believe intimacy with a person other than a parent is disloyalty to the absent parent, whom they expect to reject them if the parent discovers the child's growing affection for the substitute caregiver (James, 1994). Children harboring negative expectations of others often subject parents or caregivers to numerous tests of their commitment: Will parents or caregivers reject them if they behave in negative or outrageous ways?

It is particularly important to encourage parents or other caregivers to develop ideas and theories about the roots of this provocation, as well as about other aspects of the child's presentation. Asking parents or foster parents to reflect on the impact of the child's behavior on themselves (e.g., "When she treats me as if I don't even matter to her, I feel as though I don't want anything to do with her") often helps them generate ideas about the functions of the child's behavior, especially when the therapist follows up with probes and questions, (e.g., "I wonder why she doesn't want you to have anything to do with her? What purpose would that serve?"). The therapist can offer tentative theories about the particular dynamics underlying the child's seemingly counterproductive behaviors and hypothesize about their adaptive value, at least in the short term (e.g., "As she gets closer to you, it's really frightening for her. She's scared of getting too close to you because people hurt her [or rejected her] when she got close to them in the past. Now she expects the same, so she tries to push you away because she doesn't want to be hurt again. So in a way all the temper tantrums, screaming, and saying she hates you and wants to go back to her parents, makes sense—she has to drive you away to feel more comfortable and less vulnerable"). It is important to ask caregivers if these hypotheses ring true for them and to encourage their own theory-building abilities, especially as therapists are usually not immediately available when caregivers must respond to children's confusing, puzzling, and sometimes taxing behavior. Therapists can encourage caregivers to take a bit of time to reflect on the behavior and its possible meaning and function, rather than doing the first thing that comes to mind. Subsequent debriefing sessions with the therapist, in which caregivers have an opportunity to process the incident and reflect on the child's motivations and other possible explanations, are of real value in helping them develop these abilities. It also allows caregivers to ventilate their own feelings of frustration, confusion, and resentment in a safe and accepting atmosphere.

Spending sufficient time elucidating these pathogenic processes serves several functions. First, it ensures that parents do not personalize children's defiant and oppositional behaviors (e.g., "She wouldn't be doing these awful things if I was a better foster parent."), which in turn increases the chances of parents' responding in ways that reinforce the child's negative expectations. Inappropriate displays of anger or rejection just fuel the child's provocative behaviors, thereby setting up a vicious cycle that may ultimately lead to placement breakdown and further crystallization of negative IWM/IS.

Second, parental or caregiver ability to think about the child's behavior and mind, develop theories about why the child is thinking or behaving in this manner, and empathically communicate these thoughts to the child, promotes the child's emerging ability to think about his or her mind and the minds of others, that is, the reflective thinking we described in Chapter 2, and emotional and behavioral self-regulation. Caregivers who can observe and listen to the child closely and develop working hypotheses about the underlying meaning of the child's statements and behaviors need to communicate their understanding to the child. Helping these children accurately identify and articulate their feelings is often an essential task of caregivers. Maltreated children's ability in this area may be so compromised that they have difficulty in expressing even basic feelings.

Caregivers can do several things to help such children. They can make simple statements that reflect a child's feelings (e.g., "You're really angry at me!") so that children learn the verbal labels that correspond to these internal states. Caregivers can also model the appropriate expression of their own feelings (e.g., "Boy, I got scared when that guy nearly hit our car!"). They can encourage children to begin expressing their feelings (e.g., "I wonder how you felt when your dad didn't show up for the visit. You must have felt ___________" [pausing while waiting for the child to respond]). Therapists can teach caregivers to present theories to children about why they may be behaving in these seemingly inexplicable ways (e.g., "I wonder if you're behaving like this to see if I'm going to kick you out like your mom did"); such statements about the past help children explain and make sense of current experiences and facilitate behavioral and emotional self-regulation and impulse control (Schofield & Beek, 2005).

Promoting Behavioral and Emotional Self-Regulation

We have already described a number of strategies parents and caregivers can use to help children develop more adaptive behavioral and emotional self-regulation skills. These include assisting children to verbally express their feelings and internal state and to engage in reflective thinking, and providing them with firm and consistent limits on inappropriate behavior.

We offer a few more comments to round out this discussion. It is very easy to give up when faced with a child who thwarts any attempt at closeness or intimacy and whose behavior remains refractory to typical child management strategies that work with other children. Parents should tell the child directly that they are setting limits and consequences because they want to ensure that the child learns how to behave appropriately. Parents should also emphasize that these measures, which seem draconian, are based on their deep commitment to the child. Parental failure to effectively limit the more negative aspects of a child's behavior not only results in a further deterioration of the child's behavior, but also leads to the child's interpretation that a lack of action or ineffectiveness is more proof the parent does not care about his or her welfare. In the child's mind, if parents truly cared, they would expend the effort necessary to manage the problematic behavior.

Although parents must establish and maintain firm and consistent limits, they must also avoid unnecessary power struggles with children. They need to identify the truly important areas in which they will impose limits, such as those pertaining to safety issues. For example, allowing school-age children to defy age-appropriate curfews may place them at risk for harm and conveys the notion that parents' commitment to their welfare is tenuous. Yet rigidly insisting that children eat all the food on their plates often leads to protracted arguments, which in turn provide children with considerable attention. If a child does not eat everything in a prescribed time, parents can simply remove the plate and inform the child of the time of the next meal.

We have already discussed how parents or caregivers may benefit enormously from concrete suggestions and advice from the therapist concerning behavior management strategies. Sessions covering these topics can occur in the office or in the home setting to provide hands-on teaching and guidance. For their part, parents or caregivers must willingly work as part of the treatment team, openly communicating information about the child and their own struggles, and willingly seeking help and guidance as required (James, 1994).

Promoting Family Membership

Parents or caregivers must make concerted efforts to include children in mutually positive and pleasurable experiences and activities to counter their deep mistrust and fears of closeness and intimacy, especially in a family context (James, 1994). Children and caregivers must begin to enjoy each other's company and have some fun together. Participating in these activities helps children to learn that interpersonal relationships can be rewarding. For adult caregivers who derive little satisfaction from negative, hostile, and sometimes even outrageous behavior on the child's part, such experiences may counter disenchantment and reinforce their efforts to engage the child. Although parents and caregivers can often readily arrange such experiences, therapists may need to help some parents and children to identify activities that they might find mutually pleasurable. James (1994, p. 73) provides several good suggestions. Positive cognitive experiences may include going to a museum or carrying out a building project together. Pleasurable emotional experiences include both parties caring for a pet or watching an emotional movie. They may also share spiritual experiences, such as attending church together. Other shared fun activities may include playing simple board games at home, joint participation in sports, or reading to each other. With the therapist's guidance, parents and children can usually think of things that might be mutually enjoyable. Subsequently, the therapist can encourage the parent and child to review the activity, emphasizing its positive aspects. The therapist may ask each to identify aspects he or she liked most. Participants can retain souvenirs of these activities or outings (e.g., a movie ticket stub or a photograph of the child and parent playing catch) and keep them in a special place in the home. Souvenirs are concrete reminders of shared good times, especially helpful when parent and child later become pessimistic about the chances that their relationship will ever work.

Some parents, especially those who may have contributed to the child's maltreatment, encounter real difficulty with such tasks. They may have little motivation or expect the child to reject their overtures. The therapist can help by encouraging them to begin thinking of brief activities in which there is a reasonable chance that the parent and child will have fun together. Again, the therapist must consult closely with both concerning the choice of activities. Asking them to participate in more intense and prolonged activities, such as completing a science project together, is often too threatening, and both may refuse to participate. However, success with limited activities may start the process of instilling hope that the parent and child can relate better. Then the therapist can encourage them to try longer activities with each other.

In addition, some parents do not have the skills needed to interact positively or play appropriately with a child. Here, the first step may be for the parent to observe the therapist and child in the playroom doing typical activities such as board games, painting, or playing with dolls and trucks. This play models specific ways to interact with the child. Then the parent might be invited into the playroom to play with the child and the therapist. These joint sessions provide opportunities for the therapist to model healthy and appropriate interactions and to give the parent concrete tips regarding his or her interactional style with the child. Do not assume that a parent knows how to interact in seemingly simple activities such as drawing or building with blocks. Some with minimal skills in this area are threatened by the thought of playing with their child. They are relieved and supported by the therapist's guidance and suggestions. The therapist may serve as a mediator if things go wrong, leading the child and parent through a problem-solving process. When parents are more confident, the therapist leaves the room and watches via a one-way mirror or videotape of the interaction. Afterward, the therapist gives feedback, emphasizing the parent's strengths and capabilities. Watching segments of videotapes enables parents to become more sensitive to their child's cues and better able to make appropriate interventions.

These strategies are somewhat reminiscent of parent–child interaction therapy (PCIT), which focuses on decreasing externalizing behavior, increasing positive parent behaviors, and enhancing the quality of the parent–child relationship (Hembree-Kigin & McNeil, 1995). The children are usually 4–12 years of age. In the child-directed interaction component, the parent is taught to praise, reflect, imitate, describe, and show enthusiasm when playing with the child. The therapist observes the interactions via a one-way mirror and gives the parent directions, prompts, and instructions via an FM-signal audio reception device the parent wears. The parent-directed interaction focuses on improving the parent's disciplinary practices. The therapist instructs the parent to give the child commands and instructions. Typically, six sessions are devoted to the child-directed interaction and six more to the parent-directed interaction. There is a considerable body of empirical evidence that PCIT is an efficacious treatment for physically abusive parents (for reviews, see Chadwick Center for Children and Families, 2004; Chaffin et al., 2004; Saunders et al., 2004). For example, one outcome evaluation study found a decrease in abuse risk from pre- to posttreatment for dyads with and without a history of maltreatment, a decrease in child behavior problems, and a decrease in parental stress (Timmer, Urquiza, Zebell, & McGrath, 2005).

James (1994) describes other useful strategies designed to increase the child's sense of belonging to the family. These include the adult's making verbal references that emphasize the child's tie to the family and more concrete demonstrations, such as having a new family picture taken together (for a child placed with an adoptive or foster family or a child just returned to a parent from foster care), selecting a special place for the child at the dinner table, or purchasing a gift for the child's room.

Many maltreated children are permanently removed from parental care, and they must have alternate supports before they can acknowledge their parents' inability or unwillingness to provide the love and care they deserve and can accept this loss (James, 1994). These children often have difficulty in openly acknowledging that their parents cannot care for them or may not even love them. They can be overwhelmed by feelings of abandonment if they acknowledge their parents' lack of commitment, especially if they are without connections to other adults. Consequently, they may deny a parent's ongoing difficulties, adamantly maintain that the parent will change for the better, and present an overidealized portrayal of the parent that runs counter to the painful reality of the parent's actual deficits and failings.

Alternate caregivers like foster parents can become frustrated with the child's use of these defensive strategies, particularly if their strenuous efforts to make the child feel wanted and cared for are met with hostility, defiance, and more negative behavior. The therapist may play a significant role in educating caregivers about the function of defenses, such as overidealization, and in explaining how the child's negative behavior may be a test of the caregiver's commitment. Caregivers should not argue with a child who steadfastly maintains that parents have now resolved all the problems responsible for the child's removal from the home. Instead, caregivers should empathize with the underlying fear or anxiety that drives the child to make such assertions, even when confronted with clear evidence that the parents still have many difficulties. Caregivers who identify all of a parent's glaring deficits and foibles and try to convince the child that the parent is unfit will probably engender even more resistance. The therapist should teach the foster parent how to empathize with some of the child's underlying feelings. This empathy may be communicated through statements like "It would make you very happy if your mom stopped drinking and took you home again" in response to a child who expects to go home again soon because her mother has surmounted long-standing problems with alcoholism. Establishment of even a limited connection with an alternate caregiver begins to attenuate the child's profound sense of abandonment. Along with the alternate caregiver's ability to convey a deep understanding of, and empathy for, the child's plight, such a connection helps the child to acknowledge the significance of personal loss and begin expressing intense feelings of rage, sadness, and grief. By normalizing these feelings, helping the child find appropriate words rather than acting out the feelings through aggressive or destructive behavior, and maintaining firm and consistent limits on any negative behavior, the caregiver helps the child through the grieving process and strengthens the child's ability to self-regulate feelings and behavior.

Enlisting the cooperation of the parent whose loss the child is mourning may facilitate recovery. Specifically, child and parent may benefit from joint sessions in which the parent gives the child explicit permission to form a close relationship with alternate caregivers and assures the child that he or she will not be threatened by the child's close relationship with new parental figures. For children who believe that their negative behavior in the foster home will break down the placement and result in their returning home, a clear and unequivocal message from a parent may contribute to a decrease in the negative behavior. These discussions are difficult for children; they may require some individual sessions to express sentiments about the loss, to formulate questions for the parent (e.g., "Why did you give me up?" "Why couldn't you take care of me?"), and to decide how they want to say goodbye. Parents may also need some preliminary individual sessions with the therapist to express grief and anger about losing the child and to rehearse what they will say. Of course, some parents vehemently oppose losing their parental rights. They are unwilling or unable to give their child explicit permission to become close to another individual, and they may even blame the child for what has happened. Other parents who have lost parental rights are so egocentric or dependent on their child that they cannot let go and allow the youngster to establish alternate relationships. Joint sessions would be contraindicated with such parents.

Promoting Self-Esteem and a Sense of Self

In Chapter 1 we pointed out that many maltreated children do not have a solid sense of self. Again, James (1994) provides some good suggestions about how to help children establish a sense of self and identity. As well as being applicable to therapy sessions, a number of her suggestions can be used by parents and caregivers. Caregivers can make comments about the child's uniqueness and solicit the child's opinions about personal feelings, thoughts, and bodily experiences. Extensive or in-depth discussions about these opinions or the child's dislikes and likes contribute to the child's further differentiation of self.

Caregivers must also be astute observers of any strengths the child exhibits and then identify them for the youngster. However, we often caution parents or caregivers from using fulsome, lengthy accounts when describing strengths to their children. Some children with very low self-esteem are extremely skeptical of such positive statements and harbor strong doubts about the other person's sincerity. We have worked with children who have intentionally failed or began to engage in more negative behavior in order to prove to caregivers that their glowing descriptions are false and to reduce the expectations for even greater achievements in the future. Instead, caregivers should point out in behavioral terms what the child has done well without overelaboration or exaggeration. As we discuss in Chapter 10, caregivers can also arrange or provide opportunities for children to learn new skills and try new experiences. Some children are very hesitant to participate, as they expect to inevitably fail. Caregivers have to balance their empathy for these fears with gently encouraging, and sometimes even insisting, the child try something new. Of course, it is important to propose activities in which there is a good chance that the child will enjoy them and attain some success.

Providing Ongoing Support to the Parents or Caregivers

Parenting and caring for maltreated children with significant symptomatology can be exhausting, frustrating, and daunting. Parents and caregivers faced with this challenge deserve enormous amounts of support and assistance. There are other ways therapists can provide this support besides giving advice and guidance concerning behavior management and strengthening the parent–child relationship.

First, the therapist should normalize and validate some of the parent's reactions to the child. The child who responds to parental overtures of caring and love with increased hostility, defiance, or even rejection poses a real threat to many parents, especially to those who want a mutually reciprocal and intimate relationship with the child. These parents not only become angry but also begin to question their skills and worth as parents and individuals. Consequently, they may feel like giving up and having the child removed from their home. Foster parents sometimes complain that they feel "sucked dry." Compounding these feelings is the disruption of the entire family and the incessant demands from others to "do something" to bring the child's behavior under control. Therapists should also encourage caregivers to respond to the needs of other children in the family. Sometimes these children receive less active parenting because of the very high demands of the maltreated child.

Having an opportunity to articulate these feelings and frustrations can alleviate a parent's distress. In particular, participating in a support group with other parents or caregivers facing similar challenges and frustrations may attenuate the parent's sense of isolation. Preparing parents for their child's possible behavioral regressions as a function of upcoming events (e.g., court appearance) and helping them develop plans to cope with these contingencies decrease parents' feelings of powerlessness. Although time-consuming, regular consultation with these caregivers usually results in an improvement in the care the child receives. Parents also benefit from some respite care—for instance, having the child spend one weekend per month with another family. Again, the therapist should advocate for the provision of this service, if it is required.

WORKING WITH TEACHERS

The therapist who involves teachers in the treatment plan, as well as working with parents and other caregivers, has a better chance of helping maltreated school-age children recover. Teachers have much contact with children and often see and experience difficulties firsthand. They are in an excellent position to help remediate some of these problems.

In Chapter 4 we discussed the importance of gathering information from teachers during the assessment. The therapist should request their continued involvement in the treatment phase. Teachers usually appreciate an offer by the therapist to visit the school and meet with staff. Like the child's parents or caregivers, teachers may be frustrated and exhausted from dealing with extremely difficult behavior. However, the therapist should not portray him- or herself as the "expert" who dictates how teachers should manage the child.

Instead, the therapist must be willing to work cooperatively and collaboratively. The therapist must realize that school personnel probably already have valuable insights and ideas about the child and how best to help.

Given the sensitivity of information concerning the child's history and current circumstances, the therapist must be prudent when deciding how much to share. Therapists should have discussed this issue with the child's parents or legal guardians and obtained explicit permission regarding the information they may communicate before they talk or meet with teachers. The child, particularly an older one, should be informed that the therapist wishes to meet with his or her teachers so that everyone can work together on the child's behalf.

One of the first things a therapist might do is to provide teachers with some information regarding the reasons for the child's behavior, including a description of those historical and current factors and pathogenic processes that have contributed to the child's functioning, and realistic expectations about the child's prognosis and rate of change. Although the therapist may help the teacher understand that change will not be immediate, an overpessimistic attitude may set up a detrimental self-fulfilling prophecy. Teachers with a solid understanding of the basis of the problem behavior may begin to see the child from a different perspective and are less likely to personalize the child's reactions.

Therapists should encourage teachers to limit any physical aggression or sexually inappropriate behavior firmly and consistently. They should work with the therapist to develop some concrete strategies. Some teachers with whom we have worked have agreed to institute daily "check-ins" with these children. The teacher spends 5 to 10 minutes alone with the child near the beginning of the school day to review classroom expectations, identify situations that might pose problems during the day, and discuss possible coping strategies. Therapists should assist teachers who deal with extremely anxious children by reviewing the rationale and basic procedures of common techniques such as thought stopping and relaxation training. During daily check-ins, the teacher might remind and encourage the child to use these techniques.

The teacher may intervene in other ways. Some sexually or physically abused children indiscriminately discuss details of their victimization with schoolmates or in front of the entire class. The teacher should learn to curtail these discussions quickly and then talk privately with the child about the most appropriate times and contexts for such discussions. Teachers should encourage maltreated children to participate in school activities and follow a regular classroom routine. These activities will demonstrate to the children that they still can function and cope with the daily demands of life, despite their abuse or neglect. Excessive sympathy by the teacher often results in making fewer demands of the child, which just reinforces feelings of low self-esteem, helplessness, and inadequacy and promotes a pattern of underachievement or behavioral problems.

By maintaining regular contact with the teacher, the therapist gains valuable information about the child's functioning and any changes that may be necessary in the treatment plan to better meet the child's needs (e.g., slowing the pace of introducing abuse-related stimuli in treatment sessions). The teacher should alert the therapist to special circumstances or events in school that may be stressful to the child, such as the initiation of a sex education program in the classroom. The therapist who is alerted to such an event may raise the issue in therapy and help prepare the child. The therapist and teacher should collaboratively develop an intervention plan for use in the classroom if, for instance, the sexually abused child begins to feel anxious and distressed during a sex education program.

There should be regular and frequent contact between the therapist and teacher to maintain this high degree of cooperation, This contact is especially important for those children who present serious problems in the classroom. Many whose behavior is out of control are reassured when they know that the therapist and teacher talk with one another regularly.

Ten-year-old Bob had been sexually and physically abused by his natural mother and her common-law partner. Bob had forceably engaged other children in sexual behavior and was oppositional, defiant, and sometimes physically aggressive in the classroom. He was aware that his therapist called his teacher at the same time on the same day every week. Bob derived a great deal of comfort and security from the knowledge that two significant adults were communicating openly and frequently about his welfare. He realized that they were working together to help him. This was the first time Bob had adults in his life who worked together as a team and showed enough commitment to take time to talk with each other about him predictably and consistently. He always asked his teacher, just after the scheduled phone call, whether she had talked to the therapist, and he asked the same of the therapist in their weekly sessions. Bob appeared visibly relieved when assured by both that they had indeed talked with each other about him, even if part of their discussion had been devoted to some of his negative behavior.

Finally, a teacher often has ongoing contact with the child's parents. The therapist and teacher should ensure that they are providing the parents with consistent information and suggestions. Some parents are extremely difficult to deal with. In such cases, the therapist might be able to provide the teacher with ideas about how to best handle these interactions.

WORKING WITH CHILD WELFARE PERSONNEL AND THE LEGAL SYSTEM

Although child welfare workers and lawyers do not have as frequent contact with a maltreated child as parents, foster parents, other caregivers, and teachers do, their involvement can powerfully impact on the child's life. Many maltreated children and their families have contact with child protective services at some time during the children's growing years. The contact may arise through investigation of reports of abuse and neglect, provision of support to children and families, or removal of children from their families under child protection legislation. Any therapist involved in clinical work with maltreated youngsters and their families will need to work with these professionals to optimize the benefits to children.

An important role therapists play in the child welfare system is that of advocate for their young clients and their families. A child welfare worker will usually have to make a number of decisions that have a profound effect on a child's life. Should the child remain in care or be returned to the family? Is the child a suitable candidate for adoption? The therapist, with detailed knowledge of the child, can provide the child welfare worker with valuable information and opinions on these and other issues, especially if the therapist has known the child for a long time. For a child who has gone through multiple foster homes and seen a parade of child welfare workers come and go, the therapist may be one of the most consistent figures in the child's life and can therefore play an especially important advocacy role.

There are other areas in which therapists can be advocates for their child clients. The therapist must notify the child welfare worker about any significant concerns regarding a child's safety. We mentioned earlier that participating in therapy can elicit children's anger, which in turn may place them at risk if parents are unprepared to cope with such strong feelings. Therapists should thoroughly familiarize themselves with their jurisdiction's legal statutes concerning abuse and neglect, as well as reporting requirements and protocols. They may have to advocate for the provision of other services, such as in-home parenting guidance. The therapist also will soon encounter some of the broader systemic obstacles that impede children's recovery (e.g., long court delays, scattered and limited resources for parents). Although advocating on a case-by-case basis is necessary, therapists must remember that some of these larger problems will be solved only by concerted action and widespread pressure for change.

Therapists should expect child welfare workers and lawyers to seek their opinions and should make themselves available for consultation by promptly returning phone calls and providing timely, concise reports. Excessively lengthy reports replete with technical jargon usually are not useful. Furthermore, a therapist's report in which its limitations pertaining to the conclusions are openly acknowledged and a balanced perspective on a case is maintained is generally better received and more highly regarded by other professionals, as well as the courts. Although some professionals may take exception to others' opinions that do not confirm their own beliefs, therapists must state their opinions honestly and remember that in many cases there are no easy or clear-cut answers. Rather than offering an unequivocal opinion that may not be supported by the data, therapists instead should describe the advantages and disadvantages of a particular course of action. Such an approach may also alleviate the anxiety of a therapist who feels discomfort at becoming an agent of the courts or of the child welfare system. Therapists must realize that although they may have some specialized knowledge about a child, they do not have all the answers and that others also have useful and important information. This realization may help novice therapists, who often believe that they must provide an unequivocal opinion or recommendation to a court and that the entire responsibility for decision making rests with them.

The therapist's close involvement with child welfare workers and the courts may generate considerable anxiety or resistance in some abusive and neglectful families. The latter may feel threatened by disclosing information to the therapist. The therapist should address this issue before therapy begins, clearly informing parents of the limits of confidentiality and the conditions that would compel him or her to contact child welfare authorities without the family's permission. Parents and therapists should discuss other situations in which information will be shared and negotiate the manner in which it will be done. Child welfare workers should be included in these discussions at some point so that all relevant parties can reach an agreement. Despite this preparation, therapists must realize that some parents may refuse to bring themselves or their children back to therapy after a therapist has shared what parents consider to be damaging information with child welfare authorities or the courts. If the child involved is old enough, the therapist should discuss with him or her the fact that the therapist will be meeting with a child welfare worker. This is an opportunity for them to talk about the child's progress in therapy, the remaining issues that need to be addressed, and any recommendations to the child and family about intervention. We have found that alerting the child to these meetings often provides a greater focus for discussions. Sometimes children who are reluctant to speak with a child welfare worker will express their opinions in no uncertain terms to their therapists about such issues as the possibility of returning home. The child may be more motivated to express opinions about these matters if the therapist expresses a willingness to act as spokesperson for the child in settings such as case conferences or court hearings where the child will not be present, even if the therapist's opinions are different from the child's. The therapist must be honest in identifying any areas of disagreement with the child concerning these issues. Although the child may be quite upset with, for example, the therapist's decision to recommend that the child not return home, such disagreement often provokes even more discussion that facilitates the child's active examination and consideration of these issues.

Convening regular case conferences is a good way to ensure open communication with child welfare workers and others. A case manager, typically the child welfare worker, should be appointed for particularly complex cases. One duty of the case manager is to facilitate a coordinated approach to intervention and delivery of services, including such items as scheduling and arranging case conferences.

When we began to work with them, we quickly learned that we had to devote significant time to communicating with child welfare workers and collaterals such as teachers or other therapists. Our subsequent experiences have reinforced our initial impression that contact with collaterals is time-consuming and often imposes many demands on therapists. However, it is critically important. Therapists who believe they can work in total isolation from others and confine all their efforts to a weekly 50-minute session are missing the mark. Although clinicians must pay particular attention to many aspects of the actual therapy with their young clients, they must not lose sight of the fact that other individuals, such as natural parents, foster parents, teachers, and child welfare workers, often have as much or even greater influence on a child. It is only by recognizing the significance of these people and their potential roles as allies and by incorporating them into the treatment program that we can maximize the benefits of psychotherapy. This notion is well articulated by Cicchetti and Toth (1995): "Therapy with a maltreated child cannot be limited to the confines of the playroom, but must transcend the safety of the office to confront and impact the factors that may continue to assault the child in his or her daily life" (p. 55).

CHAPTER SEVEN

The Therapeutic Relationship

Peter, an 11-year-old boy, was referred to a therapist because his stepfather had sexually abused him from the ages of 7 to 9. When he was 10 years old, Peter disclosed to his mother that his stepfather had engaged him in numerous episodes of oral sex and mutual masturbation and that they had viewed pornographic videos together. He was referred to therapy because of his preoccupation with sexual matters. Peter was bothered by frequent sexual fantasies, including having sexual intercourse with other children and babies. There had also been several occasions when he initiated oral sex with younger children. Peter refused to complete any academic work and was in danger of failing the school year. He was defiant and oppositional with his teacher and his mother; the latter was becoming increasingly frustrated with her inability to manage Peter's behavior. He associated with adolescent boys who had an unsavory reputation in the community, stayed out late at night, and began to lie and engage in petty theft. The assessment also revealed that Peter exhibited some features of PTSD, including sleep difficulties and nightmares, hypervigilance, poor concentration, and startle reactions.

The clinician who initially assessed Peter referred him to another clinician for therapy because she did not believe she had the skills needed to help this youngster and his mother. When the therapist introduced himself in the waiting room, Peter avoided all eye contact and reluctantly and weakly shook the therapist's hand. He accompanied the therapist to his office but remained 10 feet behind as they walked down the hall.

For the first 30 minutes of the meeting, Peter responded to all inquiries with one- or two-word answers, looking at his watch, cradling his head in his arms, and periodically shutting his eyes. He explained to the therapist that he was "sleepy" because he had slept at a friend's home the night before the appointment and got little sleep. He claimed not to know whether he had any problems to address in therapy and on several occasions asked if he could leave. Overall, Peter seemed indifferent to the therapist and the possibility of receiving assistance for his serious problems. After an hour with this seemingly unresponsive youngster, the therapist felt a certain degree of frustration about Peter's lack of interest in his efforts to help him and his own inability to form any connection with the youngster. In addition, the therapist felt that he had done "all the work" and was exhausted by the hour's end. He anticipated the next session with Peter with some anxiety and trepidation.

Unfortunately, this experience is not uncommon for therapists who treat maltreated children, especially those exposed to severe and long-standing abuse and neglect and who now manifest serious developmental effects. For example, a close reading of Peter's assessment report prepared by the first clinician revealed that besides sexually assaulting him, his stepfather had met none of Peter's needs for nurturance and attention from a paternal figure. His mother reported to the first clinician that Peter had "chosen" this man, an acquaintance of the family, as his father when he was 6 years old. Peter had started to call the man "Dad" before he and Peter's mother began dating. As a young boy and even before meeting his future stepfather, Peter had talked incessantly about wanting a father with whom he could play sports. The only time his stepfather gave him any attention, however, was during the sexual assaults. The assessment also indicated that Peter blamed his mother for not having known about these assaults and for not protecting him. His mistrust of her was compounded when she sought employment outside their community immediately after his disclosure, leaving him for several weeks with two alcoholic caretakers. His mother revealed to Peter's therapist that she had always felt overwhelmed by the demands of single parenting. She had been depressed for much of her son's infancy and toddlerhood. She described parenting in these early years as "going through the motions" and acknowledged that she frequently rejected Peter's attempts to obtain her attention and affection. On occasion she hit him or angrily rebuffed his efforts to interact with her, while at the same time applying few consistent limits on Peter's behavior. Given this history and experience with others, why would a youngster like Peter put himself in the vulnerable position of becoming close to someone, especially a male therapist? Why would he talk to a therapist, or anyone, about embarrassing problems such as his sexual behavior and fantasies when others had been so unhelpful in the past?

Let us now consider another 11-year-old boy, Derek. He too had been referred to the therapist after assessment by another clinician.

Derek had been sexually assaulted once by an adolescent male babysitter who lived next door. The next day, Derek disclosed this episode to his parents, who in turn quickly notified the police. Derek provided a clear disclosure to the police, and when confronted, the babysitter quickly admitted his guilt. Throughout the whole episode, Derek had the full support of his parents.

Derek was referred to a therapist because of some anxiety-related symptoms, including nightmares and intrusive memories of the assault. Although he appeared somewhat anxious in the therapist's waiting room, Derek readily shook hands. Derek accompanied the therapist to his office without any undue hesitation or reluctance, walked beside the therapist, and chatted about how he had been to the same hospital several years earlier after falling off a bike.

In this initial interview, Derek readily responded to the therapist's questions, maintained good eye contact, and displayed a wide range of affects, including his sadness about having been assaulted by this older boy who, in the past, had been kind to him. He quickly identified his recurrent nightmares and other PTSD symptoms (intrusive memories of the assault, impaired concentration) as the primary problems he wanted to address and was enthusiastic about returning for another appointment to begin work on these problems.

Before this isolated assault, Derek had the good fortune of living with parents who consistently afforded him excellent care. Given this history, Derek entered therapy with the expectation that the therapist, like everyone else in his life, would treat him respectfully and provide the help and support he needed at this time. Although he was somewhat nervous at the beginning of the interview, his anxiety soon abated after the therapist provided a clear description of his role and of the therapeutic process. After a short course of therapy, Derek's frightening dreams and intrusive memories disappeared. Although Derek and the therapist established a positive therapeutic alliance in the first session, much of the intervention focused on providing the boy with cognitive-behavioral strategies to cope with his symptoms. In contrast, therapy with Peter was a long and sometimes arduous process. Among a diverse array of interventions, the clinician strategically used the therapeutic relationship to counteract Peter's longstanding feelings of mistrust and betrayal by others.

These two boys and their initial presentations in therapy illustrate the two major perspectives on the relationship of child and clinician in child therapy as described by Shirk and Karver (2003). As we reported in Chapter 5, clinicians can directly use the therapeutic relationship to change important pathogenic processes, such as IMWs/IS. The other perspective emphasizes the use of the relationship as a means to an end (Shirk & Saiz, 1992). The child's positive feelings for the therapist allow the child to accept the therapist as someone who will assist in resolving emotional or behavioral difficulties. The relationship promotes the child's participation and collaboration in specific therapeutic tasks or interventions. Derek's progress in therapy exemplifies the use of a therapeutic alliance. His positive feelings toward the therapist and the therapeutic process enabled him to quickly and actively learn and implement cognitive-behavioral strategies that reduced his anxiety and alleviated his distress. The therapist did not have to use the therapeutic relationship as a primary mechanism of change to help this young boy, as he did with Peter.

This chapter is divided into two major sections. In the first, we review and describe different strategies to engage children in the psychotherapeutic process, including those who form a therapeutic relationship with relative ease. We also discuss engagement strategies for children whose abilities to establish and maintain relationships have been deleteriously and significantly affected by maltreatment. In the second section, we describe aspects of the therapeutic relationship for use in the middle phase of therapy, especially to remediate the effects of insecure attachments and negative IWMs/IS.

THE ENGAGEMENT PHASE OF THERAPY

The Therapist as a "Secure Base"

Bowlby (1988b) argues that the therapist assumes the role of a secure attachment figure as the client begins to sense safety and predictability in the therapeutic process. By inspiring trust in his or her availability and responsiveness to clients, the therapist provides a secure base from which children can confidently explore their internal world, including their IWMs/IS. Sensing safety and feeling increasingly confident that the therapist will meet his or her needs for comfort and empathy, the maltreated child may more readily raise and confront challenging and distressing issues. The establishment of this secure base is similar to the notion of the therapeutic alliance. In each conceptualization, qualities of the relationship between child and therapist facilitate the child's active participation in treatment. Moreover, as we shall see later, a therapist who establishes him- or herself as a secure base may be contributing an essential ingredient to the process whereby IMWs/IS begin to change. This may be especially relevant for children with an insecure/disorganized classification where there has been a failure to derive a coherent strategy for obtaining basic protection from the parent (Cassidy & Mohr, 2001).

Promoting the therapist as a secure base often runs throughout the course of therapy. However, the therapist must pay particular attention to it in the first stage, using some of the strategies described below to begin engaging the child in a therapeutic relationship. The therapist must be aware that forming a relationship wherein the child can begin to feel a sense of safety, regularity, and commitment is sometimes a slow and gradual process. There is no one intervention or therapeutic technique that suddenly turns these children around and dissolves the strong barriers of mistrust and avoidance they have developed over many years to protect themselves. James (1994) eloquently articulated this sentiment:

> Children who have learned not to trust adults and who are intimacy-avoidant may not show signs of relationship development with the therapist for many months. It is a fairly common occurrence in work with attachment disturbance that the clinician becomes suddenly, rather than gradually, aware that the child experiences sufficient relational support to begin deeper work. This sudden "opening up" may be understood as the child responding to a specific clinical intervention or technique, rather than as the child having developed emotional readiness.
>
> It is an error, though tempting, to consider such a clinical occurrence a "breakthrough." The phenomenon may appear to be an instant shift caused by a specific action or event: a wall of "resistance" that the child or therapist shatters, splits apart, or bursts through. The process leading to children being able to trust their therapist, allowing themselves to be vulnerable and revealing tender feelings can be likened to the slow, complex development of a critical mass of emotional safety, not a sudden breakthrough. (pp. 61–62)

If the child feels somewhat secure and safe with the therapist, the therapeutic relationship may deepen. It will then provide more examples of the child's maladaptive IWM/IS, other feelings and cognitions related to the maltreatment, and further opportunities for intervention.

Orienting the Child to the Purpose, Process, and Structure of Therapy Sessions

The therapist must orient a child to the therapeutic environment and to the purposes and process of therapy. This orientation is necessary to help the child form a therapeutic alliance so the work of therapy can proceed: the child and therapist must reach some agreement or consensus about the reasons for therapy sessions and how they will be conducted. Furthermore, this phase is an opportunity to empathize with the child's affects, including feelings associated with being brought to treatment or activated by initial discussions of the maltreatment itself. The orientation sets a tone of predictability and regularity for the therapeutic process, thereby attenuating some of the child's anxiety. By paying careful attention to this phase and being exquisitely sensitive to the child's ongoing reactions, the therapist begins to function as a secure base, which provides a solid foundation for the therapeutic alliance. But there may be another benefit: the therapist is beginning to provide evidence that he or she is different from others who have hurt or victimized the youngster, thereby activating a process that may modify skewed and biased IWMs/IS.

Chapter 4 described strategies to orient the child to the assessment process, and they can be applied to this phase of treatment. The clinician may have completed an evaluation of a particular child and reviewed the assessment results with the child and family. In the first therapy session, the therapist should briefly review this information, reiterating the consensus reached in the feedback session regarding the youngster's participation in treatment and the treatment goals.

When a therapist begins therapy with a child who was assessed by another clinician and whom he or she is meeting for the first time, the therapist should ask the child why he or she was brought to see the therapist, and empathize with the child's fear or anger about attending therapy. The therapist should explore and clarify any of the child's fantasies about participating in therapy and quickly correct them to alleviate anxiety. It is well worth the time to review the initial assessment results with the child to establish an agreement about the child's participation in treatment. The clinician must take into account the child's developmental and cognitive abilities when deciding how much information to share. As we advocated in Chapter 4, the therapist should clearly and directly inform the child that he or she knows the child has been maltreated and that the maltreatment is a primary reason for participation in therapy. Besides setting expectations for the work of therapy, the therapist who talks directly about the child's victimization conveys an expectation that the child will eventually be able to handle this topic and begins to desensitize the youngster. A direct account of why the child was referred to therapy serves to counter his or her expectation that adults will be dishonest.

What might the therapist say to the child about the purpose of therapy? The child requires a clear and simple explanation. The explanation might be something like this: "I help kids figure out how they feel about being beaten up by their dad [or whatever expression may be appropriate to the specific form of maltreatment] and what they think about it. Sometimes kids feel really upset or mixed up about what happened to them. I try to help them think of other ways of letting out their feelings about what happened." Of course, the language must be appropriate to the child's developmental level. The therapist can refer to some of the child's specific difficulties as potential targets of intervention and must be prudent not to give any false reassurances, such as by saying that therapy will make the youngster "forget" the maltreatment. Children should be reassured that talking about these matters is often difficult, even for adults, and that the therapist understands that this anxiety and will not force them to deal with material before they are ready. The therapist can tell the child that he or she has many different ways of helping children "get out" their feelings and thoughts about their experiences in safe ways. Ultimately, the child has control over what is shared with the therapist. Such statements communicate respect for the child's need to get to know the therapist better and to feel a measure of safety in the therapist's presence, thereby reassuring an anxious or frightened child. Telling a child that the therapist sees other children who have gone through similar experiences also reduces the sense of isolation and stigmatization many maltreated children feel.

In addition to orienting the child to the purpose of therapy, the therapist must talk with the child about the process and structure of therapy. Even young children can benefit from brief and simple explanations of what therapy is about, that is, the process. For those who will be participating in therapy in which heavy emphasis is placed on direct verbalization, therapists should give a brief rationale of the benefits of talking about the maltreatment. The clinician can say that talking provides alternate means for expressing feelings, rather than acting them out in ways that cause the child and others trouble. Talking about the maltreatment gives children an opportunity to think differently about what has happened to them, such as reformulating the belief that they were responsible for their victimization, and helps them to eventually feel less anxious. The clinician should say that the child can use whatever words or terminology the child prefers and give permission to the child to state when he or she is not yet ready to talk about or deal with certain topics. Children who will be participating in more indirect methods of intervention deserve a simple explanation of this approach. For example, the clinician can say, "Sometimes the way kids play tells us what's bothering them. Playing also helps us think of some new ways you can use to feel better about what happened to you."

Besides setting the expectation that there is work to be done in therapy, these brief descriptions alleviate anxiety about the therapeutic process. In Chapter 4 we described how some sexually or physically abused children expect similar treatment from a therapist. They deserve and require honest explanations of the treatment process, and in particular that the therapist will treat them with the respect and dignity. The therapist must be especially sensitive to situations or interventions that replicate aspects of the original maltreatment, being sure to draw contextual distinctions for the child. For example, the therapist can reassure the child that talking about sexual matters behind closed doors with an adult will not be the initial stage of a process in which the child will be sexually abused. Drawing this distinction not only attenuates anxiety, but also modifies the child's IWM/IS in a more positive direction—"Not everyone is going to hurt me."

The therapist must also educate the child about the structure of the sessions, thereby allaying anticipatory anxiety and fears about treatment by providing a sense of predictability about what will happen from session to session. This approach may be particularly reassuring for those anxious children who have lived in unpredictable, chaotic environments where they developed the belief that all adults are untrustworthy, unreliable figures. Although the therapist's actual actions and behavior are critical in establishing and maintaining predictability, the therapist should begin the process in the first session by explaining the structure of therapy (e.g., locale, duration of sessions), as described in Chapter 4.

The child must be informed about the therapist's contact with parents or caregivers. Usually, the therapist meets regularly with these individuals to assist them in helping the child and inform them of the child's progress. In addition, the therapist can say that although he or she will not disclose information without notifying the child first, there are limits on confidentiality. For example, the therapist will not keep secrets about someone hurting the child or if the child is at risk for self-harm or harming others. Besides talking with the parents privately, the therapist might have the child present during discussions with them about the youngster's progress.

Predictability, Consistency, and Safety in the Therapy Sessions and Therapeutic Relationship

Many maltreated children have models of other people as inconsistent, unreliable, and dangerous individuals, which in turn are detriments to the child's participation in therapy. Furthermore, the child who believes that the therapist cannot keep him or her safe from acting out overwhelming feelings will be reluctant to address salient aspects of the maltreatment. "Opening up" may overwhelm a child's frail emotional and behavioral self-regulatory abilities, increasing the risk for deterioration in behavior and functioning. Some regression in the child's behavior may occur (e.g., enuresis, physical aggression), or the child may begin to complain of being bothered by intrusive thoughts or nightmares when flooded with feelings and memories associated with the victimization. It will be safer to avoid these issues and not express them if the child has little confidence in the adult's ability to limit this acting out.

The therapist can develop an atmosphere of predictability and safety in various ways. Clinicians should schedule sessions at the same time and on the same day(s) during the week and use the same therapy room or playroom, along with the same toys and/or equipment. Switching from one office to another or having different toys available from week to week may erode any trust the child is beginning to develop in the therapist. The clinician might set up a special box or folder to hold the child's art or other therapy productions. Taking the folder out at approximately the same time in each session and then putting it in its special place at the end of the session reinforces constancy and predictability. Other rituals serve the same purpose. Some children enjoy and experience reassurance from the same ritual greeting every week, such as a special handshake (Friedrich, 1990). Others hide under a table in the waiting room while the therapist feigns ignorance of their whereabouts and then expresses happiness and pleasure when "finding" them. Yet other children must play the same game or engage in the same activity at the beginning or end of each session. These opening and closing rituals provide predictability and regularity and are concrete markers or cues for different aspects of the child's and therapist's participation in the therapy session. For example, playing a simple board game like checkers may be the stimulus to discuss the past week. Closing rituals include putting away toys and equipment, turning off the lights, and closing the door. These actions symbolize the child's attempt to contain the material elicited and processed in that particular therapy session; they also allow the child to move to the routine demands and tasks of everyday life.

Therapists can impose similar regularity and predictability on other aspects of the therapeutic relationship. They should avoid or minimize cancellations or changes in appointment times as much as possible, because such changes may elicit feelings of disappointment or rage in a child. These extreme reactions are the result of the child's perception that people are again treating him or her unreliably. Because some changes or cancellations are unavoidable, the therapist should clearly explain the reasons and emphasize that they have nothing to do with the therapist's feelings for the youngster. A therapist's extended vacation may be a particularly difficult time. To alleviate anxiety arising from the belief that the child will never see the therapist again, the therapist can give the child a copy of a calendar on which the date of the next therapy session is clearly identified. Showing the child a map of the therapist's intended destination may also attenuate distress and confusion about the therapist's whereabouts. These strategies begin to alleviate the child's fear that the therapist may reject or forget the youngster. They also promote the internalization of the mental representation of the therapist as a reliable and consistent figure, especially when the child finds that the therapist has returned as promised.

PROMOTING OBJECT CONSTANCY

Maltreated children exposed to a great deal of inconsistency and neglect sometimes have great difficulty in maintaining an image of the therapist or even the therapy room in their minds (i.e., object constancy). They believe they will never see the therapist again or that the therapist will change significantly in personality or behavior from one session to another. There are several concrete strategies to help children cope with anxiety generated between weekly sessions. A calendar can show the child the date of the next weekly session. An appointment slip with the therapist's and child's names on it serves the same purpose; the child takes the slip home as a reminder that another appointment is scheduled. Sometimes a child can benefit by taking home a small object as a "souvenir" of the therapist and the therapy sessions. The child brings the object, such as a pencil, back to the next session and exchanges it for another small token. It is unwise to allow the child to take home toys from the therapy room, particularly if other clients regularly use them or if a certain toy is associated with significant issues or feelings for the child. In the latter situation, taking the toy home may escalate anxiety or acting out at home. The toy should be left in the therapy room to contain these feelings. Another prop we have used are photographs of the child and ourselves. The child can take the photograph home as a concrete reminder of the relationship and its importance to each participant. Some children are reassured by receiving pictures of their names drawn in fancy calligraphy by the therapist, and others put one of their drawings on the therapist's wall to remind the therapist of them during the week, thereby gaining reassurance that the therapist will not forget about them.

We can also enlist parents or other caregivers as effective collaborators in interventions to help children who have problems with object constancy.

Joan, an 8-year-old girl, had been removed from her mother's care because of psychological maltreatment, especially verbal abuse, neglect, and frequent episodes during which she was abandoned for prolonged periods and left to fend for herself. Her mother had been diagnosed with a bipolar illness. After being placed in foster care and beginning school, Joan's behavior in the classroom began to undergo a notable deterioration near the end of each school day. She became defiant and oppositional and had great difficulty in concentrating on academic tasks. She subsequently revealed to her therapist that she was afraid her foster mother would not pick her up at the end of the school day as promised. The child worried that her foster mother might forget about her, even though the foster mother had never failed to pick her up and in fact usually arrived a few minutes before dismissal. She also anticipated that her foster mother's personality might change so drastically between the morning and the end of the school day that she would abuse Joan (a reflection of her exposure to her mother's bipolar illness). To promote and consolidate Joan's belief that her foster mother would be reliable, predictable, and caring, the therapist recommended that the foster mother arrange to have a picture taken of her and Joan doing a positive activity. The foster mother subsequently arranged for such a photograph, and Joan's teacher permitted her to tape it prominently on her desk. The therapist instructed Joan to look at the picture each time she began to feel worried about her foster mother's commitment and to think of the times when she had appeared at school at the appointed time. This strategy resulted in a significant decrease in Joan's anxiety.

Young children require such concrete cues and reminders so that these more abstract concepts become relevant and meaningful, a theme to which we will return repeatedly throughout the rest of the book.

DEALING WITH PROVOCATIVE BEHAVIOR

Early in therapy, some maltreated children begin to test whether the therapist will provide them with a measure of safety and protection. Is the therapist someone who will protect the child from acting out strong feelings in provocative, dangerous, and unhealthy ways? Is the therapist someone who will react to provocations with firm yet appropriate responses? Sometimes telling children about basic rules (e.g., "We aren't allowed to hurt each other or break anything in the room") diminishes their anxiety about being permitted to act out strong feelings and urges in whatever way they desire. However, providing children with an elaborate set of rules may constitute a challenge to those who need to test the therapist. Interactions in the engagement phase characterized primarily by contention and conflict detract from the therapist's efforts to form a therapeutic alliance. It is usually more beneficial to present a minimum of rules and then deal with further incidents and infractions as they arise.

Children use varied and often creative ways to test limits. Some engage in daredevil and reckless behavior, such as climbing up the shelves of the play therapy room. When confronted with this behavior, the therapist should quickly and firmly insist that the child stop, pointing out the potential dangers to the child's safety and emphasizing that the therapist does not want the child to be hurt. The therapist should show a willingness to take the steps necessary to ensure the child's safety and should suggest alternate behaviors, such as helping the child stand on a chair to reach for a toy on an upper shelf. Many of these children have never had parents or caregivers who were this solicitous about their welfare, and the therapist's actions not only are concrete demonstrations of caring and commitment, but constitute discrepant information that may counter archaic IWMs/IS. Still other children become physically aggressive or try to engage the therapist in sexual behavior to determine whether the therapist will physically or sexually abuse them. Although we discuss this issue more in depth in subsequent sections of this chapter, it is important to note here that the therapist should curtail any such behavior quickly and in a straightforward and matter-of-fact way.

PHYSICAL CONTACT WITH ABUSED AND NEGLECTED CHILDREN

The therapist should exercise considerable caution in touching an abused or maltreated child. Such a gesture, although well intended, may be misinterpreted by the child as a sexual advance or physical threat. Some maltreated children are extraordinarily sensitive to any form of touching by an adult and are primed by their past histories to interpret such actions as precursors to overt physical or sexual abuse. Young victims who have experienced long-standing sexual molestation may be unable to discriminate between sexual and nonsexual touching. However, some children crave physical contact with the therapist because of their chronic histories of psychological and emotional neglect and exhibit the indiscriminate friendliness we discussed earlier. In the case of the child deprived of physical affection, the therapist must introduce other forms of positive interaction, such as a special handshake. The child's indiscriminate physical contact must be limited. The therapist's failure to stop such behavior places the child at future risk for exploitation by adults who prey on dependent children.

Some sexually abused children have learned to gain attention and affection from others primarily through sexual means, and they make direct sexual advances toward the therapist. Therapists must quickly and effectively curtail these indiscriminate advances. Sexual advances may also be a test of the therapist's boundaries and whether he or she will respond sexually to the child (Van de Putte, 1995). Furthermore, allowing this behavior just escalates the child's anxiety and places the therapist in jeopardy of being accused of improper conduct. The therapist should explain that he or she knows that the child had a relationship with an adult involving sexual activity and that sexual feelings in general are normal. However, the therapist must be emphatic in asserting that the relationship between the child and the therapist will never include this kind of contact. In this new relationship, they will communicate by means of talking and playing, and the child should understand that he or she has no need to use sexual behavior to establish a nurturing relationship with an adult. The therapist can teach the sexualized child more appropriate forms of physical contact, such as a handshake. Children's sexualized behavior sometimes generates intense feelings and reactions in the therapist. Chapter 12 describes strategies available to therapists in coping with their own emotions and issues elicited by this demanding and difficult clinical work.

COUNTERING REGRESSIVE BEHAVIOR

During the engagement phase, some maltreated children recount many details of their victimization. Doing this may elicit painful memories and feelings that threaten to overwhelm their fragile self-regulatory capacities. Consequently, their symptoms may increase or they may begin to show even more regressive behavior. Although we discuss this topic in more detail in Chapter 8, we note here that the therapist must structure sessions tightly and control their pace to ensure that these youngsters are not overwhelmed. The therapist can restrict these discussions to a limited portion of each session and request that the child deal with only one memory or issue per discussion. The rest of the session should be devoted to less intense activities such as nondirective play (James, 1994).

Ten minutes or so should be reserved at the end of each session to ensure that the child is behaving more maturely before leaving. It is undesirable for a child who has been acting like an infant and demanding feedings from a baby bottle to leave the session in that state and then have to cope with classroom demands. The therapist might tell the child that this part of the session is over and the play must now stop. At the same time, he or she can encourage more mature behavior, such as having the child help clean up the playroom. The therapist and child can discuss the demands to be faced in the next several hours and how the child can best meet them. Allowing a child to leave a session in a highly regressed or distressed state is a real disservice. Some closure at the end of each therapy session is necessary to promote adaptive functioning in the everyday world. Again, closing rituals help by symbolically containing the sensitive and painful therapeutic material elicited in the session. For example, as described earlier, the child might place art productions in a special folder and "pack it away" until the next session.

Being Empathic about the Child's Affective Expression

By articulating an understanding of the child's feelings, the therapist begins modifying the child's expectation that others will be insensitive and unaware of his or her internal states. The therapist might start this process in the first session. Because of various factors, including fears and expectations of being maltreated, the child may be highly anxious during the first several sessions. By commenting simply and directly about the anxiety (e.g., "It's scary when you think that you might have to talk about what happened to you") and explaining the reasons for therapy and what will transpire during sessions, the therapist not only clarifies the therapeutic process and expectations for participation, but demonstrates sensitivity to the child's fears and anxiety. Other types of therapist behavior reinforce an understanding and appreciation of the child's plight. With a highly anxious child, the therapist might leave the office or playroom door ajar so that the child feels a sense of safety (i.e., the child feels he or she can readily escape or that others outside will be able to monitor therapist and child interaction to ensure the child's safety), while at the same time verbalizing these underlying affects. We have already talked about maintaining appropriate physical distance from the child so as not to elicit even more anxiety about possible further physical or sexual abuse. Therapists should be careful that they do not "corner" or tower over their young clients, actions that merely reinforce children's vulnerability and powerlessness. Having a supportive adult or parent present for the initial therapy sessions also allows a child to relax. The therapist encourages the adult to gradually leave the room as the child begins feeling more comfortable in the therapist's presence.

Even when setting limits on physically aggressive or sexually inappropriate behavior, the therapist can still convey an understanding of the child's internal world. The key is to validate the child's underlying affects while assisting him or her to develop more appropriate ways of expressing these feelings. For example, the therapist might comment about the normalcy of the intense rage and anger of a child who attempts to break toys while talking about his or her physical abuse. At the same time, the therapist must quickly intervene to stop this destructive behavior and propose other ways to ventilate the rage. Likewise, the therapist should convey the notion that sexual feelings are normal and that the child is not perverted or depraved, while placing firm and consistent limits on inappropriate expression of the sexual feelings. These strategies allow the child to begin thinking of the therapist as someone who not only accepts his or her feelings but also cares enough to ensure that the child will not act them out harmfully or inappropriately.

As well as promoting modifications of the child's IWM/IS, the therapist's sensitivity and attunement to the child's affective states facilitates the development of internal state language, theory of mind, and reflective functioning. Chapter 2 reviewed the role of these essential components for adaptive emotional and behavioral self-regulation. Hughes (2004) offers a rich description of these processes:

> The child's affective response to the experience is being co-regulated by the parent's affective response, and the child's attention is being held by the parent's attentive stance. As parents respond to their child's affective states, nonverbally and verbally, they mark the affect with an empathic, congruent response, which creates within the child a secondary representation of the original raw affect and leads to the capacity for reflective thought (Fonagy,

> Gergely, Jurist, & Target, 2002). They are also providing words for them to be able to gradually identify and more fully express their inner life. (p. 266)

The therapist's empathic responses and emotional attunement, central themes that are woven into the remaining chapters, represent basic mechanisms of change.

The Role of Play in the Engagement Phase

For children who are particularly frightened of therapy or more direct interactions with the therapist, play often provides a medium through which they can begin to communicate with and relate to the therapist. The second half of this chapter is devoted to a more detailed discussion of the use of the therapeutic relationship with these avoidant children. However, we think it is appropriate to make several comments here about the use of play in the engagement phase.

Nonverbal interactions may help the child become more comfortable with the therapist. Rather than subjecting the child to direct questions and inquiries, the therapist should follow the child's lead and pace during these play activities. The therapist conveys sensitivity and empathy to the child's feelings by mirroring the child's body language and/or vocal quality (Hughes, 2004). The therapist also demonstrates interest and encourages the development of verbal expression by reflecting or paraphrasing the child's statements (Brady & Friedrich, 1982) and by asking questions, even about mundane issues, that convey a genuine interest in the child's world. A choice of play activities or materials gives the child a sense of control over what happens during therapy sessions, thereby increasing the child's sense of safety. Initially, children may choose activities in which they are confident they will meet with some success. Sometimes these activities may be characteristic of a much younger child's play because the youngster expects that success is possible only with simple and unsophisticated materials and failure is inevitable with anything more difficult. Although therapists should allow this activity for a time, they should gently encourage the child to try an activity that will challenge his or her abilities. However, the activity must be one that is likely to bring the child some success. There is also a fine line between pushing a child too strenuously to the point of eliciting overwhelming anxiety and allowing the child to repeat activities with little or no therapeutic purpose. The latter does nothing to raise the child's self-esteem or make therapy a profitable or positive experience.

Let us return now to 11-year-old Peter, whom we introduced at the beginning of this chapter.

By the second session, the therapist and Peter agreed he should come to therapy to work on some of his problems but that he needed an opportunity to get to know the therapist better before he would discuss or address these issues. Peter quite readily agreed to spend several sessions with the therapist in the playroom in order to "check out" what therapy would be like. During the first therapy session, Peter played with large building blocks that much younger children typically use. He built extremely simple constructions and resisted gentle suggestions to build something more complicated. He eventually found a checkers game and commented that he was quite a good player. However, he refused an invitation to play the game but reluctantly agreed to play in the next therapy session. In fact, Peter was quite an astute player, but he commented about making stupid moves and stated several times that he knew he was going to lose. The therapist empathized with his fears of losing and feelings of inadequacy, which resulted in a more extended discussion of Peter's concerns that everyone thought he was stupid. He believed that his substandard school performance was incontrovertible proof of poor cognitive abilities.

In the third play therapy session, the therapist suggested they play Chinese checkers, a game with which Peter was unfamiliar. Peter immediately insisted he would never be able to learn the game. However, he agreed that, at a minimum, he would listen to the therapist's explanations and then decide whether he wanted to play. Although still anxious, he finally agreed to play a game. Despite losing, Peter made a number of good moves. The therapist commented on how quickly Peter caught on to the game, cited some of these moves as concrete evidence of his ability, and overall spoke of his confidence that Peter's game would improve. Peter agreed to play a second game and in fact won, which left him obviously pleased.

These initial sessions allowed Peter to begin establishing a therapeutic alliance in which he began to feel safe, accepted, and validated. Rather than laughing at his initial attempts to play the new game, the therapist gave gentle encouragement and instruction that resulted in some success. Peter encountered his first successes in the playroom, which made his participation in therapy more appealing. Furthermore, Peter actually had some fun with this adult who, although conscious not to overwhelm him with too much attention, given Peter's fears of closeness and intimacy, maintained a warm and accepting attitude. This stance reinforced the attraction of the therapist and the therapy process for this young boy. Scrutiny of interactions between Peter and the therapist revealed a number of the therapist ingredients identified by Ackerman and Hilsenroth (2003) as facilitative of a positive therapeutic alliance: warmth, confidence, being interested and open, encouraging the expression of feelings and reflecting on them, and empathy.

These qualities and interventions not only began to engender a positive therapeutic alliance but constituted change processes themselves, First, the therapist's sensitivity to Peter's deep sense of insecurity and inadequacy and his permitting Peter some control over the play activities began to diminish Peter's expectation that adults, particularly men, would subject him to further abuse, humiliation, and degradation. Second, by giving voice to Peter's underlying feelings of inadequacy, the therapist helped this boy to understand his own internal life, and he modeled and encouraged Peter in the use of words to express feelings, rather than dysregulated patterns of aggression and defiance.

TEACHING NEGLECTED CHILDREN HOW TO PLAY

As just mentioned, these initial play therapy sessions should be fun so as to encourage the child's interest in participating in therapy. Similarly, the child must experience some degree of success, even if it is with activities such as simple board games. Successes counter feelings of stigmatization and personal failure that often accompany the beginning of the therapeutic process. However, some maltreated children encounter serious difficulty in succeeding with even simple play activities. Typically, these are children subjected to profound deprivation and neglect who never learned how to play. When brought into the playroom, they are unimaginative, inhibited, confused, and unable to use toys or equipment purposefully. Rather than allowing a child to stand immobilized, thereby compounding feelings of failure and inadequacy, the therapist must take the initiative and teach the child how to play. For example, the therapist can teach the child to use paints, building blocks, or other simple materials. The therapist might model the activity and then gently encourage the child to begin participating along with the therapist, while reinforcing the child's attempts to take some initiative in the play.

Over the years, we have formed the clinical impression that children who have been severely physically or psychologically neglected are often preoccupied with food. They frequently worry that they will not get sufficient food and engage in behavior like hyperphagia (increased food intake), stealing, and hoarding food. There is some support for this observation in the literature. Demb (1991) identified a subsample of children in foster care because of parental substance abuse. Their foster mothers reported that they had an excessive appetite for food. Furthermore, the consumption had a driven quality, and there was an apparent lack of satiety, as well as frequent eating to the point of gastric pain or vomiting if food intake was not externally limited. We wonder if food is equated with psychological nurturance for some children raised in environments characterized by emotional and physical deprivation. Clinicians can profitably incorporate food into the treatment plan of severely deprived children. Children respond positively to small snacks at the beginning or end of each session in the early phase of treatment. Food serves as evidence that the therapist is sensitive to the child's needs and demonstrates commitment to the youngster. Food may also bring clinical issues into prominence during sessions. For example, the child may devour a snack voraciously and angrily demand more. This behavior may be an opportunity for the therapist to articulate the child's anger, which is elicited when the youngster is "not getting enough," and his or her disappointment when the therapist cannot meet all of the child's massive needs.

THE MIDDLE PHASE OF THERAPY

The middle phase offers the therapist more opportunities to modify the child's IWM/IS. Here we discuss the use of the therapeutic relationship as a tool to help children who display a number of features of different attachment organizations. Our ideas and thoughts build on an earlier article (Pearce & Pezzot-Pearce, 1994) and the first edition of this book (Pearce & Pezzot-Pearce, 1997) and are derived from some of the basic tenets and ideas of attachment theory. We begin with a review of strategies that clinicians can use within the context of the therapeutic relationship with children who show characteristics of an avoidant attachment organization, including those who also have features of a disorganized attachment. We conclude the chapter with a review of other considerations in treating children with insecure attachments.

Children with an Avoidant/Disorganized Attachment Organization

Children with an avoidant/disorganized attachment organization fear further rejection or maltreatment from attachment figures and block information about their own feelings and emotions. We have seen children display elements of this avoidance in the therapeutic relationship. For example, a child may play quite independently, rarely inviting the therapist to join in. The therapist is on the sidelines, watching rather than participating. The child makes little eye contact and maintains considerable psychological distance. Expecting the therapist to hurt, reject, or disappoint him or her as others have previously, the child avoids interactions as a protection from the consequences of a close relationship. Peter's indifference to the therapist in the initial sessions probably reflects this strategy. He did not want to become involved because his previous experiences with other people, especially his mother and stepfather, generated expectations that he would be hurt again and that others would not recognize or alleviate his distress. Peter also avoided acknowledging and expressing his intense and sometimes conflicting feelings, or needs for comfort and assistance. These represented understandable reactions to his expectation that sensitive caregiving would not be forthcoming in response to any distress he might show.

The child engages in other interactional patterns to avoid a truly reciprocal or close relationship with the therapist. By behaving in a controlling, omnipotent fashion in therapy sessions, the child feels mastery and control over the interaction wherein even more maltreatment is expected (Cassidy & Mohr, 2001; Hughes, 2004). For example, the child chooses the play materials and activities and relegates the therapist to a minor role. This pattern is often characteristic of children with a disorganized attachment classification. As we reviewed earlier, a disorganized classification is assigned as an additional code to one of the organized classifications, and Peter's social relationships and representations of relationships are consistent with an avoidant/disorganized classification. We return to a description of some other early sessions in Peter's therapy that illustrate these patterns.

After participating in several sessions during which he insisted on playing Chinese checkers (and winning many games, which probably facilitated engagement), Peter began to engage in dramatic play for several months. Peter's relationship with the therapist during these sessions reflected his reluctance to become engaged in a relationship marked by reciprocal interaction. Despite the therapist's request to become more involved in the play, Peter adamantly told the therapist that his role was to be the audience. He was to sit quietly while Peter pretended he was "Superman," but also had to provide him, on cue, with praise and approval for his strength and power. As Superman, Peter portrayed himself as a powerful figure who could fend off all attackers that inevitably returned to assault other characters in the play. He placed much emphasis on his physical prowess, rolling up his sleeves, flexing his muscles, pretending to pick up objects such as cars and buildings, and protecting weaker and more vulnerable individuals.

Peter repeatedly insisted on enacting this play scenario and rigidly enforced the therapist's minimal involvement for many weeks. The therapeutic relationship underwent a significant change when Peter asked the therapist to play the role of the "bad guy." This play, which lasted for approximately 2 months, invariably began in each session with Peter telling the therapist to think of increasingly devious ways of abducting or hurting small plastic animal figures. These figures were usually defenseless creatures like puppies or birds. As Superman, Peter "rescued" the animals from the therapist, who always had to portray a menacing and dangerous figure. This play culminated in a session during which Peter introduced interpersonal disputes in the play as targets worthy of Superman's intervention. Once, Peter used small dolls and a dollhouse to enact a quarrel between a boy and his mother. As Superman, Peter intervened and essentially acted like a referee to help the two individuals resolve the dispute.

There are several important and salient aspects of Peter's play. The interaction with the therapist at the beginning was minimal. Moreover, Peter placed the therapist on the periphery by maintaining strict control over what the therapist could do and say, as he expected that the interaction might lead to aversive or harmful consequences, which reflected elements of the controlling–punitive disorganized attachment pattern. After engaging in this play in which he gained some control and mastery, Peter felt a greater sense of safety and security in the therapist's presence. He then began to involve the therapist more actively in the play, although Peter was still in charge and continued to protect himself from the therapist, who remained the "bad guy."

The content of Peter's play is also significant. His portrayal of the world as a malevolent, threatening place where people are repeatedly assaulted in such an invariant sequence reflects his history of maltreatment and is characteristic of posttraumatic play. It is also similar to the "chaotic" stories told by youngsters with a controlling–disorganized attachment classification. In the guise of Superman, Peter attempted to use the play to gain a sense of control over these traumatic events.

The therapist can use several strategies to counteract the child's fear of establishing and maintaining a close therapeutic relationship. First, the therapist must respect the child's reliance on the defensive use of avoidance. Insisting prematurely that the child openly and directly express feelings may lead to a rapid escalation of anxiety to the point where avoidance becomes even more entrenched. Likewise, confronting the child too quickly with demands for closeness, such as pressing for a full and detailed disclosure of the maltreatment, may also result in a deterioration of behavior. Feeling so threatened, the child may become even more oppositional, defiant, or outrageous so as to alienate the therapist.

Allowing children a large measure of control in choosing play materials and activities in the initial sessions also attenuates their anxiety. If the therapist had insisted upon directing or controlling the play at this early stage, Peter's anxiety might have escalated quite significantly, given his expectation that the risk for being reabused increases as a function of a relationship in which people insist on strict compliance with their demands. His attempts to control the therapeutic relationship may have become even more pronounced to avert any further abuse. In the past, closeness with another male, his stepfather, was associated with some disastrous consequences. By having a sense of control and safety, the youngster may begin regarding the therapist in a more positive light. Here is someone who understands the child's fear of intimacy and closeness. This person is willing to gradually establish a relationship in a manner that does not threaten to overwhelm the youngster with anxiety and fear. This may well be the start of the process whereby negative IWMs/IS are modified.

As in the engagement stage, it is critically important for the therapist to follow through with any promises made to the child. For example, in one early play session in which he pretended to be Superman, Peter wished aloud that he had a red cape. To show his trustworthiness and commitment, the therapist told Peter that he would bring some red cloth for a cape to the next session. When Peter entered the playroom the next week and found the cloth, he looked at the therapist and exclaimed, "You really did it!" The therapist responded that Peter was surprised that somebody would follow through with a promise, and Peter agreed that this was indeed the case. In response to inquiries about people who had disappointed him in the past, Peter identified his stepfather. Although unwilling to talk about the sexual assaults in this session, Peter told the therapist that before his stepfather and mother married, he had promised to participate in sports activities with Peter but later reneged on his promise. While recounting this incident, Peter looked and sounded sad. Although he did not pursue the matter any further in the session, Peter quietly agreed with the therapist's statement about how sad and disappointed he felt and looked. This particular interaction between Peter and the therapist was a springboard from which they could discuss other salient aspects of relationships that had not met his needs and was the first occasion when Peter acknowledged feelings of loss. It was followed in the months ahead with more direct discussions of these and other feelings.

This episode was another example of the therapist helping Peter begin to understand his feelings, which previously were a source of real confusion, and to develop more appropriate ways of expressing them, rather than by being aggressive. Peter talked about his sadness, especially in response to the therapist's empathic remarks. This helped promote his growing confidence that the therapist would ensure that he did not lose control when he became upset in sessions or become reckless or destructive. Consequently, Peter became more engaged in a therapeutic process that helped him to develop these internal controls. Therapy had now become a safer endeavor, and Peter had come to see the therapist as a secure base from which he could explore these previously frightening themes.

The therapist's empathic response to these concerns demonstrated that he was listening keenly to Peter and making a concentrated effort to understand what Peter was trying to say. Bringing the material for the cape constituted concrete evidence of the therapist's commitment to helping him, and both this gesture and the therapist's empathy offered information about social relationships discrepant from the evidence that served as the basis of his IWM/IS. The therapist's sensitivity and his follow-through with the promise to Peter the week before were two examples of many actions the therapist would repeat over time. They helped this boy reformulate his expectations of others so that he would no longer approach new social relationships with the fear, apprehension, and pessimism that were reflected in his emotionally distant and sometimes defiant and oppositional manner of relating.

Of course, there are occasions when we fail to empathize with a child's feelings or interpret them accurately. There are a number of reasons for this failure, such as that none of us are infallible or omniscient, our clients sometimes express what is bothering them in obtuse ways, especially if their expressive language abilities are poor, and a myriad of other reasons. Such failures, inevitable in the course of therapy, offer another opportunity to help children modify their IWMs/IS.

In one session Peter complained loudly about a substitute teacher who he believed was being unfair to him, a perception associated with a marked increase in his defiant and oppositional behavior at school that followed a period in which Peter's behavior had shown some significant improvement. The therapist immediately focused on helping Peter identify strategies he could use to curtail his defiance in the classroom, to which Peter responded with a mixture of frustration and exasperation: "You're not even listening to me!" In his rush to help his young client return to a better level of functioning, the therapist had not listened to what Peter was trying to articulate—that is, his feelings of sadness and rejection stemming from his perception that the new teacher did not like him. Once he finally caught on, the therapist apologized to Peter and empathized with the anger and frustration activated by the therapist's insensitivity, commenting, "You got really mad when I didn't try to understand what you were telling me." The apology and simple statement affirmed the accuracy of Peter's perception that the therapist had not picked up on his feelings, and the empathic response to his anger further consolidated Peter's understanding of his inner life and use of words to express his feelings.

The therapist wanted to help Peter relate this incident to other past situations and draw out differences so as to counter his expectation that others will react insensitively to his expressions of feelings. The therapist wondered aloud if other people in the past had not understood what Peter was telling them. Peter recounted several incidents when his mother and stepfather had either ignored or misinterpreted his expressions of strong affect, and sometimes had even hit him. In response to the therapist's inquiry about whether his parents had ever expressed any regret or apologies for their insensitivity, Peter could not recall any, but when asked, he described accurately the therapist's apology and added that the therapist knew he was mad because he didn't understand what Peter was telling him. He agreed with the therapist's following statement: "So even though I made a mistake and didn't understand what you were saying, I said I was sorry and knew you were angry with me. Although everybody makes mistakes with other people at times, some people figure out they screwed up and they mean it when they say they're sorry. I guess everyone isn't like your parents, who had trouble doing that."

Chapter 10 describes cognitive-behavioral strategies to help children like Peter critically analyze and modify their attributions and IWMs/IS, not only in the context of the therapeutic relationship but vis-à-vis everyday relationships outside of therapy. This is often a central task of therapy, given the importance of these pathogenic processes for adaptive functioning.

At this point, the child may be more tolerant of the therapist's participation in sessions and of his or her attempts to form a relationship. Rather than taking the nondirective approach that characterized initial sessions, now the therapist should try to become more involved and interactive, albeit gradually. The intent is to expose the child to increasingly larger doses of positive interaction to ease fears of close relationships and the ensuing avoidance of interaction. Becoming a more desirable person to the child may also restimulate the child's need for other relationships of a similar nature.

Some common play themes emerge that offer further opportunities to reinforce the therapist's representation in the child's inner world as positive and helpful. The child may begin to nurture him- or herself: nursing on a baby bottle, feeding baby dolls, and taking care of sick or wounded animals or protecting them, as Peter did, from abusive and menacing adversaries are common play themes of maltreated children (Frazier & Levine, 1983; Mills & Allan, 1992). One notable aspect of this play is that the child is in control. The youngster assumes the role of the protector in the play, thereby gaining a vicarious sense of nurturance and gratification. The child cannot let the therapist nurture yet because of beliefs and expectations that adults are unresponsive, unreliable, and unwilling to care for children in this manner.

After reenacting many episodes of protecting small animals from physical danger and solving interpersonal disputes, Peter began to have Superman care for and nurture individuals in other ways. As Superman, he hosted a birthday party for his elderly grandmother, to which the therapist was invited. Using toy food, Peter prepared a banquet for everyone. However, Peter made it clear that he still regarded the world as dangerous. He announced that there were wild animals outside the house where the birthday party was held and instructed the therapist to "act scared." He went out of the house on several occasions and calmed these animals with a mere glance and a few brief words of warning.

Peter was beginning to allow himself to relate more closely to others (exemplified by inviting the therapist and imaginary grandmother to the birthday party and feeding them). However, he continued to control this interaction because he still viewed the world as dangerous and threatening: his controlling stance alleviated his anxiety activated by the prospect of being hurt again. For children like Peter, relationships are characterized by ambivalence: the child longs for nurturance and attention but remains frightened about becoming too close and therefore more vulnerable.

The therapist began to give voice to these conflicting sentiments. In his role as a guest, the therapist stated he felt "really good" when people cooked wonderful foods for him (validating Peter's desire for nurturance), but added he felt "scared" by the presence of the wild animals outside and wondered aloud whether he would be safe. He said that having someone like Superman to "take care of me" made him feel better. These comments empathized with Peter's fear of being hurt again and his desire for a strong, powerful figure who would protect him from harm. Verbally articulating or somehow identifying and expressing these feelings is an important component of treatment for the avoidant child who routinely disconnects from these affective states. By articulating them in the play, the therapist brings such feelings into consciousness and provides an opportunity for the child to ultimately gain some control over their influence. Furthermore, talking initially about these conflicted feelings as if they belonged to someone else (i.e., the therapist's role as guest at the birthday party) was more tolerable to Peter. If the therapist had brought this material out of the metaphor at an earlier stage, he might have elicited too much pain and distress. Peter might have avoided this play in subsequent sessions to protect himself from the anxiety generated by interpretations that were too direct. The therapist who expresses these conflicting feelings, either directly or via indirect metaphorical methods, is again modeling a more adaptive way of expressing them and promotes the child's growing ability to regulate behavior and affects.

The therapist should not allow the child to continue to play the role of exclusive nurturer indefinitely. The therapist must initiate interaction that demonstrates goodwill and a willingness to meet some of the child's emotional and psychological needs. For example, the therapist might offer to prepare some food for the child who is feeding a baby doll. If the child seems comfortable with such relatively nonintrusive attempts to be more nurturing, the therapist can eventually offer to feed the baby. As we have commented, children may prepare elaborate meals for themselves and the therapist. Initially the child is in charge of providing this nurturance because of minimal trust in the therapist's ability or willingness to care for the child this way; the child has to do it to make sure it gets done. The therapist might begin taking a more active role by first offering a few menu suggestions, offering to prepare one or two dishes, then preparing most, if not all, of the meal, and subsequently serving it to the child, who is treated like an honored and valued guest. These strategies may be beneficially applied to children displaying a controlling–caregiving pattern. Their sense of responsibility for the therapist's welfare may be reflected in this symbolic play, wherein they nurture, feed, and generally take care of the therapist.

Peter continued to host these birthday parties, for which he made all the preparations. After Peter assumed this exclusive role in several parties, the therapist suggested that he, as a guest, be allowed to bring one dish to the party in order to "help out," because Peter had so much work to do. Peter agreed and seemed pleased when the therapist prepared his own pretend food. Each week, the therapist suggested that he prepare more food and Peter agreed.

As the therapist began to play a greater role in the play, Peter began to invite other guests to these parties, including some small animals (the weak, defenseless creatures whom he had previously protected from all sorts of danger and harm). Peter pretended these animals had a great deal of fun at the parties and had them become increasingly interactive with the therapist. Initially, he had each animal figure physically approach the therapist, then putting each one on the therapist's arms and shoulders. While doing so, Peter portrayed them as shy and retiring. He agreed with the therapist's remark that some of them had difficulty "trusting" the therapist because they were uncertain of whether he would hurt them. Immediately after this comment from the therapist, Peter stuffed a small bunny into the sleeve of the therapist's shirt. He stated that the bunny did this because she wanted to smell him [the therapist] to get to know him better.

After several more weeks of this play, Peter began to enact a series of vignettes that were more direct reflections of his ambivalence about trusting others, particularly paternal figures. Peter called this play "father and son." He assumed the role of the son and the therapist was the father. The son demanded lots of toys from the father, who met these symbolic demands for attention, love, and nurturance. Besides the father giving the son these gifts, they had fun together on the beach and built sand castles in the sandbox. This play was an expression of Peter's longing for the idealized parent who would provide the nurturance, caring, and protection he had so sorely lacked in his early years. It was accompanied by more direct expressions of Peter's growing affection for the therapist. He began to initiate some physical contact, such as putting his hand on the therapist's shoulder. He expressed a desire to prolong the weekly sessions and once left a note in the therapy room to the therapist saying that he liked him.

However, Peter's fear and anxiety about closeness with the therapist reemerged in subsequent sessions. He began to test the therapist's commitment. Peter knocked the therapist's marker off a board game so forcefully that it flew across the room, refused to leave sessions, and was somewhat rude. Unfortunately, this behavior coincided with the beginning of the therapist's summer vacation. When the therapist explained he would see Peter one more time before a 4-week holiday break, Peter immediately and angrily responded that he never wanted to return for another session. However, he could not articulate any specific reasons for this statement. The therapist empathized with Peter's anger regarding his absence. He normalized it and said he understood why Peter was so angry about not being able to see someone he liked. When the therapist firmly told Peter that he would be returning, the boy seemed relieved but needed to take home a small souvenir to reassure himself of their relationship.

At this point, the therapist could talk directly with Peter about his fears of becoming too close to the therapist. Although intellectually aware that the reason for the 4-week break was the therapist's vacation plans, Peter expressed fear that the therapist might forget about him or no longer want to see him. Although he enjoyed his closer relationship with the therapist, it filled him with anxiety. He and the therapist talked about the differences between the way Peter was treated by his stepfather and how he was treated by the therapist. Peter and the therapist were able to identify many previous occasions when the therapist had proven his commitment to Peter. This was the first discussion of many that enabled Peter to think about and critically identify his unconscious assumption (i.e., the IS) that the therapist and others would mistreat him as his stepfather had.

When therapy resumed after the vacation, Peter could tolerate more direct discussions of the therapeutic relationship. In particular, he discussed how his fear of closeness was sometimes associated with behavior in therapy sessions that was designed to push away the therapist and test his ongoing commitment. They identified similar behavior that he used in other relationships when he expected people to reject or abuse him. The frequency of this provocative behavior declined as Peter became more cognizant of his unconscious reliance on this strategy and the IS on which it was based, and as his emotional and behavioral self-regulation capacities increased.

As we have already noted, the child's nascent belief about the reliability and trustworthiness of others may be tenuous at best. For example, the child may introduce calamities (e.g., the therapist and child are attacked by monsters) during a play episode in which the therapist is symbolically nurturing the child. For several weeks, Peter pretended that pirates attacked the father and son while they played on the beach. As the son, he took the lead in protecting them, but the pirates abruptly and unexpectedly attacked again after Peter had defeated them. This is reminiscent of the "chaotic" play of controlling–disorganized children. Catastrophes and dangers arise and, although vanquished, they emerge repeatedly. This pattern, and in particular the abrupt shifts, suggest that Peter was still having difficulty in successfully defending himself or resolving anxiety. Although he showed many features of an avoidant attachment organization, his play reflected disorganization and dysregulation of defensive strategies. Peter had to fight these adversaries to restore a sense of control and power over interactions that he still regarded with a fair measure of skepticism.

Although the therapist attempted to create a warm, positive, and accepting therapeutic environment (common factors, as described above) from the beginning of therapy with Peter, he intervened with specific strategies. As we saw, the therapist began taking more initiative to increase their positive interaction, demonstrating to Peter that others could be trusted to meet his needs, and drawing the distinction between the therapeutic relationship and previous ones where his needs went unmet and caregivers reacted to his distress by ignoring and sometimes abusing him. The therapist helped Peter identify some reasons for his avoidant pattern, the conditions in which he used it to cope with anxiety and fear about intimacy, and to critically question his assumption that others were going to hurt him as his stepfather had. The therapist began to articulate these affective states to help Peter identify and develop more appropriate ways to express his conflicting feelings about relationships. For example, talking about his fear that the therapist would forget him during the 4-week vacation and ultimately reject him was a more adaptive coping mechanism than acting out to create much-needed distance in the relationship.

Fortunately, Peter's mother was able to effect some changes in the way she parented her son. She became more consistently available to him, set firmer and more consistent limits on his defiant and oppositional behavior, and became more empathic and sensitive to his anxiety and fear. Peter's therapy included many other important components, especially interventions to reduce his proclivity to act out sexually and to modify his misattributions about why his stepfather had sexually abused him, as well as anxiety management strategies. We believe the therapeutic relationship helped this young boy overcome some of the more serious developmental effects associated with his maltreatment history. The therapeutic relationship, in both its direct and indirect forms, introduced an element of discontinuity into Peter's life and helped him modify these skewed and biased IWMs/IS, as well as facilitating emotional and behavioral self-regulation;

therapy was ultimately supported and complemented by other favorable and positive experiences in his environment.

Other Considerations in Treating Children with Insecure Attachment Organizations

DEPENDENCE AND INDISCRIMINATE BEHAVIOR

There is considerable empirical support for the notion that relatively low maternal availability is associated with the ambivalent–resistant pattern of attachment (Cassidy & Berlin, 1994). In response to a parent who is minimally or inconsistently responsive, the infant heightens emotional arousal to gain parental attention. As well, the extreme dependence of these infants can be regarded as another strategy to gain the mother's response. Goldberg (1991) described the characteristics of older children who are classified as dependent–preoccupied (ambivalent–resistant). Like infants, they are preoccupied with the parent–child relationship at the expense of other activities, notably that of exploring the environment. The child and parent seem engaged in a constant struggle for control, and the child may appear whiny and contentious. Alternatively, the child may emphasize his or her dependence with extreme coyness (e.g., whispering) or feigned helplessness.

Similar interactional qualities emerge in the therapeutic relationship. In Chapter 4 we reviewed the characteristics of a disinhibited attachment disorder, including the indiscriminate friendliness that is a hallmark of this subtype and usually associated with having been raised in a neglectful environment. Initially, the child may become overdependent on the therapist, such as in requesting the therapist's phone number or address, and evidencing great difficulty in leaving a session. However, there usually comes a point in therapy when the child realizes that the therapist cannot meet all these massive dependence needs. At this point, the rage and anger originally elicited by unrewarding interactions with primary attachment figures are directed to the therapist. The child may interpret the therapist's inability to meet these needs as yet another manifestation of the basic untrustworthiness of people and proof that he or she is unlovable and unworthy. Sometimes this anger becomes clearly apparent the first time the therapist has to cancel a session.

Jodi was an 8-year-old girl who had been exposed to serious physical and psychological neglect by her young mother from infancy to 5 years of age. When she began kindergarten, the school staff discovered Jodi's neglect and notified child welfare authorities. Jodi was removed from her mother's care, eventually made a permanent ward of the state, and placed in a residential treatment program where she was referred for individual psychotherapy.

In her first encounters with her female therapist, she wanted to sit on the therapist's lap and asked to go home with her. Jodi demanded an appointment for the following day and became angry when told that this was impossible because of the therapist's schedule. Because the therapist became ill, she had to cancel Jodi's sixth session. When therapy was resumed the next week, Jodi was hostile, answering the therapist's questions in a brusque and offhand manner. When the therapist told her she had missed Jodi the week before because of the canceled appointment, Jodi immediately shot back, "Well, I didn't miss you!" She then ordered the therapist to do certain things for her, such as getting her different toys in the playroom. When the therapist remarked that Jodi was angry because she did not see the therapist the week before, Jodi denied it. However, the frequency and intensity of her hostile and angry behavior in the session began to decrease after this comment.

Several weeks later, a case conference was convened in the cottage of the treatment facility where Jodi resided. Jodi did not want the therapist to leave the cottage when the conference was over. In fact, she again asked to go home with the therapist and became angry at the therapist's refusal. At one point, Jodi physically tried to restrain the therapist from leaving and gave her some play money to buy her acceptance and affection.

What can the therapist do to help children who exhibit extreme dependence and indiscriminate behavior? In the section on the engagement phase earlier in this chapter, we talked about giving them small tokens or "souvenirs" of the therapist and therapy sessions. The souvenirs provide them with some reassurance that the therapist still thinks about them when sessions are not being held. They also promote object constancy. The therapist can attenuate anxiety about his or her availability by adhering to a predictable appointment schedule and routine and by avoiding cancellations and scheduling changes as much as possible.

The play of many of these children is quite regressive, and the therapist may have to allow a child to engage in this behavior to compensate, at least symbolically, for early experiences of deprivation and inconsistent caregiving. Although she was 8 years old, Jodi insisted on enacting scenarios in which she was an infant. Her therapist had to care for her, preparing baby food and pretending to feed her with a spoon. The therapist's efforts to nurture a child symbolically may begin to change the child's expectations that others will be unresponsive but, of course, the therapist must enlist the help and cooperation of other significant people in the child's life in this endeavor, as they are usually the primary agents of change. Furthermore, the therapist's attempts to verbalize these underlying issues may promote the emergence of more adaptive ways for the child to express his or her needs rather than continuing to rely on regressive or provocative behavior to gain adult attention. Simple statements like "It feels really good to pretend that you are a baby and someone is always there to look after you" may be useful in promoting this kind of self-regulation.

Although the therapist wants to nurture the child, too much regression can be harmful. The child does not need to act like a baby after the therapy session is over and he or she is about to return to an elementary school classroom. As we have already discussed, the therapist should insist that the child stop this regressive behavior 5–10 minutes before the end of the session, then engaging the child in more age-appropriate conversations or play activities. These activities convey the notion that although the child may regress in the playroom, it is not beneficial to continue this behavior outside therapy sessions, especially if the child has many academic and social tasks to master. Jodi's therapist always informed her that they would have to stop their "play" 10 minutes before the end of the session. Jodi spent the last few minutes putting the doll and baby toys away while the therapist asked her about the age-appropriate activities or tasks she would confront later that day (e.g., participating in Brownies). During this time they talked informally about how Jodi would meet some of these challenges.

Similarly, therapists must be especially prudent to limit children's indiscriminate displays of physical affection, as we discussed earlier in this chapter. Allowing such behavior to continue reinforces this pattern and increases their vulnerability to being exploited or victimized. Although parents' and caregivers' management of maltreated children's problematic behavior is always a critical factor in outcome, this is especially true for children who exhibit extreme dependence and indiscriminate social behavior. Given the behavior's chronic, refractory nature and its appearance in multiple environments, parents and caregivers are in the best position to intervene. We described strategies caregivers can use in Chapter 6.

Urquiza and Winn (1994) identify other characteristics of a dependent pattern of behavior. These children are unassertive and unduly compliant, and they allow other people to make important decisions for them. In therapy, the children offer little resistance to developing a relationship with the therapist and have few opinions or issues to discuss. According to these authors, "The challenge in working with a dependent child is to generate separation and individuation, to elicit a strong and determined response from the child, and [to] help the child integrate a sense of self that is based on worth, ability, and individuality" (Urquiza & Winn, 1994, p. 83).

Therapists can help such children by encouraging them to provide opinions about different subjects, even such trivial ones as favorite television shows. They might identify an area or issue about which they may disagree with the child and then inform the child of the difference of opinion.

Some children, upon hearing the therapist's opinion, immediately change their minds and try to retract their opinions. Therapists can actively intervene by informing the child that it is perfectly acceptable for the child to hold his or her own opinion. The therapist should state that his or her regard and commitment are not contingent upon the child's holding identical views. Many interventions of this nature may be required. When these interventions are combined with the therapist's active attempts to demonstrate commitment, the child may begin to change his or her expectations that any attempt to assert a sense of self or individuality will be met with rejection or abandonment. The therapist may consolidate the child's developing individuality and assertiveness by frequently soliciting the child's choice of activities in which the youngster would like to participate. Having an opportunity to make such decisions may be quite threatening for children who fear they will evoke the displeasure or anger of the therapist if they make a wrong choice, but ultimately it may help them develop a more integrated sense of self.

SETTING LIMITS ON DEFIANT AND OPPOSITIONAL BEHAVIOR

The emergence of children's defiant, oppositional or even aggressive behavior in sessions offers the therapist a wonderful opportunity to introduce a much-needed element of discontinuity. As we have seen, precipitants of this behavior include children's perceptions that the therapist cannot meet all their massive dependence needs, deficits in self-regulatory skills necessary to cope adequately with the typical frustrations all children encounter, or misperceptions and biased interpretations of social interactions. Rather than rejecting or abusing the angry child, the therapist places appropriate limits on unacceptable behavior (e.g., attempts to hurt the therapist or destroy the office or playroom equipment). At the same time, the therapist acknowledges and empathizes with the underlying anger. Children do not feel safe in a therapeutic relationship or, for that matter, at home with their families when they can do whatever they want. The absence of boundaries and limits increases anxiety, and the children's behavior escalates to the point where they might engage in destructive or dangerous behavior. Placing appropriate limits on children demonstrates to them, in practical and concrete ways, that there are adults who care enough to help them control these troublesome feelings and urges; limits demonstrate the therapist's intent to provide safety and security for the child, both physically and emotionally (Landreth, 2002).

Limit setting also introduces the child to the notion of a reciprocal or goal-corrected partnership. The therapist who stops aggressive or destructive behavior and then engages in a dialogue wherein both participants discuss and negotiate their needs exposes the child to a novel experience. Limits teach the child more adaptive ways of handling anger, such as verbalizing feelings. The child learns that feelings are legitimate but that the youngster cannot always act as he or she pleases. For example, a child may become more oppositional near the end of each session. Rather than allowing this behavior to escalate, the therapist should help the child identify feelings elicited by the termination of the session, encourage expression of what the child might need (e.g., "I want to stay here longer"), and reach a compromise solution (e.g., taking home a small souvenir), thereby enhancing the child's self-control.

There are other benefits to limit setting. Limits on children's aggressive or destructive behavior are necessary to enable the therapist to maintain attitudes of acceptance, empathy, and warmth, as well as to ensure the child's and therapist's personal safety. Limits also define the boundaries of the therapeutic relationship and provide for the maintenance of legal, ethical, and professional standards by ensuring, for example, that the child does not exhibit any sexual behavior.

There are several general steps in setting limits with children (Ginott, 1965; Landreth, 2002). First, the therapist should acknowledge the child's feelings or wishes and help the child express them verbally: "You're really mad at me because you wish you could stay here for another hour. You really like spending time here." An empathic response like this affirms that the child has feelings, identifies them, and recognizes their validity. This response is consistent with an overall goal of affect attunement and the promotion of reflective functioning. Second, the therapist clearly and exactly states the limit on a specific act: "But therapists and kids have to leave the playroom when their time is over." Many of these children will not readily pick up on fuzzy or tenuous statements such as "I don't think it's a very good idea if you put all that paint on the wall" (Landreth, 2002). To put it bluntly, the therapist has to act like the boss at this point, just as good parents act like bosses when necessary. Third, the therapist points out acceptable alternatives: "If you're really angry about having to leave, you can say to me, 'I'm mad!' " Finally, the therapist helps the child bring out feelings of resentment that arise when restrictions are invoked: "You sure don't like having to leave and wish you could stay longer. It makes you really angry when you have to leave." Ginott (1965) recommends that limits be phrased in language that does not constitute a challenge to the child's self-respect. Limits are better heeded when stated succinctly and impersonally, such as, "Time is up for today," versus, "Your time is up and you must leave now!"

Some children will engage in the negative behavior despite the therapist's attempts to limit it. If the limit setting described above proves ineffective, the therapist presents an ultimate choice to the child, such as saying he or she will prohibit the child from using the blocks (if the child threw one). Leaving the room is another ultimate choice: "If you choose to throw the block again, you choose [not to play with the blocks anymore today] or [to leave the room] (Landreth, 2002). These statements convey the notion that it is the child's choice and that the consequence does not constitute a rejection or punishment of the child. If the child throws the block, the therapist should implement the limit but clarify (not negotiate!) the reasons for this step. Therapists can tell children they are stopping the session early because they do not want the children to engage in any more harmful, dangerous, or destructive behavior that will make them feel worse about themselves. Children must be reassured that the therapist has not "given up" and that they will see each other at their next regularly scheduled appointment. Sometimes shortening each session is effective in helping children behave more appropriately, especially those who are overstimulated by the material elicited by therapy or those with especially poor self-regulatory skills.

The therapist may become annoyed with a child's provocative behavior. Acknowledging this annoyance and then emphasizing that he or she will not reject or abuse the youngster, along with identifying the precipitants of the anger and connecting it to specific aspects of the child's behavior (e.g., "When you throw paint on me, I feel really angry"), are necessary to help a child appreciate the effects of his or her behavior on others. To disrupt the stability of the IWM/IS and to induce change, the therapist should distinguish between his or her response to the child's provocation (i.e., verbalizing the anger in a nonderogatory, nonabusive manner) and those of others who have reacted in ways that reinforced the child's mistrust of people.

Although the therapeutic relationship is a significant agent of change for many maltreated children, especially those who have incurred developmental effects because of their abuse or neglect, it is not the only one worthy of consideration. We now turn in the next three chapters to other ways of helping children recover from maltreatment.

CHAPTER EIGHT

Helping Children Express Their Feelings and Thoughts about Maltreatment

Helping children identify and acknowledge feelings related to a history of abuse and neglect is an especially important task. We need to gradually expose children to the details and stimuli associated with the maltreatment, including their feelings, so that anxiety can extinguish. Uncovering the maltreatment and bringing it into the open offers an opportunity to explore and possibly reformulate the meaning and implications of these experiences and reduces the child's reliance on maladaptive defenses such as overidealization or dissociation. Indeed, assisting children to construct trauma narratives is a central component of TF-CBT (Cohen & Deblinger, 2004).

In this chapter we describe specific techniques to help children construct and express their narratives, feelings, and thoughts about having been abused or neglected. Although we describe some of our own techniques that we believe are useful, we also draw on the work of others (e.g., Cunningham & MacFarlane, 1991; Friedrich, 1990; Gil, 1991; Gil & Johnson, 1993; James, 1989, 1994; Karp & Butler, 1996; Mandell & Damon, 1989; Shelby & Felix, 2005; Urquiza & Winn, 1994) who have developed many innovative and creative strategies.

Although exposing children to anxiety-inducing material and helping them express their feelings about victimization is a prerequisite for successful treatment, alone it is usually insufficient. Often therapy may create even more difficulties if it is unaccompanied by interventions to help children develop successful coping mechanisms. In their zeal and enthusiasm to help survivors of abuse and neglect, inexperienced or novice therapists sometimes believe their primary job is to "open up" clients. They encourage them to quickly ventilate all their feelings about abusive or neglectful experiences but pay little attention to the pacing of the process or the notion that defense mechanisms, although maladaptive in the long term, are there for a reason: They protect individuals from intense pain and anxiety. Therapy that overwhelms clients with strong feelings and provides them with no adaptive emotional and behavioral self-regulation mechanisms usually results in deterioration in functioning and erodes trust in the therapist and the therapeutic process. This principle applies to working with both adult and child survivors. Therapists must actively assist young clients to develop more appropriate ways of coping with the pain, hurt, and anxiety that emerge over the course of therapy. We address this issue in Chapter 9.

Given these similarities and the overlap in the problems of children subjected to different types of maltreatment, we present an integrated approach rather than separate chapters on the treatment of problems arising from different types of maltreatment. For example, although a number of sexually abused children present with PTSD and a considerable proportion of the treatment outcome literature has been devoted to interventions that target their symptoms, therapists must be prepared to treat PTSD in youngsters subjected to other types of maltreatment. Even though the content may be somewhat different (e.g., dreams of being raped versus dreams of being physically assaulted or witnessing a parent's assault), the treatment techniques and the underlying rationale are the same. Chapters 8, 9, and 10 discuss the three major treatment themes that confront every therapist who works with maltreated children: expressing thoughts and feelings about the abuse or neglect, developing adaptive coping mechanisms, and reformulating the meaning of the experiences. As well as describing specific techniques that have broad applicability to the sequelae of the major types of maltreatment, we review intervention strategies for more idiosyncratic problems associated with particular types of abuse and neglect, such as sexual behavior problems and dissociative disorders.

ESTs FOR MALTREATED CHILDREN WITH ANXIETY PROBLEMS

One area of empirical research that has attracted a lot of attention is the use of CBT for PTSD in children. Feeny and colleagues (2004) have prepared a comprehensive review of cognitive and behavioral treatments of PTSD in children and adolescents. Although the literature is still meager, as compared with the body of research on the efficacy of psychosocial interventions for PTSD in adults, it is growing and includes child survivors of disasters, wars, and childhood sexual abuse. Chapter 6 reviewed the literature on parental involvement in the treatment of sexually abused children, including those with PTSD and other anxiety problems. As we noted, these studies often included concurrent treatment of children, and both adult and child components used CBT (trauma-focused CBT, or TF-CBT). Studies cited in Chapter 6 have demonstrated the short- and long-term efficacy of TF-CBT programs that include both child and parent components (for reviews, see the Chadwick Center for Children and Families, 2004; Saunders et al., 2004). The child programs usually comprised a number of interventions, including exposure and anxiety-management training (described in Chapter 9). Cohen and colleagues (2004) reported, for example, that children treated with CBT demonstrated significantly greater improvements in PTSD, depression, shame, abuse-related attributions, and overall behavior problems than children who received child-centered therapy. King and colleagues (2000) randomly assigned 36 sexually abused school-age and adolescent children to a child-alone CBT treatment condition, a family-based CBT condition, or to a waiting-list control condition. Children in both the CBT conditions showed improvements in PTSD and self-reported fear and anxiety than those in the waiting-list control group. Furthermore, the children treated with CBT were significantly less likely than the children in the waiting-list group to meet diagnostic criteria for PTSD at posttreatment (40% vs. 80%, respectively). Although disentangling the specific effects of the various intervention strategies included in these outcome studies remains difficult and children subjected to other types of maltreatment are rarely included in these investigations, the results are impressive. According to Berliner (2005), "There is now ample evidence that TF-CBT is the first-line treatment for PTSD, anxiety and depression in sexually abused children and likely for children exposed to other trauma as well" (p. 103).

The conditioning paradigm we described in Chapter 2 posits that individuals with PTSD avoid anxiety-related stimuli, and consequently their anxiety does not extinguish. Therefore, a central goal of treatment is exposing them to the anxiety-inducing stimuli so that anxiety can extinguish.

Dalgleish (2004) describes the importance of exposure-based treatment:

> A central treatment component in TF-CBT has been imaginal and *in vivo* exposure, especially for PTSD. Exposure-based therapies in general involve clients systematically confronting the objects of their emotional distress within a therapeutic framework. The exposure-based element of these treatments most usually involves the client repeatedly recounting the details of the traumatic event over exposure sessions. The account is often deliv-

> ered in the present tense and most usually with emphasis on the cognitions and feelings associated with various aspects of the narrative. (p. 231)

Imaginal exposure includes repeated recounting of the traumatic memories, including discussion or play reenactiments of the trauma, whereas *in vivo* exposure consists of repeated, prolonged confrontation with trauma-related situations and objects that evoke excessive anxiety (Feeny et al., 2004). This model illustrates the relevance of developing a conceptualization of the contributions of pathogenic processes to the emergence of symptoms and their relevance for intervention.

Imaginal exposure is particularly relevant to the major theme of this chapter—helping children recount their abusive and neglectful experiences and the associated thoughts and feelings by constructing trauma narratives. Chapter 9 describes *in vivo* exposure strategies. Prolonged exposure (which includes exposure to trauma-related situations, objects, or memories) has been used effectively with a wide population of adults with chronic PTSD (Feeny et al., 2004). However, no randomized control designs have evaluated the efficacy of exposure treatments in children. Saigh (1986, 1987a, 1987b, 1987c, 1989) published a series of single-case studies of Lebanese children with war-related PTSD. Imaginal and *in vivo* exposures were effective in reducing the severity of PTSD, anxiety, and depression, as well as behavioral avoidance of trauma-related situations. However, the generalizability of these results to children who have suffered traumas other than war, such as physical or sexual abuse, may be questionable, as abuse-related trauma usually includes a strong interpersonal component (Feeny et al., 2004). Although efficacy studies have incorporated gradual exposure (see Chapter 6 for a review of the studies conducted by Cohen, Deblinger, and colleagues), treatment also included other strategies, such as anxiety management training (AMT). Consequently, it is difficult to disentangle exposure's specific and unique contribution to outcome. However, given the potential benefits of exposure techniques in the treatment of traumatized children, therapists should be well acquainted with a wide range of strategies they can employ and adapt to meet maltreated children's unique needs. We now turn to specific techniques and strategies.

DIRECT DISCUSSIONS OF THE MALTREATMENT

Recounting episodes of the maltreatment constitutes a principal means of imaginal exposure for highly anxious maltreated children. Even though the therapist has attempted to instill a sense of safety and control prior to initiating discussions of the maltreatment, children frequently become anxious while recounting their trauma narratives, even those who initially appear calm at the start of these conversations. It is usually prudent to equip them with coping skills for use within and outside of therapy sessions prior to starting to have them recount the maltreatment; we describe some of these strategies in this chapter and in Chapter 9. Although some children may never have to use these strategies, it is often difficult to accurately predict how they will react when caught up in the details of the abuse or neglect. Children who are suddenly overwhelmed by anxiety during these conversations without any coping skills to fall back on may be less willing to talk about the maltreatment or return for subsequent sessions, and their confidence in the therapist as a secure base begins to erode. Often these reactions make them feel powerless and out of control, much as they felt during their victimization; gaining control of these feelings helps them regain a sense of competence and control. In addition to teaching children coping skills, careful attention to the structure of the sessions and the use of other strategies can do much to alleviate their anxiety and facilitates their willingness to divulge details of the maltreatment.

Explaining Symptoms and the Rationale of Treatment

Using simple language, the therapist should explain the pathogenic processes responsible for the emergence of symptoms associated with PTSD or other diagnoses. Cunningham and MacFarlane (1991, pp. 149–164) describe the symptomatology of PTSD in developmentally appropriate language. Providing children with a simple explanation for some of their reactions diminishes their fear that they are crazy and reduces their feelings of anxiety, isolation, and stigmatization. This is an especially effective strategy to help children begin to understand that their current difficulties, including distress manifested in the therapy sessions, are associated with previous maltreatment experiences and not the result of some personal weakness or failing.

Therapists should describe the benefits of talking about the maltreatment to further promote the child's commitment to and participation in therapy. They should reiterate that the purpose of therapy is not to forget the victimization but to learn to master the feelings associated with it and to think differently about what happened. Although talking about these events is initially frightening and sometimes painful, the intensity of such feelings usually diminishes. Gradual exposure is often a major component of the intervention, and children need and deserve explanations regarding why they must confront these painful scenarios. These explanations are more meaningful if the therapist can put them into a context that has unique relevance to the child's life. A therapist used the following description of PTSD pathogenic processes and treatment rationale with a 10-year-old sexually abused girl. Her arousal and reexperiencing symptoms were quite prominent. She had just started diving lessons at a local pool.

"I know you're really scared right now of your dad [the perpetrator of the sexual abuse]. It's kind of like when you did that belly flop off a diving board that you told me about last week. You told me how it hurt and you were scared to go off the board again, but you did. Now think of another kid who's so scared about doing another belly flop that even being in the pool is scary for her because it's so close to the diving pool. Just looking at the diving pool or board scares her because she thinks of what happened before. Her friends call her up and ask her to go swimming, but she gets nervous—just thinking about being in the place where she did the belly flop scares her.

"You got really scared when your dad abused you, and now there are times when you get scared even though your dad doesn't live with you anymore. It's hard to go to sleep because your dad used to abuse you in your bedroom at night. Even though he's not there, being in your bedroom or even thinking about going to bed brings up those feelings and memories, just like being near the diving board scares that girl who did the belly flop. It's hard for you to get to sleep because you're really nervous, and sometimes you don't even want to think of what your dad did because it brings it all back. It's just like the girl who did the belly flop—she doesn't even want to go near the board.

"Now you told me last week that although you were a little nervous about getting back on the board, you did it and did a good dive. That was the best way of feeling better—you tried the dive again and did a good job—it wasn't as scary after that. So we're going to do the same thing. I'll help you learn how to relax and feel calmer at night so you can sleep better. The more calm nights you have, the better you'll feel. In a way, it's like I'm going to be your coach and help you get back on the board. And we'll do the same thing to help you talk more about what happened. As you get more used to talking, you'll feel less nervous and upset, just as when you did more dives and started to feel less scared about that first belly flop. I'll teach you how to relax and talk, but you'll be the one who can decide how much you want to talk about it when we meet. We'll do it gradually if that's better for you."

Pacing the Discussions and Instilling a Sense of Control and Safety

According to the conditioning paradigm described in Chapter 2, imaginal exposure (e.g., talking about the abuse or exposing children to the stimuli via other media, such as play or art) may serve as potent stimulus for the emergence of anxiety. The therapist should emphasize that he or she understands and appreciates the child's anxiety and will proceed at a pace tolerable to the child. The therapist should give the child explicit permission and guidance about controlling the pace of the discussion; they can devise ways for the child to signal the emergence of strong feelings of anxiety and the need for a break. For instance, a simple verbal statement like "This is too fast" or "I'm getting too scared now" may be adequate, or the child might give the therapist a nonverbal signal, such as holding up a hand with the palm toward the therapist. In order to make the child feel more comfortable, the therapist should have the child rehearse these statements or nonverbal signals beforehand.

Youngsters can identify the sources of their anxiety by describing "the worst thing that could happen" if they told their story, and the therapist should clarify any misconceptions (e.g., "I'll go to jail if I tell what happened to me") to attenuate their anxiety. Of course, some fears are realistic, such as children's expectations that they might become distraught when talking about their experiences. The therapist can respond that although children do indeed become upset, the child remains in control of what he or she talks about, they will proceed at the child's pace, and the therapist will ensure that the child does not inappropriately act out these strong feelings. A subsequent section of this chapter discusses techniques to normalize such affective displays. Children can also rate their anxiety about these discussions on a fear thermometer that graphically displays the intensity of the anxiety. Seeing the anxiety decrease on the thermometer's scale is concrete evidence that the child is making progress and learning to conquer his or her anxiety.

Although the therapist wants to facilitate the child's exposure to this sensitive material, a too hurried pace overwhelms the child with anxiety and results in the escalation of anxiety-based symptoms, such as greater difficulty with sleeping, or further avoidance. When the therapist attempts to discuss the maltreatment, the child may change the topic or engage in provocative or oppositional behavior to deflect attention from the maltreatment. The child becomes reluctant to attend or participate in subsequent sessions, claims the sessions are "boring," or adamantly refuses to discuss topics related to the maltreatment. The child may also deny previous claims of being bothered by his or her abusive experiences while asserting, "Everything is fine."

There are various ways a therapist can structure and plan therapy sessions to contain this anxiety. For each session, the therapist and child might agree to allot a specific length of time to direct discussion of the maltreatment. It is usually best to begin with short intervals (10–15 minutes) so the child will not be overwhelmed by anxiety that might be elicited by more prolonged discussions. In this way the child is gradually exposed to tolerable doses of the anxiety-related material. For example, it is unrealistic to ask most school-age children to engage in a continuous 45-minute discussion of their victimization, given the material's intensity and their short attention spans. As the child succeeds with brief discussions and anxiety begins to abate, the youngster and therapist should decide together how to lengthen the discussions by small increments (Urquiza & Winn, 1994). Such a strategy gives the child a sense of accomplishment. It also reinforces the child's perception that the adult is sensitive to the youngster's feelings and needs and is willing to negotiate important issues and topics. Urquiza and Winn (1994) and James (1989, 1994) advocate interspersing these direct discussions of the maltreatment with periods of play. Play periods afford children some relief from the anxiety associated with talking about the maltreatment. Not only do they not have to make eye contact with the therapist while playing with modeling clay or drawing, but they can always revert to the play activity when they do not want to say anything more. Discussions about the play activity provide a much-needed break from these intense conversations.

Kot and Tyndall-Lind (2005) present an interesting and different perspective on the frequency of play therapy sessions for child witnesses of domestic violence. They argue that clinicians should reevaluate the traditional model of weekly sessions and consider more frequent ones, including daily treatment. They suggest that such modifications allow the child to be exposed to a healthy, supportive environment on a daily basis and permit the child and therapist to have a better recollection of symbolic content in previous sessions. According to Kot and Tyndall-Lind, retraumatization is less likely to occur in this modified schedule because the nonverbal nature of play therapy alleviates the child's anxiety. Although this may be a useful modification, therapists must remain observant of any escalation in the child's anxiety associated with these more frequent sessions and make the necessary adjustments in the frequency of sessions.

Constructing a Stimulus Hierarchy

As well as negotiating the duration of direct discussions, the therapist should give the youngster significant control over the choice of topics related to the victimization. This approach is particularly important at the beginning of this phase of therapy, when children are especially anxious because they feel they might have no control over the conduct of the sessions. The therapist suggests that the child begin by choosing the topic or incident related to the maltreatment to talk about ("Why don't you choose what you'd like to talk about first?") and adds that a good place to start might be an aspect of the maltreatment that does not generate too much anxiety so that they can "work their way up" to those the child finds especially frightening. The therapist should explain that working thorough a stimulus hierarchy exposes the child to increasing doses of the anxiety-related material, with anxiety extinguishing as the child successfully addresses each topic in turn.

A variation of James's "Worry Wall" technique (James, 1989, pp. 130–131) is a useful way to construct a stimulus hierarchy. The therapist invites the child to identify his or her "biggest worry" about the maltreatment and write it down on a small card, and then asks the child, "How big is your worry?" If it is a little worry, the child is told to tack the card on the wall near the floor; conversely, if it is significant and overwhelming, the child tacks the card near the ceiling. This concretely represents the stimulus hierarchy. The child can remove a card after the anxiety associated with that particular issue diminishes; the card's changing placement on the wall or its removal serves as a concrete reminder of the child's progress.

Relaxation Exercises

Deep, diaphragmatic breathing, differential muscle relaxation techniques, and visualization are strategies children can learn to employ during imaginal or *in vivo* exposure sessions when they become especially anxious. Although not all children may need to actually use such strategies, those who have strong physiological reactions may greatly benefit. Before teaching children such techniques, the therapist should explain that they take time and practice to learn. The child should not give up after only one or two tries.

We have found that various relaxation techniques can be employed successfully during sessions to extinguish the anxiety associated with maltreatment. The therapist can cue the child to intersperse direct discussions of the maltreatment or episodes of symbolic play with these techniques. Therapists adapt the techniques to each child, with particular attention to age, cognitive capacity, and interests. Perhaps the simplest technique is to have a child focus on breathing and slow it down; the basic technique is to count breaths in and out or to simply say, "Breathe in, breathe out" slowly. Initially, the therapist should do this prompting aloud. Once children can slow their breathing, they should be shown how to use imagery to increase their relaxation and sense of calmness. Some respond well to imagining they are going down a flight of stairs. With each slow breath exhaled, they take a step down and feel more comfortable and more relaxed. Sometimes a child responds well to imagining that he or she is a big balloon; with each breath out, it deflates and becomes softer and more relaxed. Imagining that he or she is a limp rag doll can also be useful. With each breath out, the doll relaxes further and slumps over. Still other children respond to developing an imaginary scene in which they feel safe, comfortable, and calm. During relaxation, the child breathes slowly and imagines all the details and sensations described by the therapist or on a CD or tape. For example, a child may like to imagine lying on a beach on a hot day. The child is lying on a thick, comfortable towel under a large shade tree. A slight breeze is blowing; the child does not feel too hot. Gulls and other children can be heard in the distance, but the child prefers to lie comfortably under the tree. The child focuses on his or her bodily sensations in this scene and feels comfortable and safe.

Close Monitoring of the Child's Anxiety

If the child appears highly distressed and does not ask or signal the therapist for a break, the therapist should comment directly about the child's distress ("You look pretty upset right now"). The therapist should ask if the child wants a break from the discussion and encourage the child to employ relaxation techniques or other coping mechanisms. After the child is sufficiently calm, the therapist can inquire about the reasons for the distress, asking if intrusive memories (flashbacks) are occurring during the discussion, or if other reasons, such as fear of the therapist's reaction to a particularly embarrassing or sensitive detail or incident, are creating anxiety. The therapist should reassure the child that he or she understands the basis of the anxiety and does not think negatively of the youngster. For example, Peter's anxiety was alleviated to a certain degree when the therapist told him he did not think Peter was deviant for having a sexual response while being molested. Therapists can instruct children to observe the therapist's reactions to their accounts closely, paying particular attention to the therapist's facial expressions or body language that might reveal those reactions. They can encourage a child to recount more of the distressing episode or incident, again using relaxation to attenuate the anxiety if it escalates. After a minute or so of the child's account, the therapist asks the child to report his or her observations of the therapist's demeanor and whether it confirmed the child's expectation that the therapist would be disgusted or defended. This is a variant of the "trust meter" we described in Chapter 4.

Drawing the Distinction between the Verbal Expression of Feelings and Behavioral Acting Out

Some children believe that if they talk about their maltreatment, they will be so overwhelmed with anger that they will lose control and become aggressive or destructive during the session. It is important to reassure the child that the therapist will ensure safety and will not allow the youngster to exhibit such behavior, while still encouraging the child to tell "a bit" of the episode or experience. At the end of each of these segments, the therapist should point out that the child did not get out of control. This reinforces the child's growing confidence, not only in the therapist, but also in his or her own ability to regulate strong feelings and behavior.

Besides participating in verbal discussions, the child can cut out magazine pictures of people showing angry feelings and contrast them with pictures of individuals behaving aggressively, to reinforce the notion that anger does not necessarily lead to aggressive behavior (Cunningham & MacFarlane, 1991). Cunningham and MacFarlane (1991) also recommend the use puppets or role plays to illustrate concretely the difference between these two concepts. For example, the youngster enacts one scene showing a puppet displaying angry feelings in healthy ways (e.g., talking about his or her anger) and then another scene in which the characters express anger aggressively. Obviously, the therapist cannot ask children to find pictures of people acting out sexual feelings in inappropriate ways. Instead, the two might discuss what would constitute healthy and age-appropriate sexual expression for the child.

Another introductory exercise that is useful in drawing the distinction between the verbal expression of emotions and behavioral acting out is "Feelings: Where Are They in My Body?" (James, 1989, pp. 93–94). The child draws an outline of his or her body and adds a legend beside the picture that identifies the child's feelings. The child chooses colors to represent various feelings and marks their locations on the body outline using the appropriate colors. This exercise does more than help the child to distinguish among different feelings. It is a springboard for discussion about the difference between talking about feelings and acting them out, for example, using a fist to express anger. It also helps the child identify body sensations that are precipitants to inappropriate behavior, such as physical aggression or sexualized behavior.

Normalizing Affective Displays

Therapists need to normalize children's displays of affect such as crying or intense fear, and they should point out they do not think less of the child because of such reactions. In fact, they can congratulate the child for having the strength to show these feelings. The therapist should facilitate the child's general understanding of the normalcy of his or her distress and its connection to the maltreatment. This is the start of the process by which the child begins reformulating the meaning of the maltreatment experience; in other words, he or she is not "crazy," other maltreated children react similarly, and these responses reflect understandable effects of having been abused or neglected.

Some children who talk about their abuse or neglect experience such intense affects that they feel as if they are being revictimized during these discussions. The therapist can take several approaches to help them overcome these feelings. First, the therapist should identify the concrete and observable differences between the situation in which the child was abused and the therapy session in which the child recounts these episodes. For example, the therapist might point out that the perpetrator is not present; no one is hurting or even touching the child; and the child is reacting to feelings, not the actual maltreatment. Second, the therapist should remind the child of other differences between the maltreatment and the therapy session: the child is now bigger, older, and more capable of asking for help and receiving protection than he or she was at the time of the maltreatment (Urquiza & Winn, 1994). Such a strategy may diminish the child's anxiety about discussing the maltreatment. It may also start the process by which the child discards the status of a victim who is powerless to protect him- or herself against future assaults. Teaching children to make appropriate self-statements (e.g., "Even though I'm scared when I talk about the abuse, it's not happening now and I'm safe") is another useful strategy, which we discuss in detail in the next chapter.

FACILITATING AND ENCOURAGING THE CHILD'S TRAUMA NARRATIVE

The therapist should sit quietly and listen attentively as the child begins to recount his or her experiences. Interrupting the description of what happened with a barrage of questions may discourage the child from continuing. If the child hesitates while recounting these experiences, the therapist can provide gentle encouragement by making simple statements such as "Go on" or "Tell me more about that."

There are several therapeutic tasks during this phase of treatment. First, the therapist must help the child recount the details of the maltreatment, especially those that were previously denied, suppressed, or dissociated, to develop a trauma narrative that accurately represents the child's experience. The therapist might facilitate recall by asking the child to provide a moment-by-moment account after the child has given an open-ended description of the maltreatment. For example, the therapist might begin with more neutral questions regarding the maltreatment's locale (e.g., "What room did it happen in?"), the time of day (e.g., "Did it happen at night or during the day?"), and what the child or family did earlier that day. The therapist should then ask about more sensitive aspects of the maltreatment and encourage the child to describe his or her experiences before, during, and after the maltreatment, including feelings, odors, sights, body sensations, and reactions (James, 1994). The therapist can ask the child to recount the narrative in the present tense to increase the salience of the anxiety-inducing stimuli and the associated effects. This exposure-based intervention may elicit considerable anxiety in the child, and the therapist can prompt the youngster to use appropriate coping mechanisms (e.g., relaxation exercises) so that the anxiety abates and eventually extinguishes. Of course, many maltreated children do not have this verbal facility and cannot specifically articulate their experiences and feelings. We devote other sections of this chapter to techniques designed to help the child relate the experience and his or her reactions.

Second, the therapist must help the child to express the associated feelings and cognitions. Simple questions like "How did you feel when he hit you like that?" may be sufficient to facilitate expression of such sentiments. These questions give the child an opportunity to put into words the often intense and confusing feelings elicited by the victimization, thereby increasing the child's self-regulatory skills. In addition, the child's responses to these questions allow the therapist to understand and then empathize with and legitimize the child's feelings. For example, the child may talk about fears of being sexually abused in the future, which may be accompanied by nonverbal symptoms of anxiety (e.g., fidgeting, increased pressure of speech, decreased eye contact with the therapist). The therapist conveys his or her understanding with simple statements such as "You're still really scared that he might do those things again to you." Subsequent statements that normalize these feelings (e.g., "Most kids would feel really scared about that") contribute to the child's understanding that his or her reactions are normal and do not indicate deviancy, and they promote the child's reflective thinking.

It is critically important for therapists to ensure that they do not impose their own preconceptions on the child's account of the maltreatment, for instance, by assuming there were no positive aspects to the relationship between the child and perpetrator. Rather than telling a child how he or she thinks or feels about the experience, the therapist must adopt the phenomenological perspective we described in Chapter 2 in order to understand as fully as possible the child's experience and perceptions of the maltreatment. It is important to help the child express the entire range of feelings harbored toward the perpetrator, including any positive ones. If this approach was not used during the assessment phase, the therapist should begin the current inquiry by requesting the child to describe the "nice things" the perpetrator did for the youngster. Some therapists find it difficult to acknowledge that the perpetrator treated the child well in certain ways or to empathize with the child's positive feelings and possibly love for the individual. However, this attitude is critically important in helping children become aware of ambivalent and conflicting feelings so that they can ultimately express their feelings of betrayal and loss. Severe criticisms of the perpetrator may elicit even stronger feelings of loyalty, especially if the perpetrator is a parent or primary caregiver. In response to this criticism, the child may defend the perpetrator even more strenuously and ultimately minimize or deny the individual's actions. A more useful strategy is to talk about the perpetrator's behavior that hurt or angered the child rather than making more personalized comments.

Structured Activities to Help Children Talk about the Maltreatment

So far we have described therapy from one perspective. The client is a child who can talk about the maltreatment and its associated feelings, cognitions, worries, and concerns. However, many maltreated children do not have these verbal skills, or if they do, they are inhibited from talking directly about their experiences for the reasons described in earlier chapters; this precludes imaginal exposure via direct discussions and conversations. Such children may require the psychological distance inherent in play therapy techniques we describe later in this chapter. However, even verbal children who can talk about their experiences may require specific strategies to be able to provide a more comprehensive account of their feelings and experiences.

James (1989, 1994) has developed many innovative and creative techniques to help traumatized children. We have found the following particularly useful. The "Garbage Bag" technique begins with the therapist drawing a parallel between concrete pieces of garbage and the overpowering, aversive feelings associated with trauma (James, 1989, pp. 166–170). The therapist continues by explaining that keeping these feelings and thoughts secret is like carrying a bag of garbage around. The child is to get rid of each piece of "garbage" (i.e., distressing feelings and ideas about the abuse) gradually. To accomplish this, the therapist asks the child to identify each aversive or distressing event or episode related to the trauma, which the therapist quickly writes on a piece of paper. The therapist does not allow the child to elaborate on these events but does permit the child to identify aversive events other than the trauma. The purpose of writing each episode or incident on a separate piece of paper is to divide the maltreatment into more manageable bits. The pieces of paper are put in a paper grocery bag that symbolically contains the memories and feelings associated with the maltreatment. Each week the child reaches into the bag, picks out one piece of paper, and discusses that particular episode or incident. This is a variant of gradual exposure: the child's anxiety extinguishes as the youngster is exposed to particular aspects or episodes of the trauma. The child can throw the paper back into the bag and choose another if he or she is not ready to address the first topic, thereby gaining a sense of control. If the child elects to work on the first issue chosen, the therapist and child might discuss it directly or choose another method, such as drawing.

The Garbage Bag exercise illustrates one of the general underlying themes of child therapy. We need to translate abstract, psychological concepts such as affects and defenses, into forms the child can more readily understand. We advise the reader to review an article by Harter (1977), a subsequent chapter (Harter, 1983), and a more recent article by Grave and Blissett (2004) that discuss the cognitive-developmental limitations of children's understanding of emotional and psychological concepts. Grave and Blissett (2004) and Harter (1983) argue that child therapists need to concretize these ideas via visualizable symbols so the child can attach real experiences to these abstract concepts. In the Garbage Bag exercise, writing down the aversive or distressing episodes, incidents, or issues puts them in a concrete form to which the child can attach feelings and cognitions. The use of the paper bag to hold these feelings is another example of the concretization of a psychological concept; that is, the child has many feelings and issues in his or her psychological world. By symbolically emptying the garbage bag of these issues, the child has a concrete reminder that he or she is beginning to master these distressing feelings and is making real progress: The fewer pieces of "garbage" left in the bag is tangible proof of this progress.

There are other structured exercises that therapists can use to expose children to details of their maltreatment and express the associated feelings and thoughts. In their manual describing a curriculum for group psychotherapy for sexually abused children, Mandell and Damon (1989) describe several "handouts" for children to complete. The content of this material is focused on sexual abuse, but the clinician can modify it for children who have been physically abused, neglected, or psychologically maltreated. The handout "Feelings about Being Molested" (Mandell & Damon, 1989, pp. 76–77) consists of eight statements (e.g., "I would like to hide from people so I don't have to talk about it"). Children rate the intensity of these feelings on a scale ranging from "never" to "always." The handout "What Will People Think of Me?" is a sentence-completion task (Mandell & Damon, 1989, pp. 77–78). The child completes sentences such as "I worry that I am the only one who ___________." Some victimized children respond in ways that convey their sense of stigmatization, powerlessness, or betrayal. These handouts are useful in individual psychotherapy or even in the assessment phase with children who may feel more comfortable approaching these issues by writing down their responses rather than verbally communicating them. A major drawback to handouts is that the child must have the requisite reading and writing skills to complete them. Asking a child who has significant difficulty with these academic tasks to complete the forms will probably engender more frustration and increase the child's resistance to participation in therapy.

There are other ways to structure these discussions of the maltreatment. Cunningham and MacFarlane (1991, pp. 136–137) used another technique, the "Tell My Story Chart," in group therapy with children who engage in sexually inappropriate behavior. The chart has relevant inquiries about a child's own history of victimization. Areas of inquiry include the perpetrator's identity, a description of what happened, how the child felt about it, and how the abuse stopped. Children who experienced other types of maltreatment also can use this chart. They have a tangible demonstration of their progress when they mark off or place a sticker on the chart each time they answer a question. The chart also provides concrete reminders of topics that should be discussed in therapy.

Therapists can use other techniques to help affectively constricted children to express feelings. In "Feelings: Inside and Outside" (James, 1989, p. 93), the therapist gives the child a piece of paper folded in half to open like a greeting card. The youngster draws a self-portrait on the outside of the card depicting the way the child thinks everyone sees him or her. Then the child opens the paper and draws a self-portrait of the way he or she really feels "on the inside." This concrete depiction of the child's feelings serves as a springboard for discussion and further exposure. The therapist helps the child identify the "inside" feelings and attach verbal labels to them. This technique may be especially useful for those children who are having difficulty expressing the range of feelings associated with the maltreatment because of shame, embarrassment, or fear of others' reactions. It is also useful for children who manifest the problems in the development of an autonomous and integrated self we described in Chapter 1. They may have split-off or dissociated perceptions of themselves and others, have developed a false self, or demonstrate a pattern of compulsive compliance. Using this instrument, they can begin to identify different and sometimes unique aspects and characteristics of themselves, such as cognitions, feelings, attitudes, and behaviors, rather than denying them.

Specific Problems and Strategies

SEXUAL CONCERNS AND ISSUES OF SEXUALLY ABUSED CHILDREN

Some sexually abused children experience pleasurable physical feelings or sexual arousal during abusive episodes. In our experience, children are often extremely reluctant to acknowledge these reactions because of embarrassment or confusion about their origins. Likewise, some therapists have difficulty understanding how children can become sexually aroused while they are being molested. Others cannot accept the fact that children have sexual feelings or show sexual responses. If this subject was not addressed in the evaluative phase, the therapist must ask the child, in a matter-of-fact way, whether he or she experienced pleasurable physical sensations during the episode. If, in response to more general inquiries about body sensations during the sexual assault (e.g., "How did your private parts feel when he touched you there?"), the child does not indicate that he or she experienced any pleasurable feelings, the therapist should ask more pointed questions. The therapist might ask, "Did it ever feel good when he rubbed your vagina?" and acknowledge and validate positive feelings as a legitimate part of the child's experience (e.g., "When he touched your vagina like that, it felt really good. Even though you were scared and didn't like what he was doing, part of you thought it felt good. Other girls who have been touched that way have told me the same thing.") Given the acute sensitivity of this matter and the child's intense anxiety, it is often useful to provide a simple but direct explanation of sexual response physiology and how sexual arousal occurs. For example, 11-year-old Peter, whom we first discussed in Chapter 7, eventually revealed that he experienced intense feelings of pleasure when his stepfather performed oral sex on him. Besides being extremely embarrassed, Peter thought his physical reactions, especially his erections, proved he was a "pervert" and that something was wrong with his penis. While empathizing with his embarrassment, the therapist provided a simple explanation of sexual response in boys. He explained how Peter's physical reactions could be understood from this perspective. Peter was relieved when he heard that the therapist had talked with other boys who had experienced the same reaction. His ability to divulge fears and anxiety about this issue was the first step in helping Peter reformulate this specific aspect of his maltreatment. Furthermore, exposing him to this material provided some immediate relief from his concomitant anxiety.

After receiving an explanation for what to them is sometimes confusing and perplexing behavior and learning that others have shown similar behavior, children may be increasingly willing to divulge more of their concerns or symptoms. Typically, these sexual reactions elicit great embarrassment and shame. Let us return to the example of Peter.

After the therapist explained the basis of Peter's physiological response to the sexual assaults and the reasons for his premature eroticization, Peter began to talk somewhat more openly about his sexual fantasies. He revealed that he sometimes thought of having sex with babies because they were "totally helpless." Although Peter expressed revulsion and disgust with himself, the therapist maintained an attitude of acceptance and reiterated his commitment to helping Peter with this particular difficulty. Eventually, as anxiety abated, Peter could reexamine this issue productively in greater depth.

Peter's revelation of these fantasies provided some relief from his almost intolerable anxiety and shame associated with them. It also served as the first step in a process where he and the therapist could examine the fantasies, and they eventually reached a mutual understanding about their emergence (i.e., they were a result of his premature sexualization rather than an indication that he was a deviant or perverted child). Finally, they developed some strategies to help Peter gain a sense of control over the sexual fantasies.

James (1989, pp. 96–98) describes a technique, "Guess What Other Sexually Abused Kids Worry About?" that therapists can use to elicit more of the child's concerns or feelings about sexual abuse. The therapist presents the exercise as educational information about the common reactions, fears, and worries of maltreated children. The therapist tells the child to listen to what the therapist tells "other kids" and then invites the child to ask questions. James uses this technique to address the concerns sexually abused children have about their body integrity or other significant issues and concerns that were identified in the assessment. For example, the therapist might comment that many boys and girls worry about the sexual excitement they possibly experienced during episodes of molestation, thereby demonstrating that these fears and worries, which the child originally believed reflected just a personal experience, are shared by many others. This new knowledge may be a catalyst that reduces the child's sense of isolation and facilitates expression of anxieties and worries, thereby leading to anxiety diminishing and opportunities for the restructuring of any cognitive distortions or misattributions related to the experience.

NEGLECTED CHILDREN WITH LIMITED VERBAL SKILLS

The techniques described above are often useful in assisting children to talk in more detail about feelings regarding their maltreatment. However, some children, especially those exposed to significant neglect, have difficulty in verbally expressing feelings (see Chapter 1 for a review of this research). The therapist must help such children learn to identify and label feelings in general before focusing on the particular affects associated with the maltreatment. Here we review some specific techniques to teach children to express their feelings verbally. Again, we draw on the work of others. Many of these techniques have a psychoeducational orientation, and it is important to make the activities as much fun as possible. They should be interspersed with other activities, because some children quickly become bored in sessions where the focus is exclusively on these more educational tasks.

Clinicians usually have numerous opportunities to model the verbal expression of a wide range of feelings in therapy sessions. They can use them in response to the child's account of abusive or neglectful experiences or even everyday occurrences. For example, a child tells the therapist that she was picked last for a game during gym class. She recounts this in an angry tone of voice while ripping up a piece of paper, but does not use the word "angry" or "mad" to label her feelings. Simple empathic statements from the therapist like "You're really mad!" model the verbal expression of this feeling. Playing board games affords the therapist another opportunity. Besides verbally identifying the child's feelings displayed during the game (e.g., anger or disappointment over losing, happiness about winning), the therapist might articulate his or her personal feelings about winning or losing. As discussed in Chapter 7, the therapist might become angry over some aspect of the child's behavior. Rather than acting out this anger inappropriately or suppressing it, the therapist should tell the child that he or she is angry. Similarly, the therapist should express pleasure when the child accomplishes tasks and demonstrates new skills (Urquiza & Winn, 1994).

There are other specific techniques clinicians can use to teach children to identify and label their feelings. One of the simplest is to present simple drawings of facial expressions that denote different feeling states and teach the child the verbal labels corresponding to each emotion. The therapist may start with the four basic feelings—happy, sad, scared, and angry—and then add more facial expressions as the child masters the basics. The therapist can use more realistic pictures, such as magazine photographs of people, and ask the child to identify the feelings the pictures might convey. Mandell and Damon (1989, pp. 60–61) describe a technique called "Feeling Collages." Although they developed this technique for group therapy with sexually abused children, we have adapted it to individual therapy and for children subjected to other types of maltreatment. The therapist and child decide on a feeling they want to portray in the collage, such as sadness, and then look through magazines to find photographs or pictures that depict this feeling. They can generate more fun by writing a number of feeling states on paper slips, putting them all in a bag, and then having each person draw a feeling out of the bag. Without showing each other the feeling states they are to portray, both construct their own collages (or just one or two pictures). At the end, each attempts to identify the feeling states portrayed by the other individual's collage. Mandell and Damon (p. 61) also suggest that the therapist list a variety of words denoting feelings. The child must construct a collage, choosing at least one picture for each feeling listed. Again, the therapist and child try to identify the feelings depicted in one another's collages.

Mandell and Damon (1989, p. 60) describe another technique, "What Kinds of Things Make People Feel ___________?," to help children identify the precipitants of common feelings like sadness or anger. Although the technique was originally developed as a worksheet, the same principle can be incorporated in a task during which the therapist and child each draw paper slips with different feelings written on them out of a bag. Then each must verbally describe a situation that would evoke this affective state. As children become more comfortable with this task, the therapist can ask them to identify actual situations that have elicited the same feelings in them. Lists or charts of the precipitants of various feelings help them identify those people, situations, or things that evoke particular feelings, including episodes of abuse and neglect. If a child is particularly anxious about doing this, the therapist should ask the child to list the precipitants of these feelings in "other kids" before identifying idiosyncratic precipitants. Nonverbal children can act out the situation in a charade game format or even draw the situation, with the therapist verbally labeling the child's nonverbal depiction of the precipitants and affects. Mandell and Damon (pp. 61–62) developed another handout, "How I Show My Feelings," in which the child lists the ways he or she demonstrates feelings nonverbally. Again, the child with poor literacy skills can portray these nonverbal expressions of feelings by using role plays or pantomime. The therapist and child then think of words that convey the feelings displayed in the behavioral depictions.

These are just samples of creative strategies clinicians may use to help children identify and label their feelings. The therapist must remain cognizant that accomplishing this task is often a gradual and sometimes long process that runs through the entire course of therapy. The therapist who believes that this task can be accomplished after two or three sessions and working on a few handouts will be sorely disappointed. Children need repeated opportunities to practice their developing skills in this area. The therapist's efforts must support and complement parents or caregivers and others such as teachers to model, teach, and encourage the child's verbal expression of feelings and emotions.

PLAY THERAPY TECHNIQUES

Why Play Therapy?

In Chapter 4 we discussed how play serves as a medium through which children, with their less sophisticated verbal skills, can communicate their thoughts, feelings, and significant concerns. The cognitive-developmental variables among these children render play a viable and meaningful communication medium. Moreover, maltreated children are often too frightened to talk directly about their experiences. For these children, play provides a safer means of communication. But, as we argued in Chapter 5, the therapist may have to take a more directive approach, albeit one that is gradual and sensitive, for those children who strenuously attempt to avoid exposure to the cues and stimuli associated with maltreatment.

Play therapy can help children learn to articulate their feelings rather than acting them out in maladaptive ways. Transforming action into words enhances impulse control. The doll play of children with anger management problems illustrates this concept and may be replete with examples of physical aggression: in the doll play, parents physically or sexually assault their children, who in turn attain vengeance or retribution by beating or assaulting others. When confronted with these displays, the therapist should introduce more appropriate and healthy expressions of anger. The therapist can initiate this process by describing the affect of the play character (e.g., "She's really mad!"). The therapist asks the child to have the character put those feelings into words ("What could she [the character] say when she is so angry?") and how it feels to articulate the feelings. For children who encounter real difficulty in refraining from physical assaults, even in the context of pretend play, the therapist might issue a challenge in a positive and fun way: "Let's see if you can put your hands together and keep them like that while you tell him how angry you are. Let's see how long you can do that. I'm going to start timing you now."

As children are exposed to more details of the maltreatment via the play and their anxiety decreases, they become more amenable to discussing their experiences and feelings openly. Webb (1991) notes that relief of symptoms with no transition from the play to the child's life is certainly possible, especially in work with preschool children. However, school-age children who learn to tolerate and engage in more direct discussions of victimization experiences seem to gain an even greater sense of mastery over these events and a greater sense of accomplishment ("I can talk directly to another person about those painful things that happened to me"). This greater sense of mastery may be particularly true for older school-age children who are expected to rely more heavily on verbal communication skills than on symbolic play in their natural environment (e.g., the classroom).

A principal goal of play therapy is to help the child toward better verbalization. Harter (1983) describes a four-phase model of therapy that has direct relevance to this goal. In play, the child moves from an indirect expression of needs and conflicts to direct verbal expression. Harter's model is consistent with our description of the use of metaphorical play. The therapist first presents sensitive topics in an indirect and gradual way that ensures that the child's avoidance and denial are not reactivated. This gradual exposure helps extinguish the child's anxiety, and the youngster becomes increasingly able to tolerate more direct exposure to the material. In Harter's first phase, the characters within the play scenario talk to each other, with one character interpreting the other's behavior. For example, one figure might comment that another is angry or distressed about being abused. Metaphorical characters provide sufficient psychological distance to enable the child to tolerate material that would be avoided if presented more directly. In the second phase, the therapist comments on how the child is like one of the dolls. In the third phase, the therapist describes another child with the same name or a similar appearance who is struggling with the same dilemmas or difficulties. This message is still sufficiently metaphorical and indirect for the child to accept the content of the communication. Finally, the therapist makes direct comments or interpretations without resorting to metaphorical or disguised communications. Shelby and Felix (2005) describe a similar technique wherein the therapist presents a life-size drawing of a child as the focus of treatment. They suggest that avoidant children may more readily identify the fears of this fictional character, the exercise thereby desensitizing the child.

We now review in detail some of the more common play therapy techniques used with maltreated children.

Doll Play

Every playroom should be equipped with a set of bendable family dolls that represent mother, father, girl, boy, baby, grandparents, adolescents, and other adults. A dollhouse with furniture adds to the child's interest and encourages reenactment of family scenes. Life-size infant dolls, along with bottles and toy baby food, provide further opportunities for children to portray their experiences. Other useful play equipment for this work includes medical kits, soldiers, dinosaurs, and animals (wild and domestic). A variant of this approach is sandplay, or sand tray therapy, a technique originally developed by Jungian analysts. An advantage of providing a sandbox or even something less elaborate, such as a large plastic rectangular container filled with sand, is that children, especially younger ones, seem to like the tactile sensation produced by the sand. They can also hide or bury people or objects in the sand. In addition, it is a medium with which most children are familiar, having played in sandboxes or sand trays at home, at a park, or in a kindergarten classroom.

Some maltreated children play spontaneously with this equipment and quickly reenact scenarios and narratives of their own maltreatment. For example, children portray the mother or father doll spanking or even physically abusing the child doll. These assaults may occur along with oppositional or defiant behavior by the child doll, such as refusing to eat. To encourage the child to talk about affects associated with his or her maltreatment, the therapist can ask how the doll feels when being so treated, or the therapist might speak to the doll directly. Upon hearing the child's (or doll's) reply, the therapist shows empathy with the expressed sentiment via simple statements like "___________ [name of the doll] is really mad when her father hits her like that."

As discussed earlier, some children, especially neglected youngsters, cannot verbalize these affects, even in the metaphor of play. They may be without the requisite verbal skills, such as internal state language. Doll play may afford another opportunity to teach a child to label these affective states. The therapist must observe the action of the play closely to detect whether the characters are giving hints or clues about how they feel. After observing the child doll lash out at others following an assault by a parent doll, the therapist might say to the child, "The doll seems really angry." Alternatively, following Harter's (1983) model, the therapist might have another doll in the play scenario make this comment. As children become more adept at labeling feelings, the therapist addresses the doll who is assaulting the child character, saying, "When you hit ___________ [name of the child character] like that, you make ___________ feel a lot of things. You make him (her) feel ___________." At this point, the therapist hesitates, leans over in the child's direction, and whispers, "What did he make ___________ feel?" The therapist should empathize and legitimize the normalcy of the doll character's feelings just as he or she would in a more direct discussion of these experiences. Such comments convey sensitivity to the child's internal state and place the child's feelings in a broader context (e.g., "Most kids get mad when they get hit like that"). These comments also serve to lessen the child's confusion about the origin of these feelings and help to reduce feelings of isolation and stigmatization. If the therapist believes the child is ready to move on to the next stage, he or she can point out the similarity between the doll's and the child's experiences. The therapist may ask if the child, when being abused or neglected, ever felt the way the abused doll feels (stage 2 of Harter's model). This may be too premature for some children, who respond to the elicited anxiety by quickly stopping the play (play disruption) or vociferously and adamantly denying they ever felt that way. Rather than constituting evidence against the correctness of the therapist's comments, these overreactions indicate that the therapist's interpretations have generated significant anxiety and are therefore meaningful to the child (Harter, 1983). Conversely, children who show no reaction probably have not been affected in the same way, leading to the hypothesis that for them the comments may not have been relevant. If the child's anxiety escalates significantly after these interventions, the therapist should empathize directly with that anxiety (e.g., "When we start to talk about what happened to you and how you felt, it makes you pretty nervous"). The therapist may also explore fears that are related to discussing the maltreatment. It may be necessary to revert to more indirect comments to allay the child's anxiety before attempting further exposure to more direct material in subsequent sessions.

Some children will not even use the metaphor of play to communicate thoughts or feelings about their victimization; even these indirect depictions and portrayals are too threatening, and the child engages in repetitive or obsessional play to avoid such feelings. In Chapter 4 we described an assessment technique in which the therapist becomes more directive and presents maltreatment-related material via doll play. The therapist asks the child to "show what happens next." The clinician may use a similar technique in therapy sessions with children who attempt to avoid any communication about their experiences of abuse or neglect. The therapist draws the child's attention to the toys and suggests that they "make up a story about a family." Some children respond but may spend most of their time arranging and rearranging the dollhouse furniture, probably to avoid significant issues. The therapist should place limits on the time spent in this obsessional play, making comments such as, "That looks pretty good. Let's see what happens in this family."

When a child continues to avoid any play that includes content related to maltreatment, the therapist should then seriously consider becoming more directive and, using doll play, begin to gradually expose the child to some of the child's experiences of abuse. The therapist may say that he or she has made up a story about the dolls and would like the child to watch. The story should incorporate aspects of the child's own aversive experiences. However, the therapist should incorporate only those elements that the child can likely tolerate. Initial portrayals of actual episodes of the maltreatment, even in the metaphor of the play, may be too threatening and overwhelming and may render the youngster even less enthusiastic about this activity. For example, the therapist may want to start portraying a family whose members are of the same genders and ages as those of the child's family. The therapist can depict the family in a relatively neutral activity and then invite the child to "show what happens next." The child may, of course, want to stay with this neutral theme, but at least the therapist has caught the child's attention. In the next session, the therapist can present another family scenario using dolls, with a more emotionally salient element that the child can tolerate. For example, the therapist suggests that one parent is "cranky" and then asks the child to continue the action. Via the character of the child doll, the therapist asks the child how he or she feels when a parent becomes cranky and to portray what happens next. The therapist may subsequently portray the child as somewhat defiant and then ask the child to depict the parent's reactions.

We have developed story stems that incorporate features of other types of maltreatment. Again, the main goal is to gradually expose the child gradually to the disturbing material. This technique is similar to the use of a gradual and paced approach when engaging the child in direct discussions about abuse-related material. Therapists may have to take considerable time with these less threatening scenarios before the child can approach more sensitive material. Rushing through this process or forcing premature confrontation of such material can lead to the reemergence of maladaptive defenses and erode trust in the therapist as a sensitive and benevolent figure.

Some therapists, especially those trained in a purely nondirective play therapy approach, object to the purposeful introduction of abuse-related material into sessions. We can counter only by again stating that the external and internal pressures on maltreated children to avoid exploring and examining these issues, either directly or indirectly, are often enormous. They present a formidable obstacle to the child's raising these issues, which in turn reduces the opportunities for the child to undergo the necessary exposure to the feared stimuli. However, we strongly disapprove of forcing children to confront overwhelming reminders of their maltreatment without adequate preparation and support.

Puppets, Drama, and Role Playing

Like doll play, puppets, psychodrama, and role playing offer metaphorical means of communication and gradually expose a youngster to maltreatment-related material. As in doll play, the therapist can assume a role in these activities, such as introducing relevant situations into the play or drama to elicit the child's feelings and thoughts.

The child may spontaneously ask to play with the puppets (a variety of animal and human cloth puppets should be available, rather than complicated string marionettes) or to put on plays. Using the puppets, the child may enact scenarios of the original maltreatment. If the child does not verbally express the characters' feelings, the therapist, as the audience, can, at the performance's end, ask the puppets relevant questions about their feelings and thoughts. Another useful technique to engage reluctant children's participation is for the therapist to initiate a puppet show, in the same manner we described in the section on doll play. The therapist presents an opening scene and then asks the audience (i.e., the child) for help in determining what happens next. Similarly, the therapist may suggest stories for puppet plays that are relevant to the child's life and circumstances, thereby gradually introducing more emotionally salient material. The following case illustrates this approach.

Seven-year-old Tara was living in a foster home after being removed from her mother, who had severely physically abused her for a number of years. Tara presented with many features of PTSD. For the first several months of therapy she was a defiant, noncompliant, and disruptive child who would not talk about her experiences. She began to show some interest in the puppets in the therapy room, picking them up and examining them. However, when invited to present a puppet show, she adamantly declined.

The therapist decided to take the initiative and presented a puppet show to Tara. She gave Tara a "front row seat" and told her it was the very best in the house. The therapist began enacting a story about a little girl who lived with her mother but sometimes wasn't very happy. At this point the therapist stopped the action and, turning to Tara, asked her what should happen next.

Tara then became a very active participant. She suggested that the mother become an evil witch who beat the girl. At this point, the therapist invited Tara into the show and asked her to think of a character she would like to portray. Tara assumed the role of a prince, who went to elaborate lengths to ensure that the witch would not hurt anyone. He locked her in jail, threw her in a lake, and gave her magic potions that killed her. Despite these actions and precautions, the witch always escaped or, if dead, returned to life.

In the metaphor of the puppet show, the therapist and Tara talked about the girl puppet's fear and anger, the normalcy of these affects, and the girl puppet's expectation that she was powerless and could do nothing to protect herself from the witch. Tara repeated this play regularly for several months. As her anxiety decreased, she and the therapist were able to have more direct discussions of how she had been treated in a similar manner by her own mother and of her fear that she would be returned to live with her.

The puppet play gradually exposed Tara to the stimuli associated with her physical abuse, initially in a disguised form and then more openly. Her anxiety began to extinguish and the PTSD subsided. In her role as the prince, Tara achieved a sense of mastery over a frightening situation. Although initial efforts were futile (the witch always returned to life or escaped), puppet plays in later therapy sessions ended with the prince finally vanquishing the witch. Chapter 10 includes a detailed discussion of play therapy techniques that facilitate the child's building a sense of mastery over the maltreatment.

Similarly, role plays and psychodrama provide anxious children with some much-needed psychological distance from relevant themes. Just as hiding behind a puppet theater and speaking as a puppet can attenuate anxiety, dressing up in costumes and pretending to be somebody else offer the same sense of distance and relief. Face makeup, masks, or even sunglasses may contribute to the child's sense of psychological safety. James (1989, p. 195) discusses "clowning." The therapist and child, pretending to be clowns, express emotions in verbal and nonverbal ways. In an earlier article, Smith, Walsh, and Richardson (1985) describe a short-term therapeutic group in which children created a pretend identity, a clown character who was a metaphorical expression of themselves, along with life stories for their respective characters. The group constructed a story of how they came together and how they got along interpersonally. The same basic premise may be applied to individual psychotherapy. Children can participate in role plays and dramas in which they reenact relevant and sometimes painful aspects of their own histories. The therapist might suggest some relevant themes (e.g., "Let's put on a story today about a little animal who doesn't have a home"). As a character in the play, the therapist models the verbal expression of feelings or asks how the child's character feels. Furthermore, therapists should encourage and assist children to demonstrate ways in which they might protect themselves or prevent further maltreatment.

Some children are enthusiastic about the idea of videotaping puppet shows or drama productions. The advantage of this technique is that the child and therapist can view the production and discuss it in detail. For example, the therapist can stop the tape at a particularly significant or interesting juncture and ask what the child's character was feeling. They might want to look at that particular portion of the tape several times to help the child identify and label the feelings accurately and to ensure that the child is repeatedly exposed to especially threatening or anxiety-inducing material.

Other props can create a sense of safety for the child participating in these dramas and role plays, in addition to the use of makeup and costumes. Toy telephones are useful for communication with somebody the child is not yet ready or able to address directly and can easily be incorporated into the metaphor of the drama or role play.

Storytelling and Story Writing

Therapists can use stories in several different ways to help maltreated children express their experiences and feelings. Within the safe metaphor of the story, the child learns to describe feelings or discuss events, including those connected with maltreatment. Stories also help the child master past trauma. For instance, traditional fairy tales such as *Hansel and Gretel* portray child characters as victorious over punitive and frightening figures. We discuss the use of stories to attenuate feelings of powerlessness and facilitate a sense of mastery and control over aversive events and circumstances in Chapter 10.

As a means of imaginal exposure and a way to help children express feelings regarding the maltreatment, the therapist may tell stories that incorporate their experiences. The therapist may also engage in a mutual story-writing task in which the clinician provides the narrative stem (see Chapter 4). The therapist asks the child to answer questions to complete the narrative. In Chapter 2 we introduced 6-year-old Gary, who was apprehended because of severe physical abuse, neglect, and psychological maltreatment. This was a young boy who misinterpreted the actions of other children on the playground. To facilitate his exposure to the abuse-related material, the therapist began to write a story, "The Little Bear's Story." The therapist developed a brief text that constituted the story stem for each chapter, as well as questions for Gary to answer. Gary and the therapist completed a chapter each week. The therapist transcribed his answers because Gary was only 6 years old and unable to write. The first three chapters and Gary's responses to the questions at the end of each chapter follow.

Chapter 1

Once upon a time there was a little bear who lived with his mommy bear and his uncle bear in a dark, scary cave. The little bear did not like living here because sometimes his mommy and uncle were mean to him.

QUESTION: How do you think they were mean to him?

GARY'S RESPONSE: They spanked him and said bad things to him like, "You shouldn't live here."

QUESTION: How did he feel when they were mean to him?

RESPONSE: The little bear felt sad and mad.

QUESTION: How would most little bears feel when their mommy and uncle were mean to them?

RESPONSE: They would feel worried about other worser things. Lock him in a closet, scared.

Chapter 2

Sometimes this little bear would get very angry when his mommy and uncle were mean to him. When he got angry he would have big temper tantrums—he would yell, stomp his feet, and sometimes he would pick fights with the other animals who lived in the forest.

QUESTION: How did the little bear feel when he had these temper tantrums?

RESPONSE: Mad.

Chapter 3

The little bear also got really scared when he got so mad and had these temper tantrums. He was scared that everyone would hate him and that he was the worst little bear in the whole world when he got mad and had these temper tantrums. Sometimes his mommy and uncle told him he was a horrible little bear when he had a temper tantrum and that no one loved him or wanted him when he was very mad. And they would be even meaner to the little bear when he had a tantrum.

QUESTION: Do you think the little bear was a bad bear because he got so angry?

RESPONSE: No, because he didn't do anything.

The narrative stems developed by the therapist incorporated actual episodes from Gary's life, including his having been abused by his mother and her partner. Both had repeatedly told him that no one loved him when he retaliated with anger. The story stems not only exposed him to the anxiety-related themes, but also elicited even more material, such as his comment that he had been locked in the closet (which was subsequently confirmed). The therapist encouraged Gary to draw pictures to depict the scenes in each chapter. Drawing was another way for Gary to express his terror and sadness about being treated so horrifically, and to elaborate upon his trauma narrative. Allowing children to use the therapist's computer to write these stories often adds another element of interest and fun. However, with young children like Gary, the therapist did the writing and transcribed his verbal responses to the questions. Gary was pleased with the "book" he produced. Over time, as Gary became more comfortable with this material, his anxiety abated, and later he could talk more directly about his actual experiences. Gary also had the good fortune of being placed with a foster parent who provided him with excellent care and ultimately adopted him. Now a young adult, Gary is flourishing. He has a career, has close friends, and is described by his adoptive mother as a loving and caring young man.

Writing letters is a technique that, like storytelling, gives the child an opportunity to express difficult feelings. The child feels more comfortable with this exercise when he or she is informed that the letters will not be mailed. Even young children who cannot read or write can participate in this exercise. The therapist functions as the "secretary" who transcribes the child's letters. Children can write letters to the persons who hurt them, including offending parents, and to nonoffending parents or other caretakers who should have protected them. Feelings of anger, betrayal, and hurt often emerge and are sometimes associated with suspicion that the nonoffending parents had knowledge of the maltreatment while it was occurring. Letters provide a forum in which a child can safely express concerns that the caretaker could have been more supportive. Likewise, letters to the perpetrator may permit recognition and safe expression of the ambivalence a child might feel, especially when the child and perpetrator had a close relationship.

In some situations, children actually send their letters, as did Tyler, a 9-year-old boy. He had witnessed marked domestic violence and wrote a letter to his father, who was serving a lengthy prison term for the assaults. We quote the contents verbatim: "When you did what you did I felt i wanted to tear you apart. So mad and sad to see it and just one song made me cry off of Eimem 'when i'm gone' So have a great day. thanks from Tyler."

Art

Art can reflect intrapsychic as well as interpersonal events. As Harter (1977) states, art visually and concretely portrays feelings and other abstract psychological constructs that the child may have difficulty expressing verbally. Many of the assessment techniques we described in Chapter 4 have corresponding therapeutic purposes. Children can produce graphic representations of their feelings elicited by the maltreatment.

Figure 8.1 was drawn by a 7-year-old boy who had been sexually abused by his father. The therapist asked him to draw his feelings about the abuse. At the lower left of the drawing is the perpetrator, with a prominent penis, and the child is at the lower right, throwing an egg at the perpetrator's genitals. The therapist then asked the boy to draw a picture of his face, showing his feelings about the sexual abuse. He produced the angry-looking face, with dagger-like teeth, that we see at the top of Figure 8.1. These graphic representations of feelings allowed the therapist and child to label them, and the therapist was able to legitimize the normalcy of the child's rage. Asking children to draw their bodies after the maltreatment gives them an opportunity to express their concerns and worries about body integrity and health. The therapist can ask children to draw their family members or the perpetrator. The drawings may quite accurately depict their feelings of loss, sadness, or anger, as well as their ambivalence. Children's drawings of idealized wishes may allow comparison with the true reality of their lives, and drawings of troublesome dreams or thoughts may allow some concrete problem solving in management of the associated anxiety. The reader may wish to consult Chapter 4 for a more detailed review of these tasks.

FACILITATING FEELINGS ABOUT LOSSES

Maltreated children need to experience and express their feelings of loss. Failure to do so may result in reliance on maladaptive defenses such as denial, which create more problems in the long term. Memories of unfulfilling

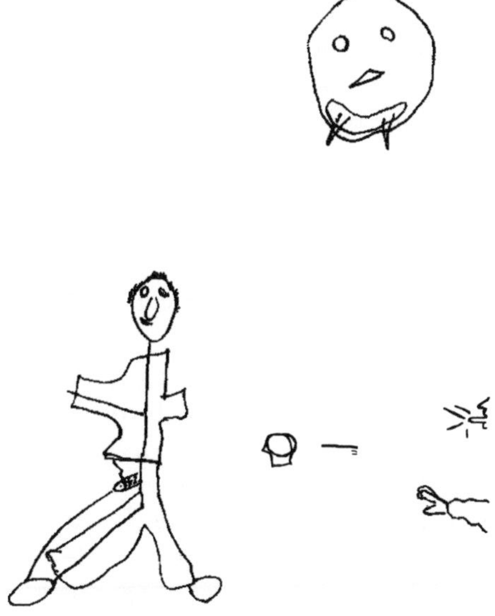

FIGURE 8.1. Seven-year-old boy's depiction of his feelings during his sexual assault.

and unsatisfying relationships with parental figures have to be described, rather than denied and repressed. For example, the child must mourn the loss of a parent that results from a legally mandated separation. The youngster must acknowledge and express the sadness and betrayal that accompany the realization that the parent was unable or unwilling to love the child in the way he or she always wanted. Obviously, examining such issues is extremely painful. The child must have alternate sources of support before he or she can acknowledge the parent's inability or unwillingness to provide the love and care the child deserves (James, 1994).

Besides defense mechanisms, there are certain cognitive-developmental factors that limit young children's ability to recognize and acknowledge ambivalence about their parents. A hallmark of the preoperational period of thought (ages 2–7 years) is the child's ability to attend to only one perceptual dimension at a time, to the exclusion of all others (Grave & Blissett, 2004). The classic example is the conservation experiment. Here the preoperational child insists that there is more water in the taller and narrower beaker than in the shorter and squatter container. The child's judgment is dominated by the perception of the single most salient perceptual feature, in this case height (Piaget, 1952, 1967). In contrast, the concrete operational child can consider more than one attribute simultaneously and can understand the reciprocal relationship between height and volume. Harter (1977) extrapolated these principles to the development of the child's understanding of emotional concepts. Just as the preoperational child can focus on only one perceptual dimension at a time, the same child has difficulty focusing on more than one emotional dimension at a time. Harter (1983) demonstrated that 4- to 12-year-old children encounter great difficulty in understanding that they can have both positive and negative feelings toward the same person. Thus, a maltreated child may have great difficulty in comprehending that he or she can both love and hate an abusive parental figure.

How can therapists facilitate the child's acknowledgment and expression of painful and sometimes conflicted feelings? Harter (1977, 1983) described a simple drawing technique that can help a child understand ambivalent feelings. The therapist draws a circle or other shape to represent the child. A line is drawn down the middle: the two halves represent two feelings, such as love and hate. The drawing provides a concrete visual symbol to which the child can attach real experiences. Such drawings help a child to recognize and better understand widely disparate feelings about the same person. Also, repetition of the drawing exercise over time in therapy serves as a concrete representation of the development of more realistic views of people or situations. Although we made the drawings in Figures 8.2a and 8.2b, they graphically represent the changes in a child's feelings about her father following an incident in which he returned to the home and not only beat her mother so severely that she was hospitalized with life-threatenting injuries, but killed the child's cat during the assault. The father had never previously been abusive to the 9-year-old girl, and she had enjoyed interactions with him during visits subsequent to a family separation some years earlier. Our first drawing (Figure 8.2a) is a graphic representation of the child's shock and anger immediately after the assault. After several months of therapy, she developed a more complex view of her feelings about her father and had she been asked to draw them, they may very well have been similar to the drawing shown in Figure 8.2b.

A therapist may use other techniques to help children express and concretize these memories and past experiences, such as asking a child to bring a photograph album to therapy sessions. Looking at pictures of family members, especially of those no longer in contact with the child, provide concrete reminders about these relationships. By reviewing the photographs, children often begin to remember specific incidents that in turn bring more significant material into consciousness. Many children in the care of child welfare authorities have been given "life books," which are compilations of mementos, photographs, and souvenirs about the child's history. They represent concrete reminders that allow children to acknowl-

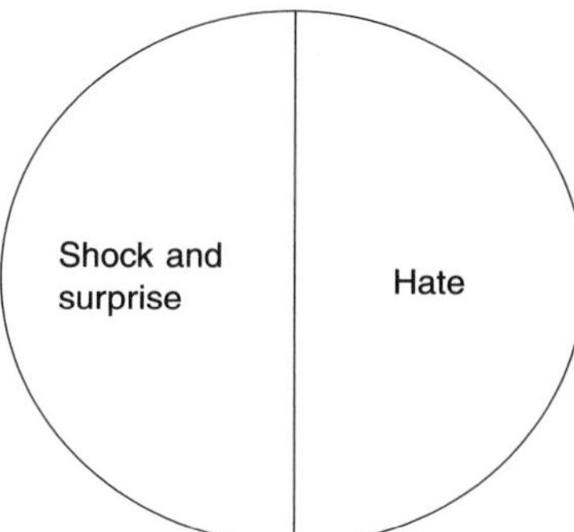

FIGURE 8.2a. Graphic representation of a child's feelings about her father immediately after traumatic event.

edge their histories more openly and directly, including the negative and painful aspects they have tried to avoid and deny. Although it is often a difficult task, the therapist and child should begin to assemble a life book, if this has not already been done. The therapist may have to gather historical information from child welfare authorities and share it with the child. Helping the child prepare simple genograms, or family trees, often clarifies some of the more confusing aspects of his or her history. It sometimes elicits even more questions, some of which cannot be answered. The creation of a family tree is another opportunity to help the child identify and express feelings of sadness, loss, and anger. These feelings may be associated with never having had, for example, a consistent father figure or even knowing his identity.

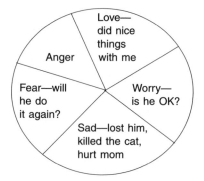

FIGURE 8.2b. Graphic representation of a child's feelings about her father after several months of therapy.

One of the most powerful exercises in uncovering these memories and feelings is to go on a "photo expedition" with the child. This procedure is particularly useful for a child with little documented history and who does not remember previous residences or placements. First, gather some relevant historical information about the child from other sources, such as child welfare records, make a list of the addresses of the child's previous residences or schools, and show them to the child. To make this exercise even more concrete and real, both might visit these locales. Obviously, the therapist must exercise extreme caution and sensitivity when deciding what information the child will receive and what sites they will visit. Giving a youngster the address of his or her biological parents whose parental rights have been terminated is not in the youngster's best interests, may contravene strict court orders prohibiting any contact between parents and child, and may constitute an invasion of the parents' privacy. It is usually best to limit information about, and subsequent expeditions to, former schools or residences. The therapist must be absolutely certain that these sites are no longer occupied by individuals with whom the child should have no contact. The therapist may teach the child how to use a simple camera, so the child can take pictures of each significant locale to place in a life book. Children usually love "field trips." They frequently begin to remember past incidents or episodes when they are at a site, such as a school they once attended, along with powerful and sometimes painful feelings. The therapist should help the child articulate these feelings and connect them to specific events, including maltreatment. Having a permanent record of these stimuli in the form of a photograph album allows the child and therapist to reexamine these issues as often as necessary.

A number of years ago one of us (TPP) treated a 12-year-old boy who had been severely neglected. His mother had committed suicide and was buried in a distant city when James was 8 years of age. His mother's death was a significant issue, and he had never seen her grave. This fact contributed to his difficulty in putting any closure to this aspect of his life. During James's treatment, my husband and children and I visited the other city for a vacation. I had offered to search for the boy's mother's grave and take a photograph of it. After considerable searching by all family members, in the cemetery where the grave was known to be, they found it and took a photograph. This photograph served as a concrete reminder of his mother's death and, although painful, did much to help James express his sadness and grief about this loss.

Cunningham and MacFarlane (1991, pp. 138–139) developed a tool they called the "Loss Timeline." Children construct a graphic representation of the losses they have experienced and their ages when these occurred. The technique may be combined with Color Your Life (James, 1989, p.

196). The child makes legends of different feelings, each associated with a different color. The child uses the colors to identify various events on the Loss Timeline. This is another visual depiction of the child's losses and the feelings associated with them.

Kagan (1986) recommends the use of games to help children who are in alternate placements express the attendant feelings. Kagan (pp. 80–92) developed "Cast Adrift," a pursuit game in which the squares graphically portray typical situations and events of being in care, such as running away from a foster home. Therapists can create games to reflect each child's particular experiences after they have gathered more information about the child's life through life books or photo expeditions. For instance, after landing on a square that says, "Removed from foster home, lose one turn," the child discusses the feelings associated with such an event.

TREATMENT OF DISSOCIATIVE DISORDERS

The major task in the treatment of dissociative phenomena is to bring feelings and experiences into the child's conscious awareness so that they may be acknowledged and explored; therefore it is relevant to this chapter, given its emphasis on helping children express feelings. The child no longer has to rely on dissociation or other defense mechanisms to guard against the overwhelming pain and anxiety associated with these experiences (Gil, 1991; James, 1989). As we have seen, dissociation is an adaptive strategy to cope with overwhelming fear and terror; if the maltreatment continues, we cannot expect children to give up dissociation (Haugaard, 2004a). The child's home and therapy session must be emotionally and physically safe living environments (Wallach & Dollinger, 1999). We have already detailed strategies clinicians and caregivers can use to promote safety, regularity, and predictability.

There are several other therapeutic strategies that can be used to treat dissociation. Gil (1991) and James (1989) advocate that therapists evaluate children's awareness of their use of dissociation and help develop a label or term they can use to communicate about it. James also suggests helping children examine the advantages and disadvantages of dissociation. The therapist explains that they have used dissociation in a creative and inventive way for protection. Silberg (1996, 2000) recommends that the therapist and child develop an agreement that the therapist will intervene when the child dissociates in therapy sessions. This agreement should include the specific actions the therapist will take (e.g., touching the child; calling his or her name). Of course, these actions must be gentle and nonintrusive to avoid eliciting even more fear or anxiety. The therapist can enlist parents or caregivers in this process by using similar methods when the child dissociates at home.

Therapists can help children to identify those situations in which they dissociate and to examine the functions of the dissociation. Were there particularly frightening aspects of the material the child was discussing in therapy that was associated with the dissociation? What was the worst aspect of this discussion? In addition to conversing with the child, the therapist can offer other ways of expressing these themes, such as in art. Exploration of the anxiety-inducing material, especially in the context of a safe psychotherapeutic environment, gradually decreases the child's anxiety and need to dissociate.

We have not had much clinical experience in treating children with dissociative identity disorder. Consequently, we refer the reader to the work of others, which provides some specific directions besides those in our earlier comments on treating dissociative phenomena (Braun, 1986; Gil, 1991; James, 1989; Kluft, 1984, 1996; Putnam, 1989). These include making a contract, with each personality a child may exhibit, to avoid harmful actions such as suicide or homicide or to meet therapy goals; working on the problems of each personality; and mapping and understanding the structure of the personality system (Braun, 1986). Gil (1991) and Putnam (1989) recommend that the therapist encourage co-consciousness and communication among the personalities. Kluft (1996) has written a valuable and detailed article describing the outpatient treatment of dissociative disorders in children, but space limitations preclude an in-depth review of this work. However, he describes the differences between the treatment of adults and the treatment of children with dissociative symptoms, the importance of creating an atmosphere of safety in which the child feels secure, fostering cooperation among the alter personalities, and teaching the child to contain strong feelings. Kluft warns therapists to refrain from exposing the child to traumatic material too prematurely; processing should proceed at a pace tolerable to the child so as to avoid significant anxieties and distress.

Both Friedrich (1990) and James (1989) caution therapists against intervening in ways that inadvertently reinforce the development of more dissociative phenomena or more numerous or complex personalities. For example, by asking leading questions of maltreated children who feel compelled to acquiesce to adult demands, the therapist may open the door to elaborated but misleading symptomatology. James also recommends that therapists work closely with other significant adults in the child's life so that they accept these phenomena but do not overreact in ways that make the child the center of attention. This is excellent advice from two experienced clinicians.

In this area clinicians seem to be divided between "believers" and "nonbelievers," with both sides expressing strong and sometimes vitriolic opinions. As clinicians, we must approach issues of dissociation and dissociative identity disorder with an open mind but evaluate the applicability of such diagnoses to our young clients in the same rigorous, comprehensive, and individualized manner that should characterize all our clinical work. Labeling a child as dissociative or "a multiple" just because these terms are in vogue does our client and our profession a great disservice. Conversely, a failure even to entertain the possibility of the presence of these phenomena results in less comprehensive and adequate service.

Whatever techniques are used, the therapist who helps children explore their histories and express the attendant feelings and issues must often use exquisite timing and clinical judgment. Knowing when to expose a child to slightly more material and when to back off are skills honed by experience, training and supervision, and a critical and rigorous examination of one's work. The therapist must have the flexibility and creativity necessary to respond to the changing and sometimes perplexing needs of these young children.

Assisting children to recount experiences of maltreatment and express their feelings is only one part of the therapeutic process. Maltreated children must also learn effective emotional and behavioral self-regulation skills to cope with painful memories and feelings. We discuss this topic in detail in the next chapter.

CHAPTER NINE

Helping the Child Develop Effective Coping Mechanisms

Abused and neglected children require help in developing mechanisms to manage their reactions to the maltreatment. The therapist can teach a highly anxious child to cope more adaptively with symptoms such as nightmares and sleep disturbances. Likewise, the physically or sexually aggressive child needs assistance to develop behavioral and emotional self-regulatory skills. In this chapter, we describe specific techniques for anxiety-related problems (PTSD, sleep disturbances, and nightmares), physical aggression, and SBPs. Given the space limitations of this book, our review must be somewhat cursory. Topics like anger management in children and, more recently, interventions for SBPs, have received considerable attention in the professional literature. We hope to give the reader a brief overview of the theoretical basis and a description of these and other commonly used techniques.

TREATMENT OF ANXIETY PROBLEMS

In Chapter 1 we reviewed the internalizing problems associated with a history of maltreatment. PTSD and other anxiety-related symptoms are among the most common disturbances in self-regulation manifested by maltreated children and generate a great deal of distress and suffering for them and their parents or caregivers. Manifestations of increased arousal associated with PTSD include sleep disturbance, hypervigilance, difficulty in concentrating, and outbursts of anger or irritability. Dreams, flashbacks, and psychological and physiological distress associated with exposure to external or internal cues that resemble or symbolize an aspect of the traumatic event are examples of reexperiencing phenomena. Helping a child learn effective ways of coping with these and other symptoms is often a central task of treatment. Chapter 8 reviewed the promising outcome research on multicomponent CBT programs for maltreated children with PTSD and other internalizing problems, and we focused on imaginal exposure as a major strategy. We now continue our discussion of other interventions, many of them derived from CBT, to reduce the often debilitating effects of anxiety.

Relaxation Exercises

In Chapter 8 we described standard techniques, such as breathing and relaxation training, to help children reduce the anxiety they experience during imaginal exposure in direct discussions of the maltreatment or during symbolic play. The therapist, besides incorporating and using these techniques in therapy sessions, should instruct and guide children with significant anxiety problems to employ such techniques in other environments. For example, children who have been sexually abused in their bedrooms at night may develop PTSD symptoms associated with bedtime routines (going to bed exposes the traumatized child to the actual anxiety-related stimuli, such as the physical aspects of the bedroom or being alone in the room). They subsequently develop symptoms such as reluctance or even avoidance of bedtime routines, difficulty in falling asleep, or frightening dreams. Although this *in vivo* exposure is necessary for anxiety to extinguish, children often need specific coping mechanisms to employ during the exposure so that anxiety does not overwhelm them.

The therapist can teach children to use these relaxation exercises at bedtime; the therapist can then record an audiotape or CD wherein he or she describes the various steps in the relaxation procedures. The child takes the tape or CD home and uses it there. Sometimes children enjoy working with the therapist to develop a recording that describes one of the imaginary, calming scenes we referred to in Chapter 8. Listening to the tape or CD while in bed may diminish the child's anxiety. The child can use other techniques such as diaphragmatic breathing and balloon imagery, described in Chapter 8, in almost any situation in which he or she feels anxious and overwhelmed. Other people around the child may not even realize that the youngster is consciously working at calming him- or herself.

To ensure children that use these techniques, parental support and involvement, especially with younger children, is critical. Therapists should teach relaxation exercises to parents or caregivers so that they know the proper technique for the child to use. This also allows them to cue the child to initiate the exercise when they notice the child is becoming anxious. A parent's offering to do the relaxation exercises with the child often decreases the resistance, normalizes the procedure, and demonstrates concretely the parent's commitment to helping the child. Furthermore, parents can use the exercises to diminish their own anxiety, which in turn may have positive effects on their responses to their children. Enlisting the assistance and support of teachers is also important for those children who experience significant anxiety in the classroom or on the playground. Like parents, they can unobtrusively signal the child that this might be a good time to start using diaphragmatic breathing or other relaxation techniques.

Visualization

Visualization is useful in assisting children to master unpleasant or frightening dreams. The therapist asks the child to recount or draw the frightening dream and then to visualize a scenario that transforms the frightening content into something more benign. For example, the child might visualize having a magic wand that changes a monster into a positive and friendly figure. Depending on the sophistication of the child's verbal and cognitive skills, detailed scenarios may be developed that incorporate this sense of mastery, and drawing and art are adjunctive strategies to visualization. The child draws the dream sequence using a cartoon-like format in which the frames of the cartoon depict the dream's progression. The youngster develops new scenes or frames, in which the child controls or vanquishes the monster or other frightening figures or scenarios, and tacks the cartoon on the wall near his or her bed. Just before going to bed, the child looks at this sequence, particularly the positive outcomes, as an aid in visualizing the new outcome. To further diminish anxiety, the therapist directs the child to use deep breathing or other relaxation exercises while visualizing the new dream.

Children can symbolically contain other frightening dreams or nightmares by drawing a picture of the dream and then putting it in a box. The youngster tapes the box shut to ensure that the dream does not "escape." The therapist encourages the child to "open up the box" (i.e., examine the maltreatment-related material symbolized by the dream) when he or she feels more comfortable, thereby exposing the child to the anxiety-inducing stimuli. This process is similar to James's (1989) "Garbage Bag" technique, which we reviewed earlier. However, keeping dreams locked up forever may reinforce the child's belief that this material is so threatening it can never be examined and must be avoided. When feeling less anxious, the child might pull a different aspect of the dream (each aspect is graphically displayed on a separate piece of paper) from the box in each therapy session and examine it.

Rituals

Other techniques also rely on the concretization of abstract psychological concepts. For example, some children with increased arousal become hypervigilant. They may fear that the perpetrator will break into their homes and reassault them. Terrorized children may harbor this fear even when they know the perpetrator is incarcerated. These children constantly monitor their environments and are acutely sensitive to any stimuli (e.g., unexplained noises) that they might interpret as evidence they are again in danger. We have had children "freeze" their perpetrators to reinforce the belief that they are now safe. The child constructs a small figure of the perpetrator from clay or other modeling material, takes it home, and places it in a container of water so that it is totally covered. The container is frozen, and the block of ice with the figure is removed from the mold and placed back in the freezer. When feeling particularly anxious about the perpetrator escaping, the child goes to the freezer and looks at the perpetrator entrapped in the block of ice. Concurrently, the child uses self-statements (detailed below) as a reminder that the perpetrator can no longer hurt the child. This strategy may be useful for children with sleep disturbances associated with the expectation that the perpetrator will return at night and reassault them. They can spend several minutes just before going to bed looking at the block of ice while using relaxation exercises.

Other children make up their own rituals to instill a sense of safety. They tour the house to make sure that the doors and windows are locked, or they check under beds and in closets. Some insist on sleeping with their parents. We try to discourage the latter as much as possible because it inadvertently conveys the notion that the child is unable to master the anxiety. Moreover, sharing their sleeping arrangements sometimes engenders frustration in parents, who are thereby deprived of privacy. However, children who are absolutely insistent can be accommodated initially by sleeping on the parents' bedroom floor in a sleeping bag or on a small cot, but not in the parental bed. Each night the parents encourage the child to move the makeshift bed a little farther from the parents' room: out of the bedroom, into the hallway, and eventually into the child's room. The use of a nightlight, particularly one the child has chosen, can reduce some of this bedtime anxiety, as can relaxing and soothing experiences such as having a hot bath or listening to music or a story read by a parent.

CBT Techniques: Self-Statements

CBT techniques can help children master anxiety-related symptoms such as intrusive memories and thoughts. Any reader unfamiliar with CBT should review standard texts in the field (e.g., Kendall & Braswell, 1993) for its theoretical underpinnings and detailed descriptions of specific techniques. Cohen and Deblinger (2004) offer the following succinct summary of CBT:

> Cognitive-behavioral therapy (CBT) is based on the premise that symptoms develop and are maintained, at least in part, by conditioned and learned behavioral responses as well as maladaptive cognitions (Brewin, 1989). The model emphasizes the interdependence of thoughts, behaviors, feelings as well as physiological responses. Thus, interventions designed to target any one of these areas of functioning are expected to indirectly impact on adjustment in the other areas of functioning as well. (p. 49)

The cognitive component of CBT is based on the premise that irrational or maladaptive attitudes or beliefs, thoughts, or maladaptive cognitive processing operations contribute to problematic behavior. Another quote expresses this conceptualization well:

> The aim of therapy is to help the child to identify possible cognitive deficits and distortions, to reality-test them, and then, either to teach new thinking skills or to challenge irrational thoughts and beliefs and replace them with more rational thinking. (Grave & Blissett, 2004, p. 402)

A major class of interventions within the CBT domain is self-instructional training. According to Kendall and Braswell (1993), "Self-instructions are self-directed statements that provide a thinking strategy for children with deficits in this area and serve as a guide for the child to follow through the process of problem solving" (p. 124). A central theoretical notion inherent in self-instructional training is the relationship between behavior and language (Ronen, 1997). We argued in Chapter 2 that the development of internal state language aids in the child's regulation of behavior and emotion. Vygotsky (as cited in Kendall & Braswell, 1993, p. 10) postulated that a crucial step in a child's ability to control behavior voluntarily occurs when the child internalizes verbal commands. The influence of self-talk or self-statements is clear when we think about learning to perform a new task or skill. We may even talk to ourselves aloud (overt self-statements) to provide ourselves with guidance and direction (e.g., "Now I have to press this key in order to call up the information on the computer"). Then we move on to covert self-talk or self-statements whereby we "quit talking out loud and begin to think the instructions to ourselves" (Kendall & Braswell, 1993, p. 184).

Let us now return to the problem of intrusive thoughts and memories ("flashbacks") associated with PTSD of maltreated children. They are often frightening and distressing because children feel they have little, if any, control over such episodes. Self-statements are an especially useful technique to diminish or eradicate this anxiety. A number of studies included in the outcome research we reviewed in Chapter 6 incorporated self-statements and thought replacement in the AMT component of treatment packages (e.g., Cohen & Mannarino, 1998b). AMT includes cognitive restructuring, which attempts to identify and change distorted attributions, schemas, and interpretations of the trauma. Similar to the situation with exposure techniques, there has been little work investigating the unique effects of AMT with children. In one study, four school-age children with PTSD received 10 sessions of AMT (Farrell, Hains, & Davies, 1998). Clinicians taught the children self-monitoring, restructuring of dysfunctional cognitions, and relaxation exercises, and they educated them about emotions. The children applied these skills to trauma-related, anxiety-provoking situations through role play and *in vivo* exposure exercises. At posttreatment, all children showed large decreases in PTSD, and three remained below clinical levels at the 3-month follow-up. Levels of general anxiety and depression also decreased. As we have already stated, it is difficult to draw any conclusions about the specific and unique contributions of more adaptive self-statements to outcome, as these techniques are applied in conjunction with other strategies (e.g., relaxation exercises in the Farrell et al., 1998, study). Theoretically, however, teaching children to replace distorted statements about themselves or the maltreatment with more accurate self-statements is appropriate, given CBT's emphasis on the relationship between cognitions and behavior (Cohen & Mannarino, 1998b).

As we reviewed in the previous chapter, one of the first things a therapist can do is to provide a simple yet direct explanation of the PTSD and make it clear that many other children have experienced similar reactions. The therapist can teach the child to use self-talk or self-statements to reduce anxiety, such as "What happened to me is over and this is just a flashback" or "This has happened to other kids too—I'm not crazy!"

Self-statements can be combined with other techniques to counter anxiety. In Chapter 7 we briefly introduced 11-year-old Derek, who was sexually assaulted once by an adolescent male babysitter. He was referred to therapy because of anxiety-related symptoms, including nightmares. Derek was bothered by intrusive memories of the sexual assault, particularly of the scene in the bathroom, where he had been forced to perform oral sex on the adolescent babysitter. The bathroom served as an external stimulus that quickly elicited his anxiety, which was reflected in intrusive memories and a sense of reliving the experience. In Derek's words, sometimes just being in the bathroom made him feel as if "it was happening all over again."

To assist Derek, the therapist suggested he say, "Stop!" to himself as soon as he became aware of the intrusive memory of the assault. The therapist and Derek developed a self-statement he could use after telling himself to stop: "This is just my memory—I'm not really being abused again!" He combined the self-statement with simple muscle and diaphragmatic breathing exercises. Other self-statements incorporated the fact that Derek had prevented further occurrences of the abuse by quickly disclosing the incident to his parents the day after it happened ("I took action, and it didn't happen again!"). The therapist suggested that Derek visualize himself as the major league baseball player he especially admired to reinforce and consolidate his growing sense of mastery over the situation. Visualization served as a concrete reminder to Derek of his own excellent athletic abilities and that the sexual assault had not diminished in any way his outstanding performance in baseball and other sports. The salience of the visualization and self-statements about his mastery and numerous other strengths increased after Derek placed a baseball card of his hero in the bathroom. This card served as a concrete prompt for him to "stop and think" and was a cue for visualizing his own substantial strengths that had not been deleteriously affected by the assault. Given his excellent adjustment prior to the assault, the support afforded by his family, and his active participation in treatment, Derek's PTSD symptoms disappeared in 6 weeks.

Some children have been so severely abused and terrorized that they experience overwhelming and debilitating anxiety that deleteriously affects many areas of their functioning. Anxiety that generalizes to different stimuli in their environments is now pervasive. These children begin to avoid such stimuli to reduce their discomfort. Ecological interventions that target a number of different symptoms in different environments frequently require the collaboration of other significant people in the child's life. This approach is characterized by the following case.

Steve was a 13-year-old boy who, from 9 to 12 years of age, had been sexually abused by his father. The abuse was horrific and had included anal rape on numerous occasions. The father also used physical violence to gain his son's compliance and ensure his silence; he threatened to kill Steve and his mother if he ever disclosed. Steve disclosed the abuse several months after his parents separated and the father left the home. The police subsequently charged his father with a number of counts of sexual assault, and the court issued an order prohibiting contact between Steve and his father.

Steve exhibited symptoms of PTSD when he was seen in the initial assessment. He had frequent dreams of the abuse and many flashbacks of the incidents. He also showed symptoms of increased arousal, including disrupted sleep and difficulty in concentrating in the classroom. Steve was especially hypervigilant, constantly monitoring his environment to make sure that his father was not following him or lurking around the home. His anxiety had escalated to the point that he was terrified to leave his home. He would not go outside and refused to attend school. Steve claimed that he saw his father near the school grounds after his dad had been charged, and he believed his father would attack him because he had disclosed. His father's threats to kill him and the physical violence to which Steve had been subjected gave these fears a solid basis in reality. Steve was terrified of leaving his mother at home because his father had also threatened to kill her. Witnessing several episodes of marital violence had exacerbated Steve's anxiety.

Interventions incorporated many of the elements we have described in this chapter. Relaxation exercises resulted in an improvement in Steve's sleep. The therapist focused on helping him leave his home to return to school. To initiate the process of gradual *in vivo* exposure and desensitization, the therapist instructed Steve to spend 3 minutes on his front steps several times each day while engaging in deep breathing and muscle relaxation exercises. Steve insisted on keeping the front door fully open so he could get into the house immediately if his father appeared. The amount of time spent outside and the distance from his front door (which he finally allowed to be closed) increased and continued to be paired with relaxation. With his therapist's help, Steve began to develop self-statements emphasizing his progress and mastery of the anxiety (e.g., "I'm now halfway down the block—I'm doing really well!"). Other self-statements, which focused on concrete strategies he could use to protect himself if his dad ever appeared, began to counter feelings of powerlessness (e.g., "I'll run right into the house, lock all the doors, and tell Mom"). After several weeks, Steve could walk around the block and approach his school, a short distance from his home.

Steve required further practice with these techniques before he could resume classes. In particular, he identified those situations at school that quickly evoked strong feelings of anxiety (e.g., being outside on the school grounds). Not only was he instructed to use relaxation techniques in these situations, but he and his therapist devised "a plan of action" to use if his father ever came to school: Steve would go immediately to the school office and tell the staff of his father's presence. Steve and the therapist had previously rehearsed what to say if this situation arose. Self-statements, such as "I know what to do now if he ever shows up," helped decrease Steve's anxiety. Fortunately, the school vice-principal agreed to be part of the treatment team. Not only was she willing to talk with Steve when he became especially anxious, but together they developed a specific plan that she or her designate would implement if Steve's father ever came to the school (e.g., calling the police to report that the father had broken the no-contact order). However, she did not give excessive attention to Steve because of the concern that this could inadvertently reinforce his expressions of distress. These plans attenuated some of Steve's anxiety and increased his feelings of mastery and control over a terrifying environment.

This case example highlights the need to involve significant people in the child's life in the treatment program. In addition to the vice-principal's being involved, Steve's mother played a critical role in assuring him she could protect herself. There were times when she had to be firm, such as insisting that he attend school even when he was anxious. Remaining at home would have done nothing to help Steve surmount his anxiety. Moreover, these strategies were only one component of treatment. The therapist helped Steve to articulate his rage, sadness, and feelings of betrayal, as well as to reformulate the meaning of these experiences.

TREATMENT OF PHYSICAL AGGRESSION AND SBPs

Preliminary Considerations

Our review of the effects of maltreatment indicates that physical aggression is not an uncommon symptom in abused or neglected children, who often require intensive assistance to prevent them from victimizing others and to learn healthier ways to express their angry feelings, in turn making it easier for them to establish more rewarding interpersonal relationships. This is a broad topic, and we can only highlight some of the more important approaches and techniques. We rely primarily on a CBT approach. Besides the work by Kendall and Braswell (1993), the reader may want to refer to the descriptions of anger management programs prepared by Lochman, White, and Wayland (1991), as well as a review of anger management control techniques for children (Stern & Fodor, 1989). We have also pointed out that sexualized behavior is another of the common sequelae of childhood sexual abuse. Children with clinically significant SBPs need the same intensive help as physically aggressive youngsters. There are some valuable resources the reader may wish to consult for detailed descriptions of treatment approaches (Bonner, 2004; Bonner et al., 2000; Cunningham & MacFarlane, 1991; Friedrich, 1990; Gil & Johnson, 1993; MacFarlane & Cunningham, 1988). In this section we review the application of CBT principles to treat physical aggression and SBPs exhibited by some maltreated children. Chapter 6 described the critical role parents play in this process, especially in supervising and limiting their children's inappropriate behaviors.

Therapists who work with maltreated children who have externalizing behaviors quickly confront a central issue: What are the therapist's values and beliefs regarding physical and sexual aggression? It is important to address this issue, because these values invariably affect one's clinical work. For example, one of our basic values in working with children who present significant problems with physical aggression is the importance of introducing nonaggressive and noncoercive means of conflict resolution. Therapists who do not introduce the child to alternate means of expressing anger may convey a tacit approval of the child's continued reliance on physical aggression. Such a misconception may lead to serious consequences for the child and others. For those children with poor behavioral and emotional self-regulation, therapy that encourages only catharsis does not serve recovery well. We strongly recommend that the reader review an article by Ryan (1989) for a more detailed exposition of this argument. She maintains that therapists must introduce accountability into therapy by limiting the child's demonstrations of power and control that victimize others. According to Ryan, therapists must confront a child's irrational thinking (e.g., "I'm going to kill the person who abused me") and offer rational alternatives to aggressive displays. Given our adherence to the value of nonaggressive ways of resolving conflict, we work actively and strategically in therapy to promote the same approach in children. Therapists should describe the underlying beliefs that guide their treatment planning when discussing recommendations and the proposed therapy plan with parents or caregivers, who need this information to give informed consent to treatment.

The issue of values becomes even more contentious when the therapist talks with children about the difference between "healthy" sexuality and "inappropriate" expression of sexual feelings. Although therapists must examine and identify their own values, they must also consult closely with parents or caregivers about their values and what they want conveyed to the child. Chapter 6 described strategies therapists can use to help parents clarify their values about sexuality and sexual behavior and what they want to convey to their children. If therapists promote one set of values and the child is exposed to a different or even a contrary set at home, the child is placed in an untenable position that undermines the parent's authority.

Therapists must be especially sensitive to religious or cultural variables that may play a significant role in the development and maintenance of sexual mores in the family, attempting to seek an agreement with parents about what is acceptable sexual expression for their child. However, we should note that sensitivity and respect for parental values concerning sexuality does not always translate into the therapist's wholehearted endorsement or acceptance of such values. On a few occasions, we reached a fundamental disagreement with a family. One set of parents believed that sexual behaviors, thoughts, or feelings constituted incontrovertible proof of sin. They believed that even raising the issue of sexuality would further eroticize their child, and they would not permit any discussion of the child's sexuality during sessions. These parents maintained this stance despite long and protracted discussions with the therapist and clear evidence that their son was increasingly making sexually aggressive advances toward younger children. Eventually the therapist had no choice but to withdraw from the case because of this fundamental difference in values. He notified child welfare authorities, given the real risk the boy posed to other children and the parents' refusal to permit the therapist to address it directly.

Clinicians sometimes struggle with the problem of how to treat child victims who exhibit "victimizing" behavior (physical or sexual aggression directed to other people). Their reluctance to address this behavior actively may result more from their greater experience and familiarity with treating survivors rather than with treating those who exhibit aggressive or exploitive behavior. Moreover, clinicians may not understand that a child's aggressive behavior may reflect unresolved issues engendered by the maltreatment. Unfortunately, the traditional division of clinicians into those who treat adult survivors and those who treat perpetrators has done little to encourage the development of a service-delivery approach for children that integrates features of both domains. Intervening with both victimization issues and physical aggression and SBPs is consistent with our philosophy of providing comprehensive treatment services. A clinician's failure to intervene when a child shows physical or sexual aggression may reflect inadvertent collusion with the child's reliance on this behavior. It places other children at risk and does little to help the youngster develop adaptive behavioral and emotional self-regulatory skills (Cunningham & MacFarlane, 1991). Conversely, the failure to address relevant victimization issues precludes an opportunity for the child to recover from the maltreatment. To provide truly comprehensive services for the different facets of the maltreated child's functioning and adaptation, the therapist must be ready and able to attend to both sets of problems.

A related question that sometimes arises concerns the timing and sequencing of interventions for a child who exhibits both internalizing and externalizing behaviors. In what order should they be addressed? Should each of the issues be addressed in a discrete phase of treatment, or can they be examined simultaneously? There is no hard-and-fast rule. The therapist must use clinical judgment about the timing of interventions pertinent to each broad class of problems. For example, a maltreated child who engages in serious physical or sexual aggression toward others will probably require immediate and intensive intervention to stop this behavior so as to ensure the safety of others, to start developing self-regulation, and to contain the child's own anxiety about behaving so inappropriately. Gil and Johnson (1993) and James (1989) commented that in many cases these problems might be addressed simultaneously, rather than separately in different phases of therapy. For example, children can articulate, in role plays, the feelings associated with having been abused, and then those associated with behaving aggressively toward others (Gil & Johnson, 1993). Eventually, the therapist can show the child the connection between his or her feelings of inadequacy and helplessness, which were engendered by the victimization, and his or her subsequent development of aggressive strategies. Even within one session, therapist and child may address the victimization issues and still have time to spend on the victimizing issues.

ESTs for Maltreated Children with Externalizing Problems

In Chapter 8 we briefly mentioned studies that reported significantly greater decreases in overall behavior problems in sexually abused children who had received CBT than youngsters who had been treated with child-centered therapy (Cohen et al., 2004). Because parents also participated in treatment and the CBT program included a number of different elements, it is again difficult to draw any firm conclusions about the relative impact of these specific interventions. Deblinger and her colleagues also reported significant decreases at posttreatment in externalizing behaviors of sexually abused school-age children treated with CBT (Deblinger et al., 1996) and at a 2-year follow-up (Deblinger, Steer, & Lippmann, 1999). In particular, those mothers who either were treated by themselves or in conjunction with their children, rated their offspring as showing significantly fewer externalizing behaviors on the CBCL, as compared with children in the child-only CBT condition.

Few studies have investigated the efficacy of other treatments or the impact of interventions on school-age children subjected to other types of maltreatment. In one of the few that evaluated treatments other than CBT, Downing, Jenkins, and Fisher (1988) randomly assigned 22 sexually abused children to a behavioral reinforcement group or psychodynamic therapy; the former was associated with greater reductions in general behavior problems than the psychodynamic group. Kolko (1996) compared CBT for school-age, physically abused children with family therapy and routine community services. As in the Cohen and Deblinger studies, the CBT group included sessions for children and their parents. Kolko reported that both the CBT and family therapy conditions were associated with decreases in externalizing behavior at posttreatment and at a 1-year follow-up.

Externalizing problems include SBPs, and the last decade has witnessed considerable attention to school-age children with SBPs and a corresponding attempt to determine the efficacy of various interventions. Cohen and Mannarino (1998b) and Cohen and colleagues (2005) reported that CBT for sexually abused 8- to 15-year-old children and their parents was more effective in treating sexually inappropriate behaviors than nondirective supportive therapy at posttreatment and at a 6-month follow-up, but not at a 1-year follow-up. Pithers and colleagues (1998b) also reported that a highly traumatized group of children with SBPs exhibited significantly more benefit from a CBT intervention than from an expressive therapy. However, Bonner and colleagues (2000) reported that CBT and a dynamic play therapy approach were equally effective in reducing children's SBPs at a 2-year follow-up. They attribute these results to the similarity in the goals of CBT and dynamic play therapy: assisting children to gain insight into their own behavior; increasing children's ability to observe and to appreciate other peoples' feelings, needs, and rights; helping children understand their needs and values; developing their own goals and internal resources; increasing children's ability to meet their needs in socially appropriate ways; and increasing children's connectedness to positive others and building internal strengths that support future growth (Bonner, 2004).

Helping Children Acknowledge and Discuss Their Externalizing Behavior

Children are sometimes reluctant to acknowledge behavior problems, especially sexualized behavior. However, this is a necessary first step that must occur prior to the therapist's initiating interventions. Because talking about difficulties may pose a significant threat to children's fragile self-esteem, they attempt to avoid these issues by an outright refusal to discuss them or by disruptive behavior designed to deflect the therapist's attention. One strategy we have used with some success is to help these children identify some of their strengths. The therapist might point out that although they have engaged in some inappropriate behavior, the children have many positive characteristics and can do some things well. This approach is eventually helpful in assisting highly anxious children to confront directly their problems with physical aggression or SBPs. Cunningham and MacFarlane (1991) devised a number of activities designed to bolster the self-esteem of children who molest other children. The "Me Badge" (Cunningham & MacFarlane, 1991, pp. 59, 60) is a nonthreatening exercise most children can do. The child identifies (or draw pictures of) positive characteristics on a circular piece of cardboard divided into four sections. These characteristics may include something the child likes to do, something he or she is good at doing, something the child does to help the family, and something that is very special to the child. This concrete and visual depiction may be kept near by and shown to the child as a reminder of these strengths when the child feels threatened by discussions of his or her problem behavior.

To help children acknowledge problems, "Five Things I Do Well" (Cunningham & MacFarlane, 1991, p. 73) instructs children to list five things they do well (or draw if they cannot write) on one side of a folded piece of paper. They then list five things they would like to do better on the other half. The therapist points out that everyone has strengths as well as areas that need improvement. This exercise gradually exposes children to the process of acknowledging their difficulties (by having them identify things they would "like to do better"). If they do not acknowledge problems with physical aggression or sexual behavior, the therapist might point out this lapse matter-of-factly and wonder aloud why they did not. Children might be asked to think of the "worst thing that could happen" if they were to acknowledge the problem. This approach helps them identify the source of their anxiety. By empathizing with their fears and then correcting particular distortions (e.g., the therapist will think negatively of a child if he or she becomes aware of the child's behavior), the therapist may help overcome a child's reluctance to explore these issues.

CBT techniques can counteract negative self-statements that inhibit children from engaging in an open and direct account of their difficulties. Cunningham and MacFarlane (1991, p. 55) described a strategy, "My Inner Critic," in which children are asked to identify their negative self-statements, including those related to their sexual behavior. Children with other behavioral difficulties such as physical aggression can identify the negative self-statements associated with these problems (e.g., "I'm a bad kid, and everyone hates me because I beat up other kids"). When they become aware of making these covert self-statements, they are told to visualize a stop sign. They then say "Stop!" to themselves and replace the negative self-statement with a more positive one (e.g., "I made a mistake, but I'm learning how to control my temper"). The therapist may have to prompt the use of this strategy or provide tangible reminders of the child's strengths (using the Me Badge) when the youngster becomes especially anxious. Self-statements should incorporate these strengths; the child should use them when feeling especially threatened by explorations and discussions of problem behavior (e.g., "Even though I sometimes beat up other kids, there are some things I do well—I'm good at math and there are times when I can be nice to people!").

Children need repeated practice to learn to implement this technique. The therapist can help them practice changing their negative thoughts into positive ones by presenting a variety of self-statements, including those associated with problem behavior. The children then have to replace negative thoughts with positive ones. For children who remain reluctant to acknowledge their behavior directly, the therapist can present a more detailed scenario that involves a child who also does not want to talk about embarrassing or shameful behavior. This introduces sensitive material somewhat indirectly via recounting a hypothetical child's behavior (similar to the third stage of Harter's [1983] model of therapy described in the previous chapter). The therapist asks the child to identify some negative thoughts of this other child, as well as the positive self-statements that might replace them.

Self-Monitoring

Before they are taught to control their anger, children must learn self-monitoring skills, a basic component of CBT. First, the therapist teaches them to identify their angry feelings. Some children cannot accurately recognize the point at which they begin to get angry, and they may realize they are angry only after hitting someone. Their control of these feelings may improve if they can identify their anger at an earlier point and implement helpful techniques before it escalates to the point where an aggressive outburst becomes likely. Children can identify the somatic cues to their anger (e.g., flushed face, increased muscle tension) by graphically depicting such somatic cues on an outline of their bodies. Some children may possibly identify the cognitions or self-statements that accompany their anger (e.g., "I'm so angry I'd like to knock his head off!").

Similarly, children with SBPs must learn to identify and recognize their sexual feelings. This is sometimes even more difficult than having children identify their anger. Typically, we do not talk with children about the fact they have sexual feelings. Children have an even smaller common vocabulary to describe their sexual feelings than that describing their anger, so they have fewer terms they can share with adults. These discussions are often embarrassing for children and adults. Furthermore, there is considerable debate about the role of sexual arousal in generating SBPs in preadolescent children (Hall, 1993). There is no consensus regarding whether every child with a SBP has been influenced by strong feelings of sexual arousal. Even if some are aroused, they usually do not have the words to communicate these internal feelings and experiences.

Chapter 8 described the importance of drawing the distinction between the verbal expression of feelings and behavioral acting out to reassure children that talking about the maltreatment will not lead to impulsive behaviors that place the child or others in jeopardy. Clinicians may have to reiterate this point to assist children to develop behavioral and emotional self-regulation. Therapists should help children to understand the difference between anger (a feeling) and aggression (the overt behavioral expression of this anger via physical attacks or other means). They can tell children that anger is a normal feeling experienced by all of us, but we do not have the right to express angry feelings in whatever form we desire, as in beating up someone. The same notion applies to sexual feelings: such feelings are normal, but their presence does not give us the prerogative to act them out in any way we want.

Another important self-monitoring task for many children is to learn to identify the precipitants (i.e., the situations, events, feelings, somatic cues, and cognitions) that precede the emergence of aggression or SBPs. This task is a major component of relapse prevention, the basis of which is understanding the chain of events that precede a particular pattern of behavior one wants to change. By identifying precipitants, the child can take alternate action to interrupt preceding events and initiate strategies to prevent their progression to physical or sexual aggression.

While attempting to determine if the child can identify precipitants, the therapist must remain aware of the possible limitations of this approach. First, interventions based on a relapse prevention approach were developed with adolescent and adult offenders. Can we apply this model to young children, particularly considering their cognitive and developmental differences? Are young children aware of precipitants, especially of the more abstract type, such as their cognitions and feelings? Harter (1977) noted that young children, even those in the stage of concrete operational functioning (7- to 11-year-old range), have difficulty in identifying and understanding their feelings, because affects are less directly observable. Other factors compound children's difficulty in examining internal psychological factors that influence behavior. Less sophisticated verbal skills, shorter attention spans, and embarrassment about the content of physically aggressive or sexually intrusive fantasies, as well as a corresponding reluctance to disclose these fantasies, render the identification of precipitants a difficult enterprise for young children. Moreover, although adolescent/adult models consider sexual fantasies to be significant precursors to sexualized behavior, at this point we have little empirical knowledge about the conscious, identifiable sexual fantasies of preadolescent children and what role they play in SBPs (Cunningham & MacFarlane, 1991).

How can the therapist help children identify precipitants? Asking them to "brainstorm" about all the situations that evoke anger is often useful. The list can be divided into different categories, such as "people who make me angry" and "things [events/situations] that make me angry." Children who cannot read or write can provide the therapist with a verbal report and then draw the particular precipitant. Having children identify and describe in detail a specific situation in which they became physically aggressive may assist in identifying precipitants. Precipitants to aggressive or other maladaptive behavior also include cognitions, which may have special relevance for maltreated children. In Chapter 2 we reviewed how maltreated children, many with insecure attachments and a consequent lack of basic trust in the world and other people, often misperceive and misinterpret social information and behavior as evidence of hostile threat or intent. They fail to attend to relevant cues in social situations and then react in an aggressive, externalizing manner to guard against the perceived threat and to compensate for feelings of powerlessness and inadequacy.

Gil and Johnson (1993, pp. 244–245) developed a technique called "Cartoons" to teach children with SBPs self-observation skills. Cartoons help children to identify behavior sequences, including the precipitants and consequences of sexual behavior. Children draw pictures (cartoons) of themselves in a series of frames or squares that depict the progression of a particular behavior. In the initial squares, children draw the precipitants to the problematic behavior: what they felt and thought (affective states and cognitions), what was going on before they engaged another child in sexual behavior (situational precipitants), how their bodies might have felt (somatic precipitants), and the actual event. Subsequent frames illustrate the consequences of the child's behavior: the consequences that accrued to the child (e.g., being grounded, suspended from school), the reactions of the other child, and the response of parents or caregivers. The series of frames is a visual depiction of the event from start to finish. Like many others, the technique relies on the notion that school-age children need assistance in making abstract concepts, such as cognitive, emotional, and behavioral precipitants, recognizable and tangible. We have found this to be a valuable technique in helping children with physical aggression problems and SBPs.

Self-Instructional Training and Problem Solving

After assisting the child in recognizing his or her anger or sexual feelings and identifying some precipitants of these patterns, the therapist should introduce other CBT techniques. Included are those that incorporate self-instructional training (Kendall & Braswell, 1993) and interpersonal cognitive problem solving (Spivak, Platt, & Shure, 1976). The child learns to use self-instructions and self-talk to guide him- or herself through the various steps of problem solving. In this way, the child's responses are preceded by deliberate thought, and self-regulation of emotions and behavior is enhanced. Therapists should guide the child through the steps in problem solving outlined below to prevent an episode of physical aggression. They can use the same strategy to help children refrain from engaging in inappropriate sexual behavior.

• *Initial inhibition of impulsive responses.* The youngster is taught to "stop and think" when he or she becomes conscious of the emergence of angry or sexual feelings and cognitions that precede inappropriate behavior. Other precipitants may include particular situations (e.g., teasing by other children, being alone with younger children). A common practice is to label these precipitants as "red flags" that signal potential problems. The therapist encourages the child to say "Stop!" and to follow this statement with another self-statement such as "I'm getting angry now. I'd better think about what I'm going to do next." A visual depiction of this instruction in the form of a small stop sign is a useful reminder to the child. The therapist can introduce other prompts for inhibiting the aggressive or sexual response, such as having the child count to 10 or "freezing" like a statue (Kendall & Braswell, 1993).

• *Problem definition.* Using self-talk, the child formulates a definition of the problem (e.g., "I'm getting real mad now, and I don't want to end up hitting him").

• *Choice of a goal.* Typical goals for aggressive children may be reflected in self-statements like "I'm really mad when he's teasing me. What can I do to make sure I don't hit him?" Self-statements for children with SBPs include "I'm feeling like I'd like to touch someone's private parts. What can I do to make sure I don't get in trouble?"

• *Alternative thinking.* Alternative thinking refers to the child's ability to generate multiple alternate solutions to a problem situation. These alternatives typically include physical aggression ("I could hit him") and others that are more adaptive ("I could walk away and find someone else to play with when he teases me"). Children with SBPs have devised alternate solutions such as playing a computer game or drawing (described below). In this stage, the emphasis is on generating alternatives rather than evaluating their utility.

• *Consequential thinking.* In this phase, the therapist teaches the child to evaluate the immediate and long-term consequences of the alternatives already generated. Kendall and Braswell (1993) recommended that the child evaluate the possibilities in terms of their emotional and behavioral consequences for the child and for the other person. The child asks him- or herself, "What would happen if I did this?" (referring to the behavioral consequences). Then the child evaluates the emotional consequences by asking him- or herself how the other person would feel. Based on this evaluation, the child decides on a solution and implements it. The child can also devise a backup plan.

• *Self-reward.* The therapist encourages the child to use a self-reinforcing statement to reward him- or herself for appropriate problem solving (e.g., "I did a great job—I didn't end up hitting him [or touching his private parts]!"). The child also uses self-statements to counter the frustration that may emerge if the child encounters difficulties. For example, rather than immediately giving up, the child engages in self-talk that counters the frustration and encourages persistence. Rather than saying, "Boy, I made a mistake. I'm really stupid," the child makes more useful self-statements such as, "Well, I made a mistake. It's not the end of the world, and I should try another way of doing this."

- *Practice and rehearsal.* An important component of self-instructional training and problem-solving practice is providing the child with numerous opportunities to practice these general problem-solving skills. After the therapist has walked the child through the aforementioned steps, role-playing with the child can begin. The therapist may want to choose scenarios that are not particularly difficult to solve to ensure some initial success for the child. The therapist encourages the child to rehearse the problem-solving sequence by talking out loud, and prompts if the child encounters any difficulty. As the child becomes more comfortable with the approach and attains more success, the therapist presents situations and scenarios that have greater problems. Among these are those that the youngster has identified as precipitants to aggressive displays. The therapist may then present actual scenarios that were particularly troublesome for the child in the past. For example, the therapist might play the role of another child who frequently teases this child, which may provoke the youngster to hit the other child to stop the teasing, and then again cue the child to use the problem-solving approach. The therapist should not present role-play scenarios that include sexualized interactions between the child and another person. Children find such scenarios too arousing, and their anxiety rapidly escalates. It is better to talk about these situations rather than role-play them.

Besides teaching the general process of problem solving, the therapist should assist the child in developing specific plans to cope with particularly difficult situations. If the child is having physical altercations with a certain child or group of children, the therapist and child should develop alternate ways to cope with this situation and then rehearse and practice the child's specific response. The same approach may be taken with children with SBPs. Children require specific plans to cope with those situations in which they are more likely to respond sexually. Gil and Johnson (1993) recommended that children develop substitute behaviors to distract them from sexual thoughts and feelings. These activities should be ones the child likes and finds pleasurable (e.g., video games, puzzles) and that expend energy but without body contact or physical aggression. Participating in these substitute activities with parents may motivate the child to refrain from engaging in sexual behavior (Gil & Johnson, 1993). Children need to try the problem-solving approach and practice alternative ways of responding in their real environments between sessions, reporting the results during their next session. "Homework" might consist of recounting observations of the other person's reactions to their nonaggressive stance, the success of the alternative solution, and personal feelings and reactions (e.g., pride at not hurting somebody).

The therapist can introduce a fun element and provide more opportunities to practice and rehearse the problem-solving approach and specific plans by writing different scenarios on index cards. The child and the therapist take turns choosing a card and rehearsing the steps. These same scenarios may be incorporated into a simple pursuit board game. When either lands on a specially designated square, he or she must respond to the provocative situation described on the card using the steps described above. Either person misses a turn if unable to generate alternate solutions or a specific plan. The therapist's involvement in these tasks makes them much more a shared activity and enables the therapist to model the problem-solving approach.

The therapist can return to the Cartoons exercise to convey the notion that responding differently to the precipitants results in different consequences for the child and other people. Using the original cartoon sequence that depicted the precipitants, the physical or sexual aggression, and the reactions of the other person and consequences that accrued to the child, children can draw the new strategies they would now use when confronted with the same precipitants, and the different set of consequences. The latter might include depictions of the children feeling good about themselves because of their greater self-control, their parents feeling proud of them, and the child who was hurt now displaying a happy face. They can superimpose this new strip on the original one, and flipping back and forth readily illustrates the benefits of these new strategies.

Interactions between the child and the therapist provide further opportunities to help children develop self-regulation. The therapist encourages the child to use the problem-solving approach when angry with the therapist. As reviewed in Chapter 2, some chronically abused and neglected children are not lucky enough to have had a relationship with a primary caregiver that fostered these self-regulatory skills. The therapeutic relationship can provide such a child with an opportunity to engage in a process wherein the therapist helps the child develop the capacity for self-regulation. For example, in Chapter 7 we discussed the tendency of children with insecure attachment organizations to become angry when they believe their needs are not being met. Besides helping the child inhibit impulsive responses by imposing external limits on aggressive or destructive behavior and encouraging the child to make self-statements, the therapist assists the child to articulate the problem in the relationship verbally with the therapist and to identify the associated affects (e.g., "I'm mad at you because you won't let me stay longer in the session"). Children with poor internal state language may need considerable help in identifying and expressing these feelings. The therapist then helps the child choose a goal and generate alternate solutions to the problem.

The therapist should be aware that many maltreated children, especially those whose internal state language was compromised at a very young age, require a great deal of practice to develop self-regulation. We stressed in Chapter 6 that the therapist must incorporate parents or caregivers in the treatment program. Their participation is especially important, because it is often in the home environment or community that the child exhibits externalizing behavior. Kendall and Braswell (1993) recommended that therapists encourage parents to recognize and praise children when they observe them using the problem-solving approach. Parents must be particularly attuned to those situations in which the child is likely to become aggressive or is at risk for engaging in sexually inappropriate behavior. The parent may then have to prompt the use of self-instructional skills via simple statements like "This looks like a good time to stop and think" (Kendall & Braswell, 1993, p. 189). A nonverbal prompt, such as a hand signal, may also be useful. Its added benefit is that although the child recognizes the cue, others are unaware of the significance of the communication. Parents who model the problem-solving approach in their daily lives exert a potent and positive influence on their children. Children who have lost control should be given a time-out until they have themselves under control again. The parent should present the time-out as an opportunity for the child to calm down and gain control (Kendall & Braswell, 1993). Time-outs are not used punitively, but as a means of interrupting the behavior, permitting the child to exercise control.

The various elements of self-monitoring, self-instructional training, and problem solving discussed above may appear complex and confusing to some child clients and their caregivers. Over years of working with children who have difficulties with expressing anger in particular, we have evolved a concrete model that can help clients understand the basic elements of these interventions. We call this model the "Anger Mountain" and find that children readily identify with it, particularly when they exhibit massive tantrums and rages. The therapist and child draw and color an Anger Mountain, as illustrated in Figure 9.1, and then explain it to the child's parents or caregivers.

Line *A* on the drawing of the Anger Mountain represents the current status of the child's anger and tantrums. A child may seem calm, but an apparently minor stimulus may well generate instant, soaring anger. Because

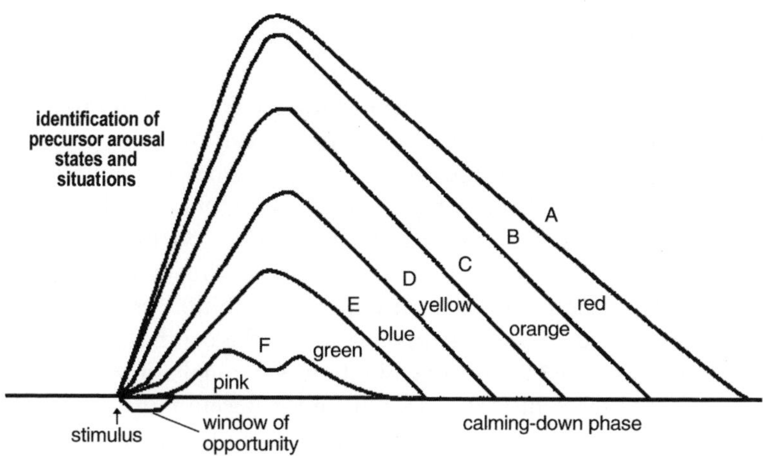

FIGURE 9.1. Anger Mountain.

of the immediacy of the child's anger, there is no time to divert the impending tantrum and manage it more thoughtfully. Furthermore, the child takes a long time to calm down. By the time the child is calm again, both child and caregivers are exhausted and feel inept and overwhelmed. To begin the intervention, the therapist instructs the child and caregivers to focus first on encouraging the child to calm down sooner. This may involve using times-outs, but instead of designating a specific length for the time-out, the parent tells the child the time-out is over only when he or she is calmer. Over time, this usually increases the probability that the child will modulate his or her reaction and calm down sooner. This is often a better approach than having the child in time-out for a set period or trying to talk the child out of the anger, as these responses sometimes inflame a tantrum further. As the child and the caregiver discover that the child can become calm more quickly, the tantrums lessen in severity, as illustrated by lines *B* through *F.* The goal is not to eliminate the anger but to moderate it so that it is manageable, as illustrated by line *F* or possibly even line *E*.

Once the child begins to learn to calm down, both the child and caregivers begin to feel less overwhelmed. A small window of opportunity to avert a tantrum then appears in the anger outburst. With parental cuing, the child begins to be aware of his or her anger, identifies the precipitants of the outbursts, and then problem solves and plans constructive ways to express it. In our experience, many children easily rate the level of their anger by using different colors on the Anger Mountain, seeing their progress as the colors change. Children feel more successful and more in control of regulating their anger.

Developing Empathy and Perspective Taking

Another important component of the cognitive-behavioral approach to anger management is the individual's ability to take the perspective of the other person (empathy). Although there are many determinants of aggressive behavior, empathy deficits have been cited as one variable associated with its emergence (Feshbach, Feshbach, Fauvre, & Ballard-Campbell, 1983). Children may avoid hurting others by becoming aware of the potentially harmful consequences of their actions. Inhibition occurs when they have a cognitive and emotional appreciation of the psychological and phys ical pain evoked by their aggression. Similarly, Cunningham and MacFarlane (1991) proposed that children with SBPs must develop an appreciation of the effects of their behavior on others. This empathic understanding contributes to their ability to stop and later refrain from the sexualized behavior.

Unfortunately, maltreated children, especially those who have suffered prolonged and serious abuse or neglect, may encounter significant difficulty in empathizing with the needs and feelings of others. In Chapter 2, we reviewed how some maltreated children's difficulty in establishing a goal-corrected partnership with a primary caretaker impairs their subsequent social relationships and reflective thinking. These relationships become characterized by an absence of reciprocity, sharing, and sensitivity to others' feelings and needs. Furthermore, a maltreated child's exposure to the psychological distress of others may be threatening, inasmuch as these reactions begin to remind the child of his or her own pain. By successfully excluding these affective states from consciousness through avoiding, ignoring, and dismissing the feelings of others, the child avoids personal distress. Such children must confront their own pain before they can acknowledge that of others.

Helping children develop empathy for others is often a slow process. Although the therapist may introduce some activities to initiate this process, children require considerable practice in honing these skills. Again, the involvement of parents or caregivers is critical. They should prompt their children to consider the consequences of their actions for other people. Chapter 7 discussed the importance of the therapist's empathic comments to facilitate the development of the child's awareness of his or her own mind and ultimately the thoughts and feelings of others. Cunningham and MacFarlane (1991) described other techniques designed to encourage a sense of empathy. The reader is well advised to review this valuable resource for creative ideas and suggestions. We briefly describe several techniques below.

The therapist can begin by helping the child to identify his or her needs in different situations before attempting to identify the needs of other people. Cunningham and MacFarlane (1991, pp. 184, 186) described an activity they call "What Would You Need If?" Children respond to questions like "What would you need if you were lost?" or "What would you need if you were caught in an elevator?" Subsequent questions deal with the needs of children who have been maltreated: "What would you need if you were physically abused?" "Sexually abused?" (Cunningham & MacFarlane, 1991, p. 184). In a subsequent exercise—"What Do They Need?"—children identify the needs of people in various situations as portrayed by magazine pictures (Cunningham & MacFarlane, 1991, p. 186). In another exercise, "Identifying the Feelings of Others" (Cunningham & MacFarlane, 1991, p. 186), they look at pictures of people in various situations and then identify the people's feelings. The therapist invites them to speculate about the possible situations and events that might have led to these affective states. This exercise is another opportunity to teach children to identify and label feelings accurately as well as to sensitize them to the feelings of others.

After these preliminary exercises, the therapist and child focus should identify common reactions of people subjected to physical aggression or intrusive sexual behavior. This may be a relatively straightforward task for children who have already acknowledged and discussed their own feelings about their victimization. By drawing on their own experiences, they can now more readily answer questions regarding the feelings of persons who have been physically or sexually assaulted. Other children may need more concrete stimuli to become familiar with the impact of maltreatment. *Good Things Can Still Happen*, produced by the National Film Board of Canada (Scully, 1992), is a particularly useful videotape. This 22-minute video depicts common reactions of boys and girls (cartoon characters in the video) who have been sexually abused. There is a pause in the video between the segments that portray these different reactions. The therapist and child can watch the video together, with the therapist asking the child to identify each character's feelings and reactions during the pauses. For those children who have not yet clearly articulated their feelings, viewing the video can reduce their sense of isolation and serve as a catalyst for more discussions about the child's reactions (e.g., "Have you ever felt like that kid in the video?"). The video also helps develop or consolidate children's appreciation for the effects of abusive behavior, including their own, on others.

Older school-age children may benefit from reading newspaper accounts of real children who have been physically or sexually abused. Again, they should attempt to identify the possible reactions and feelings of these other children. Therapists can use puppet plays to depict a character being hurt or somehow maltreated. As the audience, the child, using a puppet, indicates how the victimized character might feel.

Once the youngster becomes more comfortable with talking about physical aggression or inappropriate sexualized behavior, the therapist begins to focus on the reactions and feelings of the person the child assaulted or involved in sexual behavior. The therapist can request a verbal account of what the child did to the other person, with a particular emphasis on the youngster's perception of the other child's feelings and reactions. Children with limited verbal skills or who are reluctant or embarrassed to talk more directly about these issues can draw a picture of the incidents and of the other child's facial expressions that depict the individual's feelings. Again, the therapist must assist the child to identify and articulate these affects. Here the trick is to avoid evoking an overwhelming sense of shame or guilt about the behavior. The therapist and parents or caregivers should focus on the child's behavior, rather than personally attacking the child and conveying a sense that he or she is a replica of the perpetrator who hurt the youngster. Statements like "When you hit other kids, you're doing just what [name of perpetrator] did to you. You're turning out just like him!" erode a child's self-esteem. They transmit the notion that the child is condemned to repeat the past, only this time as the aggressor. Furthermore, these comments reduce the child's trust in the therapist and might render the youngster more unwilling to disclose this problem behavior because of fear of being insulted or condemned. Therapists need to take physical aggression or inappropriate sexual behavior seriously, but they must respectfully confront the child about these patterns and their effects on others.

Exploring the actual feelings and reactions of maltreatment victims raises a central question: "What is wrong with physical aggression (or intrusive sexual behavior)?" The child and therapist can address this issue directly by identifying as many negative consequences as possible for both the victim and the perpetrator. They can list the negative consequences for the victim on one side of a piece of paper and those for the perpetrator (e.g., loss of self-esteem, external consequences) on the other.

Therapists should attempt to convey the notion of coercion to children. They can encourage children to think of times when they felt forced to do something, including episodes from their own victimization, and then articulate the associated feelings, either verbally or through other means, such as drawing their facial expressions. The therapist should discuss how children cannot give consent, because they are not aware of many consequences of sexual behavior with others. Role plays can depict different types of coercion, in which the child portrays his or her reactions. We mentioned earlier that the therapist must avoid pretending to physically or sexually abuse the child in role plays. Such activity usually produces intense anxiety in the child; it is better to role-play this abuse more indirectly, using puppets or small dolls. The therapist can discuss the use of developmental status as a means of forcing others into inappropriate activities by referring to examples of older children using their greater knowledge to trick younger ones into sexual activities. In addition, the therapist should explain that differences in physical size might be sufficient to obtain younger children's compliance. To accentuate the potency of physical size as a way to gain compliance, we have marked a child's height on a blackboard and then invited the child to estimate the height of the child he or she abused. While the therapist assumes the child client's height, the child crouches down to the level of the other child's height. Then the child looks up at the therapist and states how it feels to be in such a position, especially if one is also being threatened. The therapist must be especially sensitive to the child's anxiety in this exercise, inasmuch as the child is in a submissive position, replicating elements of the original victimization. Before beginning the exercise, the therapist should explain its purpose and instruct the youngster to signal if he or she becomes especially anxious and needs to stop at any point. A distinction should be drawn between the current situation and those that led to past victimization by pointing out that the therapist will do nothing to hurt the youngster. As an alternative, the therapist can use dolls to represent the individuals, because doll play usually does not pose as great a threat to anxious children.

Earlier we reviewed the importance of consequential thinking in problem solving. Children can incorporate their understanding of the consequences of harmful or coercive behavior for others into self-statements (e.g., "She would probably feel really scared if I touched her private parts") and then rehearse them. A child can use these self-statements to prevent further episodes of inappropriate behavior.

Children can put empathic feelings into action once they develop an appreciation of the effects of their behavior on others. In our earlier discussion of problem solving and self-instructional training, we reviewed strategies that enable children to engage in more fulfilling and healthier interpersonal relationships. Other techniques can consolidate these skills and abilities. What Would You Do If? presents a number of scenarios to which the child is invited to respond (Cunningham & MacFarlane, 1991, pp. 201, 203); for example, "If you lost a game at school, what could someone say to make you feel better? What could you say to someone who lost a game at school?" (Cunningham & MacFarlane, 1991, p. 201). Subsequent questions focus on the child's own sexual abuse history and how others might respond to make the child feel better, and what the child might say to someone else with this history. The therapist can formulate appropriate questions for children with a history of physical abuse and neglect. Asking children to help the therapist develop these questions often consolidates their engagement in this exercise. Using the format originally developed for group therapy, each child picks and responds to a card on which one of the "What Would You Do If?" scenarios is written. A similar format may be used in individual therapy, or the therapist might create a simple pursuit board game. When either therapist or child lands on a specially designated square, he or she must pick one of the cards on which these scenarios are written. The child takes another turn as a reward for an appropriate response that displays an empathic appreciation of the needs of others.

After completion of these exercises, which focus on more general responses to others' distress, the therapist assists the child in identifying ways to make amends to the person the child hurt or victimized. In one useful technique, the child composes a letter of apology. These letters may be mailed, but only with the informed consent of the parents or legal guardians of both children. The client child should state how he or she feels about hurting the other individual and describe what happened to validate the other person's experience. The therapist encourages the child to assume responsibility for his or her actions, absolve the other person of any blame, and express some concern for that person. The therapist can act as a secretary, transcribing the dictation of those children unable to write. Discussions of the benefits that will accrue to the other individual, such as feeling validated and believed, may be useful. Children should be asked to put themselves in the other person's place and describe how they would have felt if their own perpetrators had apologized as they are now doing. It is also important to identify the benefits to the child who has apologized. These include feeling better about him- or herself because the child's guilt feelings are alleviated, as well as the realization that the child can take responsibility for his or her behavior.

Letters and discussions serve as rehearsals for actual sessions in which the child apologizes to the other child (again, of course, with the informed consent of the legal guardians of both children). This session should occur after the child has developed some genuine appreciation of the effects of his or her actions. Having a child flippantly or smugly "apologize" does nothing to validate or legitimize the other child's concerns or issues. We have treated children who have devised other creative ways of making amends to younger siblings whom they have physically assaulted or sexually abused. One 11-year-old boy decided to allow his 7-year-old brother unrestricted use of his prized baseball glove for an entire week to make amends for his physical assaults toward the younger boy. Actions like these may be the first step toward a healthier and more fulfilling relationship between the child and the other individual.

"Recording Friendly Deeds" (Cunningham & MacFarlane, 1991, pp. 198, 200) is an excellent exercise to develop positive social skills and counter negative self-esteem, especially when it is based on negative and harmful interactional patterns with others. Therapists can tell children that although their physical aggression or SBPs indicate that they made mistakes in the past, they are still able to relate in caring ways to others. This exercise is designed to provide children with proof of this statement. As a homework assignment, the child must perform a "friendly deed" a certain number of times in the week before the next session. The child records the identity of the person who is the object of the caring act, the deed itself, and the other person's response on a simple chart. Children who cannot write may depict this information in simple drawings. Having the child observe and record the other individual's reactions enhances the child's understanding that his or her actions have effects on others and that these effects can be positive and beneficial. We have asked parents or caregivers to initial each friendly deed the child completes that week, just as the parent might do for regular school homework assignments. Doing so ensures that parents become aware that their children can succeed, rather than being condemned to repeat physical or sexual aggression. The therapist should reinforce the child for completing the friendly deeds in the intervening week. The child then completes another cartoon sequence (described above) that describes the deed and the consequences, as well as the child's feelings, cognitions, and situational variables that preceded the initiation of these friendly actions. This exercise provides the child with more practice in understanding that behavior has precipitants and consequences.

CHAPTER TEN

Reformulating the Meaning of the Maltreatment

Episodes of abuse and neglect often affect a child's appraisal of the world and his or her place in it. In Chapter 2 we reviewed the important role children's attributions and broader IWMs/IS play in subsequent adaptation to maltreatment. They need an opportunity to understand what has happened to them and to critically examine and reformulate some of their assumptions about and interpretations of the experience. In this chapter, we discuss three major issues concerning the reformulation of the meaning of maltreatment. First, therapists must help children to modify misattributions and maladaptive beliefs. Second, children must attain a sense of mastery over the past maltreatment and confidence that they can reduce the likelihood of future assaults. Third, efforts have to be directed at helping youngsters develop more positive self-esteem.

ATTRIBUTION RETRAINING

We have reviewed considerable empirical support for the notion that attributions and appraisals constitute significant pathogenic processes that contribute to maltreated children's adjustment. They have particular relevance to the emergence of PTSD and other internalizing disorders, including depression and low self-esteem. Chapter 2 described a conceptualization of PTSD, which incorporates these cognitive components along with conditioning processes. Attribution retraining (AR) techniques (also called cognitive restructuring or cognitive processing) assist clients with anxiety problems to modify their attributions. This approach has proven effective with adult rape victims (Resick & Schnicke, 1993) and has been applied more recently to sexually abused children. We have already reviewed the research that found CBT for sexually abused youngsters results in better outcome than nondirective supportive treatments, and AR has figured prominently in a number of these intervention studies (e.g., Cohen & Mannarino, 2000; King et al., 2000). However, the inclusion of other treatment components, such as exposure and parent training, makes it difficult to draw any firm conclusions about AR's unique contribution to outcome, although the adult rape treatment literature indicates that cognitive processing therapy was effective by itself in treating both PTSD and depression at posttreatment and at a 6-month follow-up (Resick & Schnicke, 1992). Furthermore, given the evidence of the role of attributions in maltreated children's outcomes, there is strong support for the notion that modifying misattributions may make a significant difference. For example, Cohen and Mannarino (2000) reported that negative abuse-related attributions and lax family structure predicted posttreatment trauma symptoms in sexually abused school-age children.

We have also emphasized the influence of IWMs/IS and biased social information-processing styles as major pathogenic processes. Chapter 7 focused on the strategic use of the therapeutic relationship to change children's basic expectations about how other people will respond to them. In this chapter we describe other interventions to modify these expectations.

Modifying Attributions of Responsibility

Therapists who treat maltreated children should read Lamb's (1986) article on the issues of blame and responsibility. She points out that many therapists reassure sexually abused children that they are blameless so that the therapists can present themselves as trustworthy, helpful individuals. Lamb contends that although this view seems just and proper, it may have detrimental effects. The gist of her argument is that these statements confer victim status on children and diminish their sense of power and control. According to Lamb, sometimes sexually abused children feel they made some choices that led to a continuation of the abuse. By saying it is not their fault, the therapist removes any sense of efficacy they may have experienced and reinforces feelings of helplessness and concomitant anxiety (Celano, Hazzard, Campbell, & Lang, 2002). Lamb also maintains that simple statements such as "It's not your fault" run counter to the sense of responsibility children may have felt in these interactions. Offering premature reassurances of blamelessness may invalidate the child's phenomenological experience and erode the child's growing perception that the therapist is sensitive to feelings and issues (Friedrich, 1990).

How then do we help these children change the belief that they were responsible for the maltreatment, including those who engaged in behavior that contributed to a continuation of the sexual abuse, such as going back to the perpetrator's home or seeking extra rewards or privileges for complying with sexual activities? Therapists should point out they are not "bad children" but that they had not learned enough about the world to make the proper decisions, thereby discouraging them from making internal attributions: "Even though you made a mistake, no one has the right to abuse you" (Celano et al., 2002, p. 69). They should explain that despite a child's returning to the perpetrator's home, the adult still had ultimate responsibility for his or her actions—the adult was older, more knowledgeable, and more able to exert power and control over the child. Acknowledging that the child made a mistake by returning to the perpetrator's home may seem somewhat heartless and cruel. However, by doing so the therapist suggests that the youngster can make different decisions in the future that can reduce the risk of further exploitation.

Therapists can ameliorate internal attributions of blame (e.g., "I was abused because I was a bad kid") by stating that no matter what the child did, he or she did not deserve this kind of treatment. The therapist should coach the child to use appropriate self-statements when bothered by these internal attributions (e.g., "He was a grown-up, and he shouldn't have done those things to me"). Another effective way of concretizing this concept is to use role plays. Court scenarios are especially useful. The therapist introduces a scenario in which the child is asked to defend the perpetrator and the therapist assumes the judge's role. As the judge, the therapist asks the child for an explanation of the perpetrator's behavior—will the child attribute responsibility to the child victim or to the offender? If the child blames the victim, the judge proposes an alternate explanation. For example, the child may say that his or her acting-out behavior was the cause of the physical abuse. The judge can respond by stating that even if the child had been behaving inappropriately and needed discipline or limits, nothing would have justified that kind of treatment. Similarly, the child may refer to the physical pleasure he or she derived from the perpetrator's sexual assaults or attribute the adult's actions to the child's questions about sexuality. Again, the judge (i.e., the therapist) might remark that even though the child was curious or even aroused, these feelings did not justify the adult's behavior. This scenario may lead to a discussion of the normalcy of children's physiological/sexual arousal and that it can never be used as a rationale by adults for involving children in sexual behavior. As the judge, the therapist should explain the concept of consent and how the child did not have the requisite knowledge to agree to the perpetrator's advances. Roles may be reversed. The therapist then plays the offender or the offender's legal counsel, who presents several rationalizations for the perpetrator's behavior. The therapist gently prompts the child (as the judge) to think about what the offender is saying and whether it truly justifies the offender's actions toward the child. The child derives a sense of power and mastery by successfully countering the therapist's (i.e., the perpetrator's) arguments and rationalizations and then handing out an appropriate sentence.

Other strategies can reinforce the notion that children were not responsible for the victimization. By reviewing salient aspects of parents' historical difficulty in caring for them, children's internal attributions may change. We have requested that child welfare workers who were involved with a child at a very young age meet with the child. The welfare workers recount the reasons for their agency's involvement and describe the difficulties parents had in caring for the youngster. Although painful, these realistic portrayals also facilitate the child's acknowledgment of profound feelings of loss associated with parental inability or unwillingness to care for him or her. Usually, children must have begun the process of acknowledging parental difficulties and their own feelings of loss, and must have alternate sources of strong support (e.g., foster parents) before they can accept such sensitive historical information. Presenting this information when a child still adamantly denies the parent's problems and tenaciously clings to hope that the parent will reform, often strengthens the child's defenses of denial and avoidance.

Some children persist in maintaining that they should have physically fought the perpetrator or defended themselves from the assaults. Similarly, children who have witnessed domestic violence often believe that they should have protected the parent who was assaulted. Although therapists must empathize with children's concern for their parents, a failure to modify these unrealistic expectations leaves them with no alternate strategies that have a better chance of ensuring their continued safety and increasing a sense of mastery. Although the therapist identifies and empathizes with the child's wish to have been strong and powerful, typically underlying such fantasies, the therapist should point out sensitively that the child probably would not have been successful in defending him- or herself by this means. Wieland (1997) recommends that children draw a picture of themselves at the age of the abuse and a proportionally sized picture of the perpetrator. Inspecting the size differential offers concrete evidence of the perpetrator's greater strength and power and the child's limited ability to fight back. Of course, children need to be equipped with realistic self-protection strategies (described later in this chapter) that they can use to counteract the feelings of powerlessness and inadequacy associated with this greater awareness of their limited ability to physically fend off perpetrators.

Children deserve an explanation of the perpetrator's behavior to help make sense of it and attenuate their feelings of responsibility. As is true of every other aspect of human behavior, multiple factors contribute to abusive or neglectful behavior. However, it is probably wise to provide children with a simple and direct explanation for the perpetrator's behavior without attempting to incorporate all the causative factors or subtle influences. Presenting all these aspects would overwhelm the child with excessive information. For example, it may be helpful to say, "Your dad has a big problem with using drugs, and it's really hard for him to stop. When he uses those drugs, he has trouble making meals or making sure you get to school on time." Saying that the perpetrator is "sick" (unless the perpetrator has a demonstrable medical condition that is a significant etiological agent), although an easy explanation, often creates even more difficulties. The idea of sickness diminishes the notion that the perpetrator was responsible for his or her actions. The child may feel sorry for the perpetrator and guilty for having disclosed the assault and getting a "sick" individual into trouble. The youngster may also feel guilty about having strong feelings such as anger toward someone who is ill. Other explanations such as "She really loves you, but she has all these angry feelings too" may be incomprehensible to young children. They have difficulty understanding that people can experience opposing feelings simultaneously (i.e., love versus anger) (Harter, 1977).

Celano and colleagues (2002) comprehensively review a number of other creative AR techniques, including story metaphors, games, direct discussions, and visual illustrations. For example, the "Why List" consists of 17 possible self-blaming attributions from which the child is asked to chose any he or she may harbor (Hazzard, 1995). This is similar to the handout "I Think This Happened Because ___________" (Mandell & Damon, 1989, p. 77). Children list the reasons they think they were sexually abused and identify the reasons the perpetrator engaged in this behavior, thereby helping them articulate their attributions about the maltreatment. In both techniques, the therapist can encourage the child to critically examine the validity of these attributions.

Modifying Attributions That the Maltreatment Is Inevitable and Pervasive

Therapists must be prepared to help school-age children modify misattributions and misappraisals of others' motives by encouraging them to consider alternate explanations or attributions for interpersonal events. In Chapter 2 we reviewed research on the biased social information-processing styles of physically abused children. They are more likely than nonabused peers to make attributions of malicious intent and hostility in ambiguous social situations. For example, a child may be prone to believing that another child intentionally wanted to hurt him or her when that child accidentally bumped into him or her in a crowded school hallway. Another child without these negative expectations or IS might become annoyed, but would probably not regard the incident as a personal attack and therefore would be less likely to become belligerent or even aggressive.

Talking to school-age children abstractly about such internal psychological concepts is usually fruitless. Attributions and appraisals are sophisticated psychological concepts, and our challenge is to find ways to make them concrete and relevant for children (Grave & Blissett, 2004). A strategy we have found useful is to have children choose an actual incident in which they made such attributions and to subject them to a critical analysis. There are several steps in this process.

First, we have to help children identify situations that rapidly elicit these IS. The therapist begins by requesting the child to recount an actual interpersonal incident and then asks questions to elicit the child's expectations of how the other person was going to respond: "When you fell off your bike yesterday and scraped your knee, I wonder what you thought your foster mom was going to do?" "When you broke the window at home, what did you think your dad would do?"

The therapeutic relationship may also furnish opportunities to identify these IS. They are even more immediate and accessible than those associated with events that occurred just a few days prior to the session. For example, questions such as "When you got mad at me just now when I wouldn't let you take that toy home, what did you think I was going to do to you?" may be useful to help children more readily identify and articulate these expectations.

Second, the therapist can relink the IS to the context in which they were formed: "When your real dad got mad at you, I wonder what he did?" The therapist follows this comment by an interpretation that ties the child's current IS to these earlier interpersonal events: "Now, when your foster dad gets angry, you think he'll hurt you just like your real dad did." Interpretations offer children explanations of their sometimes confusing and inexplicable behaviors and promote their own reflective thinking. As we reviewed in Chapter 9, therapists may have to use developmentally sensitive strategies, such as "Cartoons," to facilitate children's accounts of these situations and associated feelings.

Third, it is important to differentiate the original context responsible for the IS from new situations. The major question the child confronts in this phase is whether the IS are applicable to these new situations: "Although

I got beat up when I lived with my real family, is the same thing going to happen again to me?" Children need to gather concrete examples of nonabusive, caring relationships. Using information from life books or other historical information as cues, the child can develop a list of positive interactions/relationships. The child and therapist should focus on specific and concrete evidence of the child's having been well treated, such as a birthday party organized by an otherwise neglectful parent. Some children with horrendous histories may have had few, if any, positive past experiences they can identify. The therapist may have to focus more on the here-and-now and have the child identify specific incidents of good care. A child can also identify the differences between his or her "old family" and the "new family." Besides describing the actual changes, therapists can help children do the same regarding the feelings and cognitions and/or assumptions evoked by these different experiences. For example, some severely neglected children in foster care will identify concrete changes, such as being adequately fed. The therapist asks how it feels when the child is fed and then directs a series of questions designed to help the child reformulate and modify basic assumptions about the world: "When your foster parents give you food, how do you think they feel about you? Do you think other people will feed you, or is everyone going to be like your parents, who didn't give you enough to eat?"

The therapist may also draw upon his or her interactions with the child to initiate a similar process: "When I kept the promise I made to you that we would paint this week, how did you feel? Do you think other people will keep their promises in the future?" Children might maintain a written log or record of the "friendly deeds" that others have done for them. Illiterate youngsters can draw pictures that depict these positive interpersonal experiences and bring them to therapy sessions. The therapist can use these data to introduce an element of discontinuity into the child's IWM/IS. This discontinuity begins to counter a tendency to misattribute hostile intent to others, as described in Chapter 2.

Fourth, the therapist must encourage children to test the validity of archaic IS in new situations by carefully considering the evidence for these IS and attributions. Again, the therapeutic relationship may be an opportunity for such a dialogue. For example, the therapist can ask the child, "What did you think I'd do when you tried to break that toy?" and then encourage the child to consider confirming or disconfirming evidence: "What did I really do when you tried to break it? Look at me right now. What does my face look like? How does my voice sound? Do I seem mad at you?" Follow-up questions, such as "Is everyone like your dad? Are they going to hurt you when they get angry?" consolidate the distinction between the child's "old life" and "new life."

Probably the trickiest part is enabling children to make more balanced attributions and appraisals when they are actually involved in interpersonal situations in their natural environments, because the therapist is not there to cue and guide the child. The following case illustrates some useful strategies.

Laura was a 9-year-old girl who was born in Romania and spent the first 5 years of her life in a large, understaffed orphanage. She was subjected to severe neglect and some physical abuse. A Canadian family adopted her when she was 5 years old. Soon after her arrival in Canada, she began to exhibit defiant, oppositional, and physically aggressive behavior. A clinical assessment revealed that Laura had little trust that adults would meet her needs. She expected that others were intent on hurting her and generalized this expectation to her adoptive parents and her 4-year-old sister, Jane. Laura instigated numerous quarrels and conflicts with Jane, especially when she believed Jane did not like her or was, in Laura's words, "out to get me." These negative expectations constituted significant pathogenic processes that strongly influenced her aggression toward Jane. Although the expectations and hypersensitivity were consistent with her history of neglect and abuse in Romania and were adaptive in that environment because they alerted her to possible assaults that she could take action to avoid, they negatively affected her perception of social relationships in her new life and provoked aggression and belligerence. Her aggressive or hostile responses effectively resulted in rejection by other people, notably her peers, and consolidated her negative IS.

Laura and her therapist reviewed a number of incidents when she had become angry with her sister or peers. After considerable practice, Laura became adept at identifying the attributions she made whenever she perceived (or misperceived) any minor slight. The therapist also taught her other CBT techniques, such as "stop-and-think," to use when she became aware of these misattributions so as to inhibit her from reacting aggressively.

In order to help Laura modify attributions of malicious intent, the therapist asked her to do some homework before the next session. She was to record certain details of a quarrel with a family member or peer if one occurred in the intervening week: 1. Who was involved? 2. What happened? 3. Her initial explanation of the other person's behavior (the attribution). 4. An alternative explanation.

In the following session, Laura reported she had become angry with Jane when her younger sister did not pass her a pitcher of juice at breakfast. Her first explanation attributed Jane's refusal to pass the juice to Jane's hating her. Very much to her credit, she thought of an alternate and probably more accurate explanation right at the breakfast table that precluded her usual aggressive response: The jug was too heavy and she couldn't lift it because she's only a little child.

We cannot emphasize enough that this is really hard work and can be a long and arduous process for school-age children with such entrenched beliefs and perceptions. They require much practice to make these alternative appraisals and attributions. The example offered above was just one session of many in which the therapist and Laura reviewed similar incidents and practiced rehearsing alternate explanations and responses. Moreover, these children require the support and guidance of people in their natural environments. The therapist enlisted Laura's parents as key allies in this process. They cued her to "stop-and-think," gently reminded her of the need to consider alternative explanations for other people's behavior, and even suggested some alternatives.

Countering Victimization as the Defining Characteristic of Self-Image

A child may regard the experience of victimization or maltreatment as a core component of his or her self and personality. Rather than looking at other aspects of their functioning or personality, such children tend to regard themselves solely as "victims" of abuse or neglect. Unfortunately, such a self-view exacerbates feelings of powerlessness and inadequacy and leads to even lower self-esteem. The therapist's task here is to help the child understand that he or she is not alone. Others have been victimized, survived, and even done well: maltreatment should not be the defining characteristic of the child's personality or life (James, 1989; Urquiza & Winn, 1994).

James (1989) describes some creative techniques to address this issue. Using "The List of Bad, Mean, Rotten Things That Can Happen to Kids" (James, 1989, pp. 170–172), the therapist conveys the notion to the child that "bad things happen to other kids, that what happened to them is just one of several terrible things that could have happened, and that things could be worse" (James, 1989, p. 170). In this technique the child or therapist writes on strips of paper all the negative experiences that might happen to children. The child is invited to place the strips in order, with the very worst experiences at the top and the others below in descending order of how awful the child perceives them to be. This is a particularly useful tool for group therapy, as children can compare their lists (James, 1989). They begin to view their own experiences of maltreatment in the context of a range of experiences with which children must cope. In fact, there might be other, "worse things" that could happen. James also notes that repeating the exercise at later points in treatment is a good way for the therapist and child to see how the youngster's perspective has changed.

Another technique developed by James (1989, pp. 173–175), "The Elderly Child Remembers," helps the child acknowledge the maltreatment and place it in its proper perspective. The child imagines him- or herself in the future as an elderly individual who is talking about his or her life to elderly friends. The therapist instructs the child to describe the feelings about having been abused or traumatized years ago and how the child "got stronger, and then how you went on in your life to be successful" (James, 1989, p. 174). This exercise allows children to imagine themselves as survivors of maltreatment. It introduces the possibility that they can be successful, thereby challenging expectations that they are condemned to suffer forever because of the maltreatment.

Chapter 8 described the use of life books and historical information. The therapist might point out that the child has had some happy times and has achieved some successes, although the therapist should make no attempt to deny or minimize the trauma and associated feelings the child has experienced. Photographs of the child winning an award or even just having fun with other children can support this view. The therapist can use statements like "Even though your mom didn't pay you any attention and you had to come to a foster home, these pictures show me that you've been able to do some pretty neat things." Such statements underscore the point that the child should not regard the victimization as the sole defining characteristic of his or her life. As in James's (1989) technique of "The Elderly Child Remembers," the therapist asks child to describe some of the major accomplishments and positive events the child foresees for him- or herself in the future. This exercise may be verbal or done through other means, such as drawing or role plays. It instills a sense of hope and counteracts feelings of despair, hopelessness, and depression.

Physically Abused Children's Concerns about Body Integrity

Children who have been physically assaulted may harbor fears about their health and body integrity. Some children have been scarred or disfigured (e.g., burns, scars from facial injuries). These marks serve as continual reminders of the maltreatment (Urquiza & Winn, 1994). The feelings elicited by these stimuli should be discussed directly, and the therapist should openly empathize with the child's anger, sadness, and loss connected to the assaults. Compounding children's distress is anxiety about what to say to people who ask about their obvious injuries or scars. The therapist and child should rehearse what the youngster will say; they should generate a response that will not elicit fear, rejection, pity, or even more intensive questioning. Some children may be particularly anxious about others seeing their scars, since they expect people to reject them automatically. Children can complete a homework assignment in which they observe the reactions of others to their scars or disfigurement and then recount their observations in the next session. The therapist might pose questions such as "Did everyone laugh at you?" "Did they still let you play with them?" "When kids asked you what happened and you told them what your dad did, did they laugh at you or blame you?" The therapist should encourage the child to engage in self-talk and use self-statements such as "If they don't want anything to do with me because I have a scar, then it's their problem, not mine!" and acknowledge the child's specific accomplishments despite a disfigurement, scar, or disability. This approach may help the child develop an identity that is more balanced and not based solely on body image (Urquiza & Winn, 1994).

Sexually Abused Children's Concerns about Sexuality and Sexual Functioning

Sexually assaulted children are sometimes fearful of sexually transmitted diseases such as HIV/AIDS or are concerned about their genitalia and sexual functioning. These children need prompt medical attention, including being tested for HIV and other diseases. Although stressful, a sensitive medical examination of the child's genitalia may reassure the child that there is no permanent damage. Positive test results will exacerbate the child's distress, especially if HIV is diagnosed. At this point, the therapist and child are dealing not only with the direct sequelae of the assault but also with the complex issues arising from a diagnosis of a serious illness.

We discussed in Chapter 8 how sexually assaulted children worry about their sexual adequacy and functioning. The therapist should provide direct information about sexuality, including the anatomy, purpose, and functions of the genitalia and an explanation of normal sexual response to help them reformulate their experiences. Boys should be educated about the physiological basis of reactions like erections. The difference in the size of the genitalia between the adult male perpetrator and the boy may also be a source of worry, with the child feeling in some way inadequate. Again, the therapist should provide information about sexual development and puberty to allay these concerns. This concern may also be true of boys who have been sexually abused by adult females.

In Chapter 6, we introduced 10-year-old Bob, whose mother had sexual intercourse with him. He divulged to his therapist that he was worried that something must have been wrong with his penis when he had intercourse with his mother 2 years earlier. He thought it was "too small" for his mother's vagina. He had felt his penis was being "swallowed up" and was somehow damaged when she inserted it into her. Bob feared he would never be able to satisfy a female partner sexually when he was older. His anxiety decreased when the therapist explained to him that his genitalia had not been harmed or injured in any way (this had been confirmed by an earlier medical examination). The therapist and Bob talked about puberty and its concomitant physical changes, including those of his genitalia. This discussion, combined with information about normal sexual response, alleviated some of Bob's anxiety about not being physically able to satisfy a sexual partner when he was older and reduced his feelings of powerlessness and passivity.

Bob also revealed to his therapist that he was worried that he might reexperience some of the memories of the sexual abuse when he was older and involved in a sexual relationship. Rather than discounting this fear as unrealistic, the therapist empathized with Bob's anxiety. He suggested to Bob that working hard in therapy now was the best thing he could do to minimize the likelihood of future problems. The therapist avoided giving Bob any outright guarantee that he would never have any problems in later life.

Therapy terminated approximately 2 years later. Bob, who had been placed in a foster home after he had disclosed the sexual abuse, contacted the therapist again when he was nearly 15 years old because he was having some problems with his foster father. Bob and the therapist began a short course of sessions to address this particular difficulty. The therapist took the opportunity to inquire about Bob's sexual adjustment. Bob reported that although he was not yet sexually active, he was no longer bothered by the intrusive memories of having sexual intercourse with his mother that characterized the initial phase of therapy several years earlier. Bob was hopeful his positive adjustment would continue. However, given the horrendous abuse he had suffered at the hands of his mother and her common-law partner, there is no guarantee that Bob will remain asymptomatic, especially as he moves into the next developmental stage of forming romantic and sexual relationships.

Children may worry about their sexual orientation if they were abused by someone of the same gender. Telling a child with this concern that it is nonsense does a real disservice if the youngster is indeed developing a homosexual orientation. Again, glib and easy reassurances should be avoided as much as possible. The therapist should explain the development of sexual orientation to children, emphasizing that no one, including doctors and therapists, knows all the factors that lead to a particular sexual preference. Children may refer to their own sexual excitement and arousal as "proof" that they are gay. A discussion about the basis of sexual arousal may attenuate some of this anxiety and provide a more balanced perspective on this issue. Urquiza and Winn (1994) note that children who are confused about their sexuality may feel compelled to engage in sexual relationships with members of the opposite sex to prove they are "straight." The authors recommend offering support and encouraging the child to refrain from initiating sexual relationships until he or she is emotionally and physically prepared for the experience.

BUILDING MASTERY

Maltreatment frequently engenders feelings of helplessness, powerlessness, depression, and inadequacy. Besides acknowledging these feelings, children need to move from a position of powerlessness to one of effectiveness. This change diminishes feelings of inadequacy regarding past victimizations and increases the children's confidence in protecting themselves from future assaults. The therapist has many ways of developing this sense of mastery. These methods range from indirect, metaphorical play techniques to strategies that engage the child in more direct discussions and explorations of these issues.

Posttraumatic Play and Reparative Metaphors

There has been a long tradition within the fields of psychoanalytic and psychodynamic therapy that regards children's play as an attempt to allay anxiety by mastering situations. Sigmund Freud used the term "repetition compulsion" to "describe the unconscious need to reenact early traumas in the attempt to overcome or master them" (Goldenson, 1984, p. 632). Traumatized children's play frequently reflects the repetition of these themes. For example, children who have been involved in motor vehicle accidents often reenact repeated car crashes in which the occupants are seriously injured and ultimately rescued by police. Children who have undergone painful and invasive surgeries pretend they are doctors and perform countless operations on dolls or stuffed animals, thereby converting a passively experienced event into one over which they have control. Their anxiety begins to diminish as they attain a sense of mastery. Besides providing the child with a metaphorical or symbolic way of becoming the victorious survivor who is no longer the passive victim of uncontrollable forces, play is an opportunity for the therapist to introduce more adaptive ways of mastering fears and anxieties rather than allowing reliance on strategies such as physical aggression.

Some children spontaneously begin to enact scenarios of abuse or neglect using play. They may depict it in an even more disguised form by using animal rather than human characters or by portraying the maltreatment metaphorically: the animals or humans are attacked by monsters rather than physically or sexually assaulted. After enacting the play scenario, the child uses the play to depict a solution. For example, Peter, portraying himself as Superman, was a powerful figure who rescued animals from threatening figures (Chapter 7). He used play to transform himself from a passive victim of severe and long-standing abuse into a figure who was now invincible and invulnerable to the assaults of others.

There are other children who enact the traumatic or victimizing experience in their play but cannot resolve or master the situation. Terr (1990) cautions that reenactment without resolution reinforces a sense of helplessness and of being at the mercy of forces beyond the child's control. These feelings of terror and helplessness may be accompanied by further behavioral regression. Terr argues that therapists need to intervene actively after a repeated number of these play scenarios have been acted out (8–10 sessions). Intervention is necessary to help the child assume a more active role in the play and generate alternate resolutions, thereby promoting a sense of symbolic mastery and control over the frightening or painful event.

Terr (1990) describes many useful strategies to modify posttraumatic play. These include disruptions in the actual play sequence, such as asking the child to make physical movements like standing up or taking deep breaths. Verbal statements from the therapist about the play and comments on the action may interrupt the child's self-absorption and rigid reenactment. Terr also recommends more active interventions. The therapist can modify play sequences by asking the child to take a specific role and to describe the character's perceptions and feelings. The therapist can manipulate the characters by moving them around or provide even more directive and specific prompts by asking the youngster to respond to questions like "What would happen if the little girl asked somebody for help?" The therapist might prompt the child by saying, "Let's make this little girl really powerful. Let's think of some ways she could get away from that monster. She could ____________," with the therapist turning to the child and inviting a response. Encouraging the child to differentiate between the traumatic event and current reality also allows the child to modify the play. Videotaping the play and then watching it together is another opportunity to stop the play at important junctures and encourage the child to think of ways to solve the dilemma that appears at each point.

The therapist can present play scenarios that are not as disguised as those discussed above, to expose the child to more direct representations of the maltreatment. For example, the therapist can say, "Let's make up a story about a little girl whose dad hits her a lot." Some children will enact extremely aggressive solutions to being hurt. Some clinicians argue that these actions are permissible, inasmuch as they are fantasy enactments. We have trouble with allowing children to continue using these harmful and destructive solutions, even in the metaphor of the play. Although aggressive play scenarios may increase a child's sense of mastery and power, they may also promote reliance on hurting and exploiting others in other environments. The therapist can offer alternate strategies in the context of the play to increase the child's sense of safety and personal effectiveness and to restore his or her self-esteem. The therapist might say, "Rather than hitting that monster, what could the little girl say to the monster?" or, "Is there anyone else here that the boy could ask for help?" The therapist and child can generate and present alternate strategies in a game-like format. The child might be told, "Let's think of as many ways as we can that the girl can use to protect herself from that guy who is trying to hurt her." Following the problem-solving approach outlined in Chapter 9, the therapist then encourages the child to think of the various solutions' consequences for both the perpetrator ("How do you think he'd feel if he got stabbed by a knife when he tried to hurt the girl?") and the child/hero ("How do you think she'd feel if she tried to kill him? What do you think would happen to her if she killed him?").

Storytelling may also impart messages about constructive and healthy ways to gain mastery over traumatizing events. Mills and Crowley (1986) discuss the use of therapeutic metaphors in general with children, and Davis (1990) has written a book of metaphorical stories for abused children. Useful material is included in both works. Therapists can use individually tailored metaphorical stories in storytelling to help youngsters develop adaptive responses to abusive situations. The therapist begins by recounting a metaphorical description of an abusive situation and then asks the child to "make up the ending." With Gardner's "Mutual Storytelling Technique" (Gardner, 1971), the child tells a story and the therapist repeats it with the same theme and characters. However, the therapist introduces a healthier resolution than that initially proposed by the child. Applying this technique to metaphorical stories about maltreatment, the therapist tells the story again but modifies the child's ending to propose a more constructive solution that does not rely on aggression.

Developing Realistic and Viable Self-Protection Strategies

Children may be better able to tolerate more direct discussions of anxiety-provoking issues after participating in play activities that have desensitized them to these issues and engendered confidence and feelings of mastery via fantasy. Although the therapist must allow initial fantasy attempts to emerge, the failure to introduce other means will reinforce the notion that the child must rely on fantasy measures in real-life situations. Children should have realistic expectations about their ability to care for and protect themselves, such as understanding that adults have ultimate responsibility for ensuring their safety. Moreover, the therapist needs to promote more realistic and viable strategies for the child to reduce the probability of future victimization. This knowledge may further attenuate anxiety and feelings of powerlessness. Now the child has a better idea of what he or she could actually do. For example, in Chapter 9 we described how Steve's anxiety began to decrease after he developed a specific and viable plan to implement if his father tried to reassault him.

To initiate this process, therapists should comment on the previous methods or strategies youngsters used to protect themselves during the abuse. These are often valiant attempts by young and inexperienced children to alert others to the terrifying things that are happening to them. One 5-year-old girl knocked on her bedroom wall, which adjoined her parents' bedroom, whenever her stepfather sexually abused her. She explained to her therapist that she was trying to give her mother a "sign" about what was happening. The mother recalled sometimes hearing the knocking, but usually she was so tired that she fell asleep. Therapists can tell children that they did the best they could have done, given the situation and their lack of knowledge and experience about how to deal with the traumatizing events.

A study of the characteristics of sexually abused and nonabused children's conceptions about personal body safety demonstrated the need to directly educate children about maltreatment (Miller-Perrin, Wurtele, & Kondrick, 1990). Investigators presented a vignette describing the violation of personal body safety to 25 boys and girls of ages 5–12 years who were entering a treatment program for sexual abuse victims. They were matched with a group of 25 nonabused children. The sexually abused children were more likely to describe the vignette situation as involving abuse or rape and were more likely to provide a correct definition of sexual abuse. However, 25% of the sexually abused children still could not label the situation accurately as abusive, even though they had participated in treatment for sexual assault. Only half of the sexually abused group and 28% of the nonabused group could provide a correct definition of sexual abuse. Although children need to be able to recognize and identify different situations as abusive or even neglectful, it is often a difficult for them to do so. Some situations are quite clear, as such flagrant acts of physical or sexual abuse. Others may be more ambiguous, especially for younger children. For example, because some sexually abused children have learned to equate sexualized interactions with manifestations of love and nurturance, they may not see them as exploitative.

Cognitive-developmental variables also influence children's understanding of concepts typically presented in abuse-prevention programs. Tutty (1994) prepared an excellent review of the developmental issues related to child sexual-abuse prevention. She notes that developmental factors, such as a child's difficulty in understanding abstract and subtle concepts, affect how readily the child appreciates ideas like "good touch" versus "bad touch." Teaching children to oppose the wishes of an adult, especially a familiar adult in a caretaking position, is another common task in sexual-abuse prevention programs. Here again, developmental factors affect children's understanding of the issue. Damon (1980; cited in Tutty, 1994, p.181) found that children of ages 5–6 believe that authority figures have an inherent right to be obeyed because they are larger, more powerful, stronger, and have higher status.

The empirical findings regarding the effectiveness of child sexual-abuse prevention programs are mixed (Daro, 1991). Tailoring material to a child's cognitive characteristics and learning abilities, presenting material in a stimulating and varied manner, and providing many opportunities to rehearse prevention strategies through staged interactions were all especially useful in helping children learn the concepts and skills of self-protection. Therapists should incorporate these characteristics of successful prevention programs in interventions used in individual therapy. They should present information in different and stimulating ways. For example, the therapist might write descriptions of different scenarios on cards. The therapist and child then take turns discussing each scenario and deciding whether it might constitute an act of abuse or neglect. Rather than trying to provide children, especially younger ones, with an exhaustive list of all the potentially abusive or exploitative situations they might encounter, a more useful and viable strategy is to teach them to tell an adult when a situation confuses them (Daro, 1991). The effectiveness of this simple strategy is indirectly supported by the reports of adult sexual offenders who say they are deterred by a youngster who indicates an intention to tell a specific adult about an assault (Budin & Johnson, 1989; Conte, Wolf, & Smith, 1989).

Our clinical experience has convinced us of the importance of providing children with many opportunities to rehearse what they would actually do or say in these situations. Therapists should present various situations, some of which replicate selected aspects of the child's past episodes of maltreatment, and then ask the child to respond to these situations. They can present scenarios in a more tolerable form, such as puppet plays, to children who remain particularly anxious about dealing directly with this material. Therapists can begin the play by enacting a situation in which the characters are victimized, then requesting the child to step in as the puppeteer and demonstrate an adaptive solution. They can emphasize how the child might disclose the situation to a trusted adult, including the actual words the child would use. Children should identify those adults to whom they feel they could disclose this information. We have constructed simple pursuit games in which children must answer hypothetical questions regarding personal safety when they land on specially designated squares. The scenarios might include some that deal with other aspects of personal safety (e.g., "If you got lost in a department store, what would you do?") and others that focus on victimization episodes. The therapist should develop scenarios that parallel the child's own past experiences. Participants get an extra turn if they can provide an adaptive solution to these dilemmas. Allowing each participant to take two extra turns if he or she can also role-play the response introduces more fun and provides additional practice. Again, the therapist must pay careful attention to the nature of the child's responses and intervene to correct any unrealistic or inappropriate solutions.

Another way to help children gain a sense of mastery over past victimization is to have them help others who are struggling with similar issues. This approach is particularly applicable to older school-age children who have the cognitive and verbal skills needed to participate in these projects. The knowledge that one can now help others often has a positive effect on self-esteem. This project is usually best introduced in the latter phase of therapy, when children feel better about their experiences and have learned some adaptive ways of handling their reactions. We have invited maltreated children to "help other kids who are beginning therapy" by preparing brief pamphlets that describe the common reactions and feelings associated with maltreatment. The pamphlets help children consolidate their understanding of their own reactions and raise self-esteem. We have been impressed with the enthusiasm and eagerness of children to assist others. Some have even volunteered to meet with the other child. The sharing of similar experiences is one of the great strengths of group psychotherapy. On several occasions, we have invited children to prepare a video in which they talk about their own experiences and the coping mechanisms they used. We also give them a copy of it. With explicit permission from the children and their legal guardians, we have shown these videos and pamphlets to other children, who then experienced a reduced sense of stigmatization and isolation. Of course, therapists must ensure that children who receive these productions have no knowledge of those who prepared the pamphlets or, even more important, who appear on the videos.

REPAIRING AND RESTORING SELF-ESTEEM

Helping children feel better about themselves is necessary to counteract feelings of stigmatization, inadequacy, and depression. This task often runs throughout the course of therapy. The clinician must be alert to opportunities to bolster the child's self-esteem. In Chapter 9 we described some specific strategies (e.g., "Me Badge," "Five Things I Do Well") to challenge the child's model of the self as unworthy and inadequate. We also reviewed the use of positive self-statements to counter negative ones. These strategies are particularly useful in situations in which the therapist wants to help the child explore and examine some of the more troublesome aspects of behavior and functioning. In Chapter 9 we examined strategies children might use to gain better self-control and regulation of their behavior and emotions. Such improvements have a positive effect on children's self-esteem, especially if the behavioral changes are accompanied by their greater acceptance by and involvement with other people, including peers. In this chapter, we examined how to instill in the child a sense of mastery and self-efficacy concerning past and possible future maltreatment episodes, which may also have a positive effect on self-esteem. At this point, children no longer regard themselves merely as passive victims. Changing internal attributions about the maltreatment enables children to see themselves in a different and more positive perspective.

What are some other activities that will consolidate this healthier sense of self-esteem? We again refer to the child development literature to sensitize clinicians to the developmental variables that have significant implications for our interventions.

Providing Children with Behavioral Evidence of Their Strengths

Harter (1983) describes a four-stage sequence of the development of children's concept of the self. The first stage corresponds to Piaget's preoperational stage of thought (in children 2–7 years of age). In this stage, a child defines the self by behavior and observable attributes. In the second stage, corresponding to the Piagetian concrete operational stage of thought (age 7 to early adolescence), the child begins to integrate these behavioral descriptions as trait labels (e.g., smart, popular). However, Harter notes that children at this age engage in all-or-none thinking. Thus, a child may conclude that he or she is not a good athlete because of difficulties in one or two athletic activities, despite other indicators of skill. In adolescence, abstractions emerge (third stage), and then single abstractions become further integrated into higher-order abstractions (fourth stage).

One implication of this developmental sequence is that therapists must provide the behavior evidence on which trait labels are constructed. Relying on trait labels (e.g., "You're a smart kid") may not have as great an impact as citing the specific behaviors that form the basis of such statements. When Peter began to play Chinese checkers with the therapist (see Chapter 7 for a more detailed description of this vignette), he immediately said he would never learn to play the game. The therapist empathized with his fears and provided Peter with gentle encouragement at least to try. This approach was in sharp contrast to simply telling Peter that the therapist thought he was "smart" and could do it. Peter lost the first game, but the therapist identified several of Peter's moves that showed good judgment and forethought; these statements constituted concrete evidence of Peter's intellectual ability. Peter began to request the game as a routine part of subsequent therapy sessions. The therapist often had to identify other behaviors that reflected good abilities in order to help Peter improve profoundly low self-esteem. The therapist also taught him to use self-statements that identified specific strengths and abilities whenever Peter began feeling bad about himself.

The therapist should acknowledge specific aspects of the child's participation in the therapeutic process so as to raise the child's self-esteem. Statements like "You really worked hard in therapy today. Even when you became so upset and started to cry about how your mom was never around for you, you kept on talking about it" are much more meaningful than vague and diffuse statements such as "You did well." The therapist should use examples of the child's interaction with the therapist as further evidence of progress: "When you got really mad at me today because I wouldn't let you do the finger painting, you used words to tell me how mad you were rather than trying to hit me." This content can be incorporated into the child's positive self-statements, which he or she might employ at particularly difficult moments in therapy.

Encouraging the Child to Try New Activities

The therapist should encourage the child to try new activities during therapy sessions to provide more opportunities for success. Sitting passively and allowing the child to engage in the same activity month after month just reinforces the notion that the child is incapable of doing anything else. Although Peter was somewhat resistant, the therapist gently encouraged him to try playing Chinese checkers. The trick is to suggest an activity that the therapist believes the child can handle with some success. Difficult material that the child cannot master will only provide another frustrating and demeaning experience. With younger children or those whose self-esteem is profoundly low, shorter activities may be a better choice than those that take a long time to complete. While these children wait to see if they will be successful, their anxiety will so escalate that they refuse to continue. Therapists should teach young children with little play experience how to play, such as how to use plastic building blocks or how to paint. We have successfully taught older school-age children to use the personal computer in our offices to write and compose stories or letters to their perpetrators. The process of learning to use a computer or mastering other skills (e.g., learning to operate a video camera when taping a session) enhances a child's feelings of adequacy and self-esteem.

The therapist should encourage the child to develop new interests outside therapy as well as during therapy sessions.

After being placed in a foster home, Bob expressed a strong interest in playing organized hockey, an opportunity he never had previously. However, he was anxious about joining a league because he barely knew how to skate and believed he could never match the skills of the other boys. Fortunately, his foster parents sought out a team that accepted him, and the coach gave Bob extra instruction in the fundamentals of the game, such as skating and stick handling. The therapist encouraged and supported Bob in this new activity, and they explored some of his distorted cognitions about joining a hockey team. He expected that spectators would laugh at him if he fell on the ice and that he would never get a goal. Bob was encouraged to develop alternate self-statements to use when bothered by these thoughts and to "collect the evidence" to confirm or refute these expectations (i.e., to observe the fans' reactions to any errors he made on the ice). This strategy, as well as the generous support and encouragement of his foster parents and the one-on-one instruction from his coach, contributed to Bob's persistence with hockey. His self-esteem received a real boost when he won the trophy for the most improved player at the season's end.

This concrete demonstration of Bob's ability helped challenge his initial model of himself as a passive, powerless child who could do nothing to change his life. This example also illustrates the importance of working closely with the significant people in the child's life to ensure exposure to multiple and positive experiences.

Some maltreated children, especially those who have been neglected, begin to fail dismally at school; in these cases the therapist might advocate for individual tutoring or other specialized educational services. Academic tutoring may increase children's academic skills and decrease their frustration and disruptiveness in the classroom. These improvements, in turn, promote social adjustment and counter the development of negative self-concepts (Conduct Problems Prevention Research Group, 1992). Therapists should consult closely with tutors about the children's presentations or progress in tutoring sessions.

A child can also start a scrapbook that includes drawings or even photographs of his or her new abilities and strengths so as to concretize these accomplishments. Again, therapists should emphasize the specific and observable evidence of these gains. They can instruct the child to be alert for evidence of new strengths between therapy sessions and to depict them in the scrapbook for the next session. This exercise may become a routine part of therapy, with the child identifying at least one strength per week. Therapists eventually should encourage children to look for new strengths in the social skills area, such as concrete examples of their helping other people (see Chapter 9 for a description of the "Recording Friendly Deeds" exercise). The first example of an interpersonal strength in a 9-year-old boy in foster care occurred when he got a drink of water for a younger child who was also in care. Therapists can keep a running account of the child's progress in therapy by identifying one positive thing the child does in each session or in the intervening week. The child or therapist writes this "positive" on a large piece of paper. As these positives are accumulated over the course of weeks and months, they give the child a concrete, visual record of all the things he or she has accomplished. At termination of therapy, we give children these often large sheets of paper as souvenirs of the progress and gains they have made.

Board games are useful to help children who have problems with self-esteem. Therapists can teach children games with which they are unfamiliar, so as to boost their sense of mastery and adequacy. Games should not be so complicated and involved that they take hours to complete; there should be a good chance of finishing the game in the therapy hour with, ideally, time left over for other activities. There must be a selection of games, ranging from simple ones that even young children can master to the more complex that challenge older school-age youngsters. Children who are particularly anxious about their abilities may choose to play games in which success is solely dependent on luck. While allowed to play such games initially, they should be encouraged to attempt games that have elements of skill.

Reactions to losing and winning are often accurate reflections of children's self-esteem, as is other behavior, like cheating. Some children with low self-esteem interpret losing a game as further evidence of their inadequacy or stupidity. If they do agree to play a game, they quickly begin to verbalize fears about losing. The therapist should articulate and empathize with the anxiety. The therapist can ask a child to identify the "worst thing that would happen if you lost this game." Children's common fears include fear of the therapist's reaction (e.g., "You'll think I'm dumb," "You'll laugh at me") or feeling even worse about themselves if they lose. The therapist should tell the child to observe the therapist's behavior keenly at the game's end to see if any of these expectations are fulfilled. This course is preferable to providing a blanket reassurance that the therapist will not denigrate the youngster. The therapist might suggest a few practice games before they play "for real." This approach may be especially important for particularly anxious children or those who are trying new games. The therapist can explain that some games, just like many other activities, require practice to develop proficiency. After playing several of these practice games, the therapist may be concerned that the child still lacks skills and will lose badly. Proposing that the child accept a handicap (which may not be the right choice of words for some children) is one way to avoid crushing defeats that exacerbate a child's low self-esteem. An example of such a "handicap" is for the child to have fewer board pieces to move. To ensure that the child is not insulted by this suggestion, the therapist might use the game of golf as an example, explaining how handicaps are regularly assigned to different players. In addition, the therapist says that he or she does not want to be unfair and take advantage of the child's lack of experience or practice.

Some children beg the therapist to let them win the game. The therapist should comment empathically about the child's anxiety, conveying an understanding that losing poses a real threat to the child's self-esteem. However, the therapist should also say that he or she will not throw the game. Permission to cheat reinforces children's expectations that they will never attain success through personal efforts. Consistent with the findings of developmental research reviewed above, children need concrete and authentic experiences to raise self-esteem, not experiences they know are based on dishonesty. The rest of the world, particularly other children, may not be as benevolent as the therapist and will quickly rescind invitations to participate in games after the youngster repeatedly tries to cheat. Intervening with cheating in this manner may prevent such unfortunate occurrences in the future, thereby improving the child's social skills.

Children may begin to cheat during games to preserve fragile and tenuous self-esteem in the face of losing. Again, the therapist must intervene and bring the transgression to the child's attention as soon as it is noticed. Asking if the child cheated (especially when the therapist knows it occurred) is often misguided, because the child usually denies it. Then the therapist is left in the situation of trying to decide what to do next. Therapists should present cheating as a statement of fact rather than an inquiry if they are certain the child has cheated. Therapists can help children reflect on why they may have cheated; questions regarding how the child might feel if he or she loses are often useful in identifying a need to win at any cost to preserve shaky self-esteem. The therapist should say firmly that cheating is not allowed. Not only is it not fair, but if the child cheats while playing with other children, he or she will probably be thrown out of the game. Moreover, by allowing cheating, the therapist colludes with the child's negative self-image: "If I let you cheat, what I'm really telling you is that I don't think you're able to win by yourself. I think you can win without cheating, so that's why I'm not going to allow you to do it."

There may be no choice but to end the game and refuse to play if a child persists in cheating despite these explanations and discussions. The therapist should explain this decision in terms of concern for the child: "We have to end the game now because you're continuing to cheat. I don't want you to think that this is the only way you're able to win. That wouldn't be good for you, so we're going to stop the game." The therapist might offer to play the game in the next session to provide the child with another opportunity to handle the anxiety more adaptively. Some children may attempt to change the rules in the middle of the game to ensure victory. Therapists must curtail this play and give the same rationale as that used to limit cheating. Modifications of the rules should occur before a game begins and only after both the child and therapist have discussed and reached an agreement about the proposed changes.

These interactions with the therapist are often a novel experience for children who have never heard an adult tell them he or she thinks they are capable of success. Such new expectations, and the therapist's firm yet nonpunitive stance toward behavior like cheating, constitute experiences that help children modify the IWMs/IS in a more favorable and positive direction. Therapy can be a powerful tool when it integrates skillful attention to relevant content with sensitive use of the relationship as a medium of change.

CHAPTER ELEVEN

Termination of Therapy

The termination of therapy is a process that all client children and therapists confront, but it has received insufficient thought or attention in the literature. Many maltreated children come to regard their therapists as significant figures. Ending therapy provokes strong reactions in both clients and therapists. Attending closely and carefully to the feelings and cognitions evoked in children can transform this therapy phase into one that further promotes growth. Termination offers another opportunity to help children reexamine historical issues, especially those related to loss. It is also an opportunity to develop healthy and adaptive coping mechanisms to deal with this inevitable component of human relationships.

CRITERIA FOR TERMINATION OF THERAPY

Therapy should end when the treatment goals have been met. This highlights the importance of conducting a comprehensive assessment from which realistic goals are derived. Goals guide our ongoing clinical work and serve as markers against which we evaluate the success of our interventions and whether we can begin the termination process. Of course, original treatment goals may undergo modification during therapy as children reveal more about the maltreatment and respond idiosyncratically to interventions. We advocated in Chapter 4 that therapists should reevaluate goals regularly to determine their ongoing appropriateness and the child's success in meeting them. This is especially important in long-term psychotherapy, given a possibly greater tendency for the case to drift without clear objectives or direction. Regular reviews also contribute to the child's own sense of progress and enhance self-esteem.

Some therapists believe that although treatment goals have been achieved, psychotherapy must continue in order to prevent the emergence of future psychological or behavioral symptoms. The rationale seems to be that more of a good thing will protect children from future problems. This notion that psychotherapy can effectively address issues emerging much later is misguided. Therapy can increase the probability of more adaptive future functioning via the development of healthy coping mechanisms and a reformulation of maltreatment. Participation in successful therapy also establishes the expectation in children and families that subsequent difficulties can be faced rather than ignored or denied and increases the chances that clients will not interpret a subsequent return to therapy as a personal failure to be avoided. However, issues related to the maltreatment may emerge later, albeit in somewhat different forms, as a result of subsequent life experiences (e.g., revictimization) or the individual's progression through different developmental phases. Developmental transformations of these original issues could not have been successfully treated earlier because they had not yet emerged: individuals may need another course of therapy at this later time. In Chapter 2, we reviewed the case of Chris, who reentered therapy when he began adolescence. Adolescence was a catalyst for the evocation of issues pertaining to sexual identity and homosexuality, themes related to Chris's history of sexual abuse by his father. The therapist could not have treated these specific issues when Chris began therapy at 8 years of age, inasmuch as they had not attained any prominence or significance during that developmental stage. Again, we cannot treat what has not yet emerged. Attempts to do this result, at best, in therapy with vague and diffuse goals, but at worst, in a process that wastes the time and effort of both therapist and child. A more reasonable course is to terminate but give the child and family an open invitation to recontact the therapist if future problems emerge. Through this "family practice" model (described more fully in Chapter 5), the therapist, child, and family recognize the accomplishments of the child in a course of therapy. It also acknowledges the real limits of psychotherapy in providing absolute immunity to the effects of the maltreatment throughout the remaining lifespan.

Although the major criterion for termination is the achievement of treatment objectives, changes in children's presentations in therapy may provide clues that indicate they are less dependent on therapy and that termination can be considered. Dodds (1985) describes some of these changes. For instance, interest in attending therapy sessions begins to wane. Children start to come late, miss appointments, ask to leave early, or perhaps comment that there is nothing more to talk about or nothing interesting to play. These actions may be accompanied by a greater focus than usual on matters outside therapy, such as school activities and friends. Children begin to speak of activities they would be doing if not at the therapy session. Discussions about these other matters reflect a greater interest in nontherapeutic issues, particularly if youngsters are not encountering any problems in these areas. Salient themes that characterized earlier play are often no longer present, and there is a greater emphasis on playing for the sake of playing, rather than on using it to communicate about maltreatment-related issues. Older school-age children begin to make direct statements about the therapeutic relationship. They may acknowledge the therapist's role in their recovery or comment on their sense of being heard. They spontaneously start to reminisce about past therapy events or ask directly when therapy will end. Changes in the therapist's interactions are also apparent. The therapist makes more statements that review and encapsulate past therapy events and that encourage the child to take greater risks outside therapy. If the therapist notices such changes, it may be appropriate to reevaluate the child's progress in meeting treatment goals as the first step of the termination process.

PREPARING CHILDREN FOR TERMINATION OF THERAPY

Children must receive adequate preparation for the termination of therapy whenever possible; the therapist should broach the subject with a child well ahead of the expected final session. The time needed for termination depends on factors such as the nature, intensity, and duration of the therapeutic relationship and the child's typical pace and rhythm in processing issues (Carek, 1979). Children traumatized by previous losses also need sufficient time to cope adequately with the end of therapy. Carek (1979) suggests that termination over 2–3 weeks may be adequate if the therapy has been more short-term. One or two months or more are usually necessary for children in long-term therapy (1 year or more). However, flexibility is key. Despite involvement in intensive, long-term psychotherapy, some youngsters have been disengaging for some time before termination is raised as an issue. As a rule, 4–6 weeks is adequate.

One way to approach termination is to remind youngsters of the original reasons for therapy and to inquire whether they think these still exist. The therapist remarks that treatment cannot continue forever and it is time to think about when the child might stop coming, given many improvements. The therapist discusses the reasons for termination in some depth, even if the child professes a firm understanding that termination is needed because goals are met. Given our strong orientation toward cognitive-developmental variables, we believe the therapist must provide specific and concrete examples of the youngster's gains. The therapist can contrast these with the child's condition that led to the initial therapy referral. Although we must acknowledge that the relationship is ending, we can also point out that termination is a "commencement": the child is leaving the old, but with gains so great enough that the youngster can begin something new (Allen, 1942). We sometimes use the term "graduation" with older school-age children. We explain that ending therapy is somewhat similar to leaving a valued and trusted teacher at the school year's end following successful completion of the term. Although this event is characterized by feelings of sadness, it is also a time to feel proud of one's accomplishments.

Ross (1964) recommends that therapists do not allow children to make the final decision about the actual termination date. To do so places an unfair responsibility on them and may lead to an impasse if a child sets a distant date. Many clinicians choose a termination date that coincides with another transition in the child's life, such as the end of the school year. The child may regard termination as a change similar to others in which relationships end before new ones commence. This approach seems to help children through the process. However, Sandler, Kennedy, and Tyson (1980) argue that termination of therapy at the start of school vacation may lead some children to rationalize that the separation is not final, being due solely to the vacation. This rationalization plays into their attempts to deny and avoid painful feelings of sadness and loss. Therapists must remember that there are no rigid rules regarding timing, and they must use clinical judgment to decide what best meets each child's needs.

Therapists can taper the frequency of sessions during the termination phase. This helps children become comfortable with the idea of functioning more independently without regular therapeutic assistance. For example, sessions may be biweekly at first and then less frequent as the final date approaches. If children have no opportunity to deal more independently with the challenges and problems of daily life before therapy ends, their self-confidence is eroded and they may become anxious about their ability to handle challenges without the therapists' assistance. In the termination phase, therapists should continue to encourage children to use skills that foster more independence and should provide positive feedback and reinforcement for these efforts. These measures are particularly important if independence was a central therapeutic issue in the preceding treatment.

HELPING CHILDREN EXPRESS FEELINGS ABOUT TERMINATION OF THERAPY

Children usually have ambivalent feelings about termination. They feel pleased with their accomplishments and look forward to devoting the time now occupied by therapy to other activities. They also feel sad at the prospect of no longer seeing the therapist, especially if the therapeutic relationship was a principal means of change. Termination may reelicit feelings about relationships that were evident in earlier therapy stages. For children with an insecure attachment history, dependence needs may reemerge. Children may demand more frequent sessions, ask for their therapist's home phone number, and request assistance for tasks previously handled with ease. Displays of anger, with children vehemently protesting the therapist's decision to end therapy, may accompany these demands.

Youngsters with an avoidant attachment history may rely on defenses that characterized earlier functioning. Rather than openly and directly acknowledging the sadness and loss evoked by termination, they may avoid or deny these feelings. They may even refuse to acknowledge that the relationship will end. Many maltreated children have experienced numerous losses, with people leaving their lives without explanation. They had no opportunity to express feelings of loss, abandonment, and anger. Other children resort to the same internal attributions that were apparent at the initiation of therapy, believing they have done something to anger or alienate the therapist, or feeling unworthy of the therapist's commitment.

Termination of the therapeutic relationship provides an excellent opportunity to help children consolidate their ability to cope adaptively with these feelings. Reminding children of the number of remaining sessions at each session's start counters tendencies to deny the reality of the impending termination. Therapists should encourage children to verbalize the feelings evoked by termination, and empathize with and validate their normalcy. Modeling emotional expression may occur as the therapist articulates personal feelings about ending the relationship, although not to the extent that children feel burdened. Dodds (1985) reminds us that we do not want our child clients to feel responsible for either causing our feelings or helping us deal with them. Some children feel especially hesitant to verbalize their anger because they do not want to alienate the therapist further. Telling children that anger is a normal and expected reaction to separation and loss enables them to acknowledge similar feelings.

The therapist can use other techniques besides encouraging children to verbalize feelings associated with termination. The children can draw facial expressions that depict their feelings, present puppet plays that focus on issues such as separation, or use some of the other techniques described in Chapter 8. Discussions of the common reactions of "other kids" expose children to this painful material. Children can prepare a book or pamphlet describing their experiences in therapy, including the ending phase. We must be cautious about maintaining an exclusive focus on the negative feelings connected with terminating therapy. Assisting youngsters to identify positive feelings associated with termination promotes a more balanced perspective on ending the relationship.

Although therapists involve children in discussions of the reasons for ending therapy when termination is first addressed, they will have to clarify the reasons during this phase. Children may require several explanations that therapy is ending because of their progress and not because of any personal animosity toward them. Again, it is helpful if the therapist and child review the specific changes made by the youngster. Vague statements like "You're doing a lot better!" may be virtually meaningless to a young child who needs observable evidence of improvement. The child and therapist can review the cumulative record of weekly accomplishments kept throughout the course of therapy (Chapter 10). Reminiscing about therapy provides another opportunity for children to express feelings about specific therapeutic experiences and interactions with the therapist. Reminiscing also allows some closure in the relationship and consolidates youngsters' perceptions of their gains. Confirmation that children can return to therapy if needed also attenuates some of their sense of loss and pain. A small ceremony is a concrete reminder of the relationship's importance and is a way of acknowledging and celebrating a child's growth. Children usually enjoy planning a small party for the last session. We have had children invite family members to these celebrations, which have included cake and other favorite foods. By giving the child a small gift, such as a book or a certificate to proclaim the child's participation and progress in therapy, the therapist concretely affirms the relationship's importance to both child and therapist.

During termination, children may begin to regress or show symptoms that had originally led to therapy. This behavior reflects their distress about leaving therapy. The therapist should focus on helping these youngsters express their underlying feelings, rather than interpreting the behavior as a need for further treatment and then quickly postponing termination. The problems usually disappear as children resolve their feelings about termination.

Parents or caregivers also require help during the termination phase, and therapists should encourage them to express any worries or concerns. Many fear that they or their child will not cope without regular assistance from the therapist. They may be particularly distressed if the child temporarily regresses during termination. Parents see this as evidence that the child needs more therapy. While empathizing with this anxiety, the therapist should review the progress they and their child have achieved over the course of therapy. The therapist can review possible steps should future problems arise. For example, parents also experience some alleviation of their anxiety when informed that they are welcome to recontact the therapist if necessary.

PREMATURE TERMINATIONS

Unfortunately, not every termination occurs in this planned fashion. Therapy may end unexpectedly because a family moves. The therapist should attempt to have at least one final session with the child to explain the real reason for termination and to emphasize the therapist's regard for the youngster. This session also allows the child to express some feelings about the impending separation. If having even one session is impossible, the therapist might send a short letter to the child to clarify the reasons for termination and convey best wishes for the future.

Just as in the other phases of therapy, termination evokes feelings in therapists as well as in children. We conclude this book by a consideration of this important topic.

CHAPTER TWELVE

Personal Implications for the Therapist

We now discuss the personal implications for therapists of this intense work with often very damaged, maltreated children and their families. No matter whether children demonstrate situational or long-term effects, therapists need to hear and respond to painful descriptions of traumatic events. For some, this can be a difficult and provocative experience. Lyon (1993) described the marked reactions of hospital staff members to adult patients' accounts of violence and abuse. Some reported nightmares, intrusive and repetitive images, and somatic symptoms such as headaches, nausea, and sleeplessness. The staff members' reactions to patients' accounts of victimization were intensified by their own personal histories of victimization or psychological difficulties. Lyon speculates that these reactions might be a type of secondary PTSD.

Many children with a history of an insecure attachment organization attempt to provoke therapists into rejecting or abusing them. Such responses would confirm their expectations of how others will respond to them. In several chapters of this book we described how children exhibit provocative behavior that can be hostile and outrageous and may continue unabated for lengthy periods. Others treat therapists as nonentities, as described in Chapter 7. Work with such children can be physically and emotionally exhausting and usually engenders a range of strong reactions in therapists.

COUNTERTRANSFERENCE

Countertransference is a concept that focuses on therapists' reactions to their clients. Friedrich (1990) defines countertransference as "reactions to our clients that are based, in part, on who we are and what we bring to the therapy process" (p. 269). Schowalter (1985) suggests that such reactions are more likely to occur in child therapy than in adult therapy, especially when a child client is the same age as the therapist's own child or when the client's problems are similar to those of the therapist or his or her children. Friedrich stresses that it is crucial to be aware of our own personal issues and how these may interfere with a child's therapy. During the client's therapy, the therapist must always be aware of his or her personal reactions to the client, inasmuch as these can help or hinder the therapy's progress. A therapist's reactions and issues may arise not only from early childhood roles or from early victimization but also from current relationships and possible victimization within those relationships, along with a myriad of other factors.

Reactions may be intense and varied. Feelings that are common to foster and adoptive parents and therapists in their work with damaged and maltreated children include resentment, anger, betrayal, and hurt, which often arise from daily interactions with children who cannot trust others (James, 1994). Furthermore, frustration, helplessness, and hopelessness all arise when the therapist faces a damaged child whose problems seem almost insurmountable (Pearce & Pezzot-Pearce, 1994). A therapist must be attuned to these feelings and reactions to avoid being overwhelmed and giving up. Such reactions may also provoke an array of defensive strategies in the therapist, such as denying that a child has significant problems. In either situation, therapy will not be helpful to the child.

The therapist's awareness of personal feelings and reactions and of the active strategies needed to cope with them are necessary to avoid inappropriate responses to the child. For example, a therapist may prematurely terminate therapy with a hostile and provocative child who fights the process of engaging in a working relationship. In such a situation, the therapist would probably come to anticipate therapy sessions with dread and show little enthusiasm. This reaction is particularly likely if the therapist has no understanding of the reasons for the child's provocation. In turn, the therapist's reaction would confirm for the child that he or she is bad, uninteresting, and unlovable and intensify the child's attempts to distance him- or herself from the therapist. Similarly, therapists may anticipate sessions with a lack of interest if children repeatedly exclude them from an active role in the therapy. Children may then interpret the therapists' lack of enthusiasm as proof that they are unlovable and unworthy of attention. At other times, therapists may prematurely discontinue therapy if the situation seems simply unworkable and so overwhelming that chances of improvement are slim. Alternatively, therapists may have difficulty ending therapy if children are overdependent on them, prolonging therapy well past the time when the children are making active use of the sessions and can function without them. Therapists may also extend sessions because they enjoy and very much like a particular child or feel sad about losing an enjoyable client or one with whom they identify strongly.

When faced with children who are highly distressed, particularly because of parental maltreatment, therapists may experience strong rescue fantasies. Some are so overwhelmed by such fantasies that they consider becoming a foster or adoptive parent to a maltreated child. In our experience, this reaction is often typical of therapists early in their careers. Such a step requires extremely careful consideration of the potential impact for the child, the therapist, and the therapist's family. A therapist who takes a child home in a foster care or adoptive capacity clearly cannot function as that child's therapist. Moreover, children who display serious developmental effects pose real challenges to family life. They often require 24-hour care and sometimes extraordinary structures in the home to keep them and others safe. If a therapist decides to foster or adopt, he or she, like any other parent or caregiver, must have realistic goals and be prepared for the stress, exhaustion, and turmoil that may follow. We do not want to present an overnegative picture of parenting maltreated children; many foster and adoptive parents have derived great satisfaction and rewards from raising youngsters with such histories. Our point is that despite their training, knowledge, and expertise, therapists are not immune to the challenges, demands, and concomitant reactions that others experience with these children. Therapists must be attuned to these reactions to guard against making decisions about the child and therapy that are based more on the therapist's feelings and needs than on those of the child.

Friedrich (1990) outlines reasons for therapists' troublesome reactions to their child clients' histories of sexual abuse. Some of these probably also apply to reactions to physically and emotionally abused and neglected children. Therapists might think of such children as second-class citizens who should have known better and are culpable for their own victimization. Other reactions of therapists include confusion about dominance and sexuality, blurred lines between therapists' various roles (e.g., advocate, therapist, case manager, agent of the court or of child welfare services), personal issues with sexuality or physical violence, difficulty in accepting failure, and their tendency to view a situation in unequivocal and rigid terms. The latter includes the need to see certain people, such as perpetrators, from a rigid perspective, rather than to empathize with the child's ambivalence about these individuals.

Although therapists experience many reactions and feelings that stem from their own professional and personal issues, other feelings may be evoked by the child's presentation. These reactions often provide crucial information about the motives and personality dynamics of the child. The therapist has a greater likelihood of understanding the implications of these feelings for clinical practice after extensive experience with many youngsters and a wide range of responses to child clients. For example, a therapist's intense negative reactions to a specific child may suggest that the child strongly needs to distance and provoke or ignore others. Therapists can use such reactions to generate working hypotheses about children that require validation through careful and more objective assessment and observation. They must be ready to evaluate these responses critically and use them to further enhance the progress of therapy.

COPING STRATEGIES

Given the challenging issues that maltreated children present in therapy, there are several strategies therapists might use to cope more effectively with their own reactions. Using these not only helps the therapist but maximizes the benefits of psychotherapy for the child. Below we outline some of these strategies.

Be Aware of Personal Issues

As was evident in the preceding discussion, it is crucial that the therapist be aware of individual issues concerning the child client that might impact on the therapist role. A therapist who is uncomfortable with children might be strongly advised to work in a different area, perhaps with adult survivors, especially if the therapist is aware of personal difficulty in dealing with children who are aggressive and provocative, highly dependent and clingy, markedly regressed, or self-abusive. A therapist with a strong aversion to perpetrators might be cautioned against working directly with children who display physical or sexual aggression. The strong feelings evoked by the behavior of such children may contribute to the therapist's condemnation of them in unhelpful or even destructive ways. The therapist must also be aware of any personal bias toward children who repeatedly overidealize a perpetrator. A therapist who cannot acknowledge a child's positive feelings for a perpetrator excludes an important issue from therapy.

Therapists working with maltreated children must liaise closely with child welfare services and the justice system. Although a therapist may agree to see a specific child only after child welfare workers have investigated the case, the child may make further disclosures during therapy that the therapist is compelled to report to the appropriate authorities. In addition, the therapist may have to be a source of support for children and families who are going through the process of police interviews and criminal hearings, and the therapist may also have to testify personally in criminal proceedings as well as in family court. Despite the efforts of all concerned, temporary or permanent guardianship orders may be necessary, and the therapist is often called upon to provide opinions about the type of parenting or care children require. Any therapist working with maltreated children must have a knowledge of these systems and the relevant legal statutes. Therapists must feel comfortable working with personnel in these areas, attending court and providing testimony, and participating in an adversarial legal system.

Therapists who have significant personal issues with maltreatment or sexuality should carefully evaluate whether it is appropriate for them to work with maltreated children. A therapist who is personally involved in an abusive relationship might overidentify with the child client and have trouble maintaining an objective and accurate perception of the case. The same applies to a therapist who is abusive toward his or her own children, has a personal childhood history of maltreatment, or has personal issues relating to sexual identification or sexual functioning. For example, a therapist who detests homosexuals might have extreme difficulty in responding to a young boy's concerns that he is gay because a male perpetrator sexually abused him. He or she might downplay the boy's concerns and glibly reassure the child that he is not gay without empathizing with the boy's anxiety. The therapist might criticize the child for even voicing such concerns and deter the active exploration of the boy's feelings and worries. Another therapist who has sexual difficulties may have a real problem in listening to a child's account of his or her sexual arousal. Again, the therapist's verbal and nonverbal responses may inhibit open discussion about such issues.

These are just a few examples of how a therapist's own issues might influence the conduct and course of therapy. They highlight the potential damage and disservice therapists might do to child clients if they are unaware or unwilling to examine themselves closely. There are several avenues therapists can use to address personal issues and biases. Apart from regular self-examination, they should consult with other professionals about case issues, including their personal reactions to their clients or their client's problems. These steps may be taken informally, or they might be a component of a formal supervisory relationship. Supervision is available in most agencies, but independent practitioners should ensure that consultation and/or supervision opportunities are built into their practices. Finally, therapists should consider a self-referral to therapy if issues and biases arising from personal background and/or current functioning are negatively impacting clinical work. A break from clinical practice with maltreated children may also be necessary.

Obtain Appropriate Training and Experience

Any therapist who wants to treat maltreated children effectively needs extensive knowledge and experience in areas such as general child development, the understanding of psychopathology and family functioning, assessment strategies, and therapeutic methods, including the literature on ESTs. As we advocated earlier, the field of developmental psychopathology provides an excellent conceptual framework for understanding children, the developmental tasks and challenges they face, and the multiple variables that influence developmental outcome. The practitioner must have a broad knowledge of maltreatment sequelae and the dynamics responsible for these effects, including the transactional model, along with an extensive repertoire of clinical skills. Given the complexity and demands of this work, therapists with limited and narrow training or those who are just beginning to explore this area of work should seriously evaluate whether they have the requisite skills, experience, and knowledge to function independently. One or two workshops do not provide the depth and extent of experience and knowledge required to treat these children. Novice or inexperienced therapists should seriously consider working in an agency where rigorous training and close supervision are available. Alternatively, novice therapists may contract with a skilled practitioner for training and supervision. Either approach will ultimately serve both therapists and clients well.

The extensive knowledge base and array of clinical skills discussed above are necessary to ensure that therapists can meet maltreated children's complex and diverse needs. Without a thorough understanding of the pathogenic processes underlying children's reactions, therapists may become discouraged and frustrated and begin to personalize children's negative reactions in therapy. These reactions in turn may lead to inappropriate and possibly harmful therapist behavior that reinforces maltreated children's IWMs/IS. Seeing maltreated children in therapy can be an arduous task and can negatively affect therapists' view of their own competency. A theoretical paradigm is crucial to therapists' understanding children's presentations and the process of therapy so that their sense of self-worth does not depend solely on client success, or "cures."

Set Realistic Treatment Goals

By developing a clear conceptual framework that facilitates an understanding of the child, therapists can more realistically set treatment goals. They must realize that for many children, change will be extremely slow and sometimes imperceptible. For some children, a truly positive outcome is unrealistic. The latter is the situation in the following example.

Trudy was a 12-year-old girl referred for assessment and therapy after apprehension because of severe sexual abuse by her mother, uncle, and brother. Trudy was living in a receiving group home with three siblings at the time of referral. She was highly indiscriminate, kissing strangers who came to the door and climbing into strangers' laps in shopping malls. During the assessment, Trudy appeared emotionally needy and somewhat intellectually limited. Given these characteristics, the goals in the residential treatment facility where she was later placed focused mainly on life skills. The treatment staff hoped Trudy could learn to protect herself and become less indiscriminate. They were especially worried about the possibility of early pregnancy.

Trudy engaged in therapy and benefited from it. With individual, residential, and family therapy and the ongoing involvement of child protection personnel, Trudy gave birth to her only baby after she was 18 years of age, and she avoided being abused again by family members. These were significant achievements. Once she became a mother, however, Trudy was overwhelmed by the dependence needs of her child. In addition, she chose partners who abused both her and her child, but she also had the insight to seek help for both of them. The child was eventually placed under the permanent guardianship of child welfare authorities. Despite this negative outcome approximately 12 years after the first referral, the case may still, in some ways, be considered successful. Given her indiscriminate style of relating, which placed her at risk for further victimization, without intervention Trudy would likely have been seriously hurt or killed by someone before reaching adulthood.

Although Trudy's case may seem extreme, it is not unusual. Children whose early years are replete with maltreatment may never come to truly trust other people. Forming intense and long-term relationships may be difficult. The therapist's awareness that some children will always struggle with issues of intimacy and trust is a prerequisite to establishing realistic goals. This awareness is particularly necessary in determining placements for children who cannot remain in the care of their biological families. A common attitude seen among some foster and adoptive agencies is that love alone will heal broken children. This is particularly apparent when the children are very young. Many people cannot fathom that a 2- or 3-year-old child can already have a markedly impaired capacity to trust and respond to warm caregiving. This attitude can be detrimental with children who are so damaged that they will encounter real difficulty in tolerating close relationships (James, 1994). Repeated and futile attempts at having them adopted further damage these children and engender considerable distress and conflict in the families in which they are placed.

Realize That Multiple Experiences Are Necessary to Produce Change

Therapists must recognize that in order to alter their expectations in relationships, many maltreated children require multiple exposures to attuned caregiving and sensitive responding from others, given the absence or near absence of it in their lives previously (Graziano & Wells, 1992; Pearce & Pezzot-Pearce, 1994). Experiences of this kind maximize a child's chances of recovering from maltreatment and are consistent with the basic tenets of developmental psychopathology. As we argued in Chapter 5, direct psychological treatment of maltreated children is just one component of a multifaceted strategy to reestablish the child's progress along an adaptive developmental trajectory. The therapist is not the sole "fixer" who makes children better, and a positive or negative outcome is not the therapist's sole responsibility. A positive outcome is more likely to result from the combined efforts of many people who provide the child with sensitive caring in daily interactions. They include therapists, natural parents, foster parents, adoptive parents, and teachers, among others. All must work together to offer children repeated experiences that begin to alter their IWMs/IS and facilitate the development of adaptive coping mechanisms. Therapists working with maltreated children must keep this in mind to avoid feeling discouraged, a sense of failure, and an overwhelming sense of responsibility for every aspect of those children's lives. Therapists can also advocate for and facilitate this cooperation among the individuals involved, provided they adhere to the notion of the importance of multiple experiences for recovery.

Many children require other professionally based interventions besides psychotherapy. Youngsters may display impairments across broad domains of functioning associated with the maltreatment or that have origins independent of the maltreatment but serve to moderate its impact. As therapists, we must realize that we do not possess all the skills and knowledge required to intervene effectively with this diverse set of problems. Often, one of the best steps we can take is to refer our clients to other professionals who have the expertise to intervene successfully in those areas beyond our limits of knowledge, training, or competence.

Therapists must also remember that a particular course of psychotherapy with severely maltreated children is unlikely to entirely resolve all issues, because the child's perception of the maltreatment may change as a function of different developmental stages and the diverse experiences and situations encountered subsequent to the maltreatment. A child's return to therapy several years after its termination is consistent with the family-practice orientation we described in Chapter 5 and should not necessarily be considered a treatment failure. In fact, the child's return may attest to the strength and importance of the relationship, and it is not uncommon to have maltreated children return intermittently for further work. In Chapter 2 we described Chris, who requested further contact with his previous therapist to address sexuality issues. Although these issues were related to his early abuse, they became salient with the onset of puberty. Cameron, the subject of the case history below, has maintained an ongoing, although at times sporadic, relationship with his therapist for a number of years.

Cameron was a 5-year-old child referred for counseling by his mother and child welfare worker. A stepfather had badly physically abused him. His mother had fled the home to protect Cameron, leaving behind his younger half-sister. Cameron was highly anxious and eventually required long-term therapeutic foster care placement and permanent guardianship. The latter occurred even though his mother continued to have contact with him. At various times over 13 years, Cameron attended counseling with his therapist. Initially, weekly therapy lasted approximately 1 year, followed by decreasing contact. There were several subsequent periods of no contact for 1–2 years. However, Cameron requested contact at the onset of each major developmental stage. Child welfare authorities and his therapist accommodated him, because he always used the sessions to articulate and work through issues related to his early history. Currently, Cameron sees his therapist approximately eight times a year. He successfully completed high school, lives independently, works part time, and plans a university education.

Although Cameron's requests for more therapy were appropriate and proved to be of real benefit, some therapists might interpret them as failure. This is clearly not so. With this ongoing input, Cameron did better than was expected in the initial course of therapy. This case is exceptional in that both Cameron and his therapist continued to live in the same city and all parties were agreeable to an ongoing relationship. Even when the child and a particular therapist do not resume their relationship, a course of therapy may make a child more open to later work with other therapists.

Other children call intermittently to "touch base." Attempts to reach their therapists demonstrate the strength and importance of the initial therapy work. We have received calls from adolescents and young adults we saw in therapy many years previously. Children may remember therapists' names and phone numbers. For example, one of us (TPP) received a call from a 22-year-old man who had been seen in therapy 12 years previously. For years, he had carried the therapist's business card that he was given during his last session, just before he moved to an adoptive home in a distant city.

Establish Positive Relationships with Coworkers

As work with maltreated children can be exhausting and trying, it is important to establish supportive relationships with coworkers. These relationships provide emotional support and an opportunity for case discussion and consultation. These contacts are especially important when children and their families trigger personal issues. Support is often readily available when therapists work as part of a team, particularly in programs that focus on the evaluation and treatment of maltreated children. Given that all team members face similar issues with their clients, the resulting mutual support can reduce feelings of isolation and helplessness that are often a part of this work. However, in teams in which members vie to be the most effective or competent therapist, mutual support may be minimal or absent and these feelings may very well be exacerbated.

Obtaining emotional support, supervision, and consultation may be a greater problem for independent practitioners. They find the same issues provocative but may not always have colleagues readily available for support or discussion. It is crucial that therapists make provision for regular opportunities for consultation or supervision. This contact may be achieved by contracting with a skilled therapist or by meeting regularly with several therapists for group supervision to obtain much-needed support.

Have a Sense of Humor

Work with damaged, maltreated children requires knowledge, skills, energy, and dedication. Even with these assets, therapists may be quite sobered by the issues their young clients present. It is important to retain a perspective about this work, combining it with a sense of humor. This attitude may prevent intense feelings of hopelessness and early burnout.

Humor may be used in several ways. It might be used with clients directly, although we must be careful about the timing and type of humor. We should not use it to minimize children's pain or to demean them sarcastically. Early in therapy, children may be unable to respond to humor. Progress may be evident when children start to regard the therapist's humorous comments as benign rather than negative. Further progress is evident when children begin to use humor themselves, even teasing the therapist in a playful and trusting manner.

Humor has a valuable role in a therapist's relationships with colleagues. At times, it eases tense and critical situations and provides sufficient release so that a therapist can again address difficult issues. Although they should recognize their own personal strengths and weaknesses, therapists should never be so serious that they cannot laugh at themselves. Of course, the reverse is not always ideal. A therapist who jokes constantly may become wearisome to both clients and colleagues and may trivialize the intense and significant difficulties that both face.

Limit the Number of Cases and Diversify Your Caseload

Given the intense emotional demands of this work, therapists may find it useful to limit the number of maltreated children they see, particularly when children display significant attachment difficulties and long-standing developmental effects. When the books and journal articles they read, the workshops they attend, and the cases they accept are only those involving abuse, therapists may easily become overwhelmed, emotionally fatigued, and exhausted. Other clinical interests offer diversity and enrichment that are critical in countering eventual burnout. Therapists should take care to balance their caseloads with clients who have different problems or demands. Having some variety in roles, such as being a cotherapist, supervisor, or consultant, eases the demands on therapists. These strategies are particularly important if clients provoke personal issues. Prioritizing time and workload demands can be effective strategies to prevent burnout. Setting these priorities allows therapists to remain interested and energetic, which ultimately benefits more clients. Moreover, therapists who have a breadth of different experiences and clinical knowledge, as well as specialized training in assessing and treating victims of maltreatment, may bring a more sophisticated understanding to these cases.

Run a Safe Practice

Some therapists so identify with the helping role that they assume all clients want help and will appreciate and reciprocate their kindness and involvement. This is a naive view, particularly if therapists do not consider their personal safety. Adults, some of whom are extremely hostile, usually accompany children to sessions. Although therapists often recognize that these adult clients may present a risk, many do not regard their child clients similarly. Care is needed in dealing with the adults, but it is also necessary with children, especially older ones. In our experience, although the risk of harm to the therapist is negligible, therapists should stay cognizant of several simple precautions they can use.

Risk for harm to the therapist can arise from several sources, but relatively simple techniques reduce the risk to physical safety. These may include an office design with access control, glass panels or windows near the office door (with blinds for privacy), and a buzzer or phone alarm system that the therapist can activate easily. Within the office, the therapist may place furniture so as to permit easy exit if required. Office equipment such as scissors and letter openers should be placed out of easy reach of volatile clients. It may also be worthwhile to alert other personnel if a therapist is worried about safety with a particular client: the door may be left slightly ajar, but the therapist must be careful not to compromise the client's confidentiality or privacy. Although we discussed this strategy in Chapter 7 as a way to ease a child's safety concerns, it may occasionally do the same for the therapist. Another risk is the allegation of misconduct with the child. In Chapter 7 we explained that a therapist should use caution in touching a child who might misinterpret intent because of an abusive history. Allegations of misconduct decrease with competent practice, although all therapists who work in this area are at some risk because of the nature of the problems clients present. Good case notes and documentation are not only useful in formulating a case, they also provide an element of safety in that there is a clear and comprehensive record of treatment issues and therapist's responses. Although some strategies such as a having buzzer alarm may never need to be used, they are worth the consideration and effort.

Make Use of Ongoing Educational Opportunities

Although there are formal requirements for ongoing education to maintain certification or licensing in a number of professions in many jurisdictions, in some locations this is not always the case. Regardless of existing policy, therapists do well to make use of ongoing educational opportunities, such as workshops, courses, and training and supervisory relationships. Therapists should carefully choose educational experiences to meet their needs, as identified through a careful examination of their own practices. Educational opportunities provide new ideas arising from recent research and the clinical experience of others. These new concepts augment and broaden clinical skills and stimulate fresh and creative ways of conceptualizing issues and problems; they also validate some of what the therapist already does. Educational experiences and contact and interchange with colleagues in various educational settings can help reduce the isolation that is part of the constant daily work with abused and neglected children. In addition, conferences and workshops give therapists opportunities for self-reflection away from the intense demands of clinical practice. When chosen carefully, educational opportunities are well worth the time and financial investment.

Therapists may also develop entirely different educational opportunities for themselves by assuming teaching roles. For example, therapists may provide volunteer lectures or workshops to agencies or community groups. The preparation for such activities necessarily involves serious reading and review that forces a critical examination of thinking and practice in order to accurately reflect current theoretical paradigms and good practice methods. Other therapists take on more formal educational tasks through teaching courses, presenting at professional conferences, supervising trainees, or participating in clinical practice groups where they are expected to rigorously review current literature and then lead discussion on specific topics of interest, particularly as it applies in specific case examples. Teachers and presenters are truly challenged to organize and update their thinking and practice, as not only must they prepare and present their information, but they must respond to astute and incisive questions from their listeners. In many ways, one of the best ways to hone thinking and clinical skills is through a process of explaining them to others, particularly other informed professionals.

Keep Your Personal World Healthy and Separate

Working as a therapist can become all-consuming for some people. It is crucial for therapists to maintain a personal world that is healthy and separate from their clinical work. Although this may apply to any therapist, it is particularly important for those who work in the highly demanding field of child maltreatment.

We believe it is essential for therapists to maintain personal lives in which they have other interests that replenish the interest and energy needed to deal with difficult and challenging children and families. Therapists must set priorities concerning their time and workload so their work does not significantly restrict or entirely consume the time for other pursuits and nonwork relationships. These outside interests include not only taking holidays but also leaving some weekends, evenings, or other times free. Therapists must take particular care to nurture their relationships with friends, partners, spouses, children, and families. Besides providing emotional satisfaction and support, these relationships increase their feelings of self-worth and impact positively on their professional lives. These relationships provide multiple experiences for the therapist that directly parallel those the therapist and others provide for the maltreated child. They help therapists maintain a balanced perspective about their work and offer recognition of other supports and satisfactions in their lives.

Why do we and thousands of other therapists work with abused and neglected children? There seem to be numerous reasons that would encourage clinicians to look elsewhere for professional and personal satisfaction. The stories of many children are horrifying, and some have been so damaged that the gains derived from psychotherapy and other interventions are minimal at best. However, the intellectual challenges inherent in this work have always attracted our attention. Treating these children and their families often defies easy and pat solutions. The clinician must attempt to conceptualize these cases in a comprehensive and rigorous manner and then develop and apply creative interventions.

Moreover, there are emotional rewards. Most of us are in the business because we truly want to help others. We can help many maltreated children, even when the results are not spectacular and when treatment requires intensive and long-term commitment. The rewards do not lie in helping children lead problem-free lives; that goal eludes all of us. The reward comes from assisting children to become open to the whole range of human feelings and experiences, gain some mastery over their emotions and thoughts, and put their histories of abuse or neglect in the proper perspective. At some point, a child's experiences of abuse or neglect may very well occupy a small proportion of an otherwise healthy life. Furthermore, as therapists, we often do this work without direct knowledge of the longer-term benefit that may accrue to the children with whom we have formed caring and thoughtful relationships. It may very well be that although grown clients do not always remember the content of our sessions with them when they were our child clients, they do remember that we were people who cared about them and offered a safe place for them to understand the difficult events and feelings that happened to them when they were children.

We would like to end this book with a final case example.

An 11-year-old boy who had been severely physically abused was referred for psychotherapy. Shaun had been beaten so badly by his father that he was hospitalized for 2 weeks with multiple and serious injuries. He had been beaten on many previous occasions. Over the 2-year course of therapy Shaun struggled with acknowledging his ambivalent feelings toward his father. Like many such children, he presented an overidealized depiction of his dad and minimized his own rage and sadness. Eventually he acknowledged anger and profound grief about never having had a loving father. By the end of 2 years, Shaun had made considerable progress. Although he still had some problems with interpersonal relationships, he and the therapist agreed to terminate therapy. In the final session, Shaun thanked his therapist, remarking that the therapist had helped him "become human again." When asked what he meant, Shaun stated, "You helped me feel again."

It was a compliment the therapist will never forget.

References

Aber, J. L., & Allen, J. P. (1987). The effects of maltreatment on young children's socioemotional development: An attachment theory perspective. *Developmental Psychology, 23*, 406–414.

Aber, J. L., Allen, J. P., Carlson, V., & Cicchetti, D. (1989). The effects of maltreatment on development during early childhood: Recent studies and their theoretical, clinical, and policy implications. In D. Cicchetti & V. Carlson (Eds.), *Child maltreatment: Theory and research on the causes and consequences of child abuse and neglect* (pp. 579–619). New York: Cambridge University Press.

Ablon, J. S., & Marci, C. (2004) Psychotherapy process: The missing link: Comment on Westen, Novotny, and Thompson-Brenner (2004). *Psychological Bulletin, 130*, 664–668.

Achenbach, T. M., & Rescorla, L. A. (2000). *Manual for the ASEBA Preschool Forms and Profiles.* Burlington: University of Vermont, Center for Children, Youth, and Families.

Achenbach, T. M., & Rescorla, L. A. (2001). *Manual for the ASEBA School-Age Forms and Profiles.* Burlington: University of Vermont, Center for Children, Youth, and Families.

Ackerman, S. J., & Hilsenroth, M. J. (2003). A review of therapist characteristics and techniques positively impacting the therapeutic alliance. *Clinical Psychology Review, 23*, 1–33.

Ainsworth, M. D. S. (1989). Attachments beyond infancy. *American Psychologist, 44*, 709–716.

Ainsworth, M. D. S., Blehar, M. C., Waters, E., & Wall, S. (1978). *Patterns of attachment: A psychological study of the strange situation.* Hillsdale, NJ: Erlbaum.

Ainsworth, M. D. S., & Bowlby, J. (1991). An ethological approach to personality development. *American Psychologist, 46*, 333–341.

Alessandri, S. M. (1991). Play and social behaviors in maltreated preschoolers. *Development and Psychopathology, 3*, 191–206.

Alessandri, S. M. (1992). Mother–child interactional correlates of maltreated and nonmaltreated children's play behavior. *Development and Psychopathology, 4*, 257–270.

Alexander, F., & French, R. M. (1946). *Psychoanalytic therapy.* New York: Ronald Press.

Alexander, J., & Parsons, B. V. (1982). *Functional family therapy.* Monterey, CA: Brooks/Cole.

Allen, F. H. (1942). *Psychotherapy with children.* Lincoln: University of Nebraska Press.

American Psychiatric Association. (1987). *Diagnostic and statistical manual of mental disorders* (3rd ed., rev.). Washington, DC: Author.

American Psychiatric Association. (1994). *Diagnostic and statistical manual of mental disorders* (4th ed.). Washington, DC: Author.

Asher, S. R., & Coie, J. D. (Eds.). (1990). *Peer rejection.* New York: Cambridge University Press.

Axline, V. (1964). *Dibs: In search of self.* New York: Ballantine Books.

Axline, V. (1969). *Play therapy* (rev. ed.). New York: Ballantine Books.

Barahal, R., Waterman, J., & Martin, H. (1981). The social-cognitive development of abused children. *Journal of Consulting and Clinical Psychology, 49*, 508–516.

Baron, R. M., & Kenny, D. A. (1986). The moderator–mediator variable distinction in social psychological research: Conceptual, strategic, and statistical considerations. *Journal of Personality and Social Psychology, 51*, 1173–1182.

Baxter, L. R., Schwartz, J. M., Bergman, K. S., Szuba, M. P., Guze, B. H., Mazziotta, J. C., et al. (1992). Caudate glucose metabolic rate changes with both drug and behavior therapy for obsessive compulsive disorder. *Archives of General Psychiatry, 49*, 681–689.

Beeghly, M., & Cicchetti, D. (1994). Child maltreatment, attachment and the self system: Emergence of an internal state lexicon in toddlers at high social risk. *Development and Psychopathology, 6*, 5–30.

Bellak, L. (1993). *The Thematic Apperception Test, the Children's Apperception Test, and the Senior Apperception Technique in clinical use* (5th ed.). Boston: Allyn & Bacon.

Belsky, J. (1980). Child maltreatment: An ecological integration. *American Psychologist, 35*, 320–335.

Belsky, J. (1993). Etiology of child maltreatment: A developmental–ecological analysis. *Psychological Bulletin, 114*, 413–434.

Belsky, J., Rovine, M., & Taylor, D. G. (1984). The Pennsylvania Infant and Family Development Project: III. The origins of individual differences in infant–mother attachment: Maternal and infant contributions. *Child Development, 55*, 718–728.

Bentovim, A., van Elberg, A., & Boston, P. (1988). The results of treatment. In A. Bentovim, A. Elton, J. Hildebrand, M. Tranter, & E. Vizard (Eds.), *Child sexual abuse within the family: Assessment and treatment* (pp. 252–268). London: Wright.

Berlin, N. G. (2002). Parent–child therapy and maternal projections: Tripartite psychotherapy—a new look. *American Journal of Orthopsychiatry, 72*, 204–216.

Berliner, L. (1989, November). *Evaluation and treatment of children with sexual be-*

havior problems. Paper presented at the Adolescent Offenders Conference: Prevention, Treatment and Management, Vancouver, BC.

Berliner, L. (2005). The results of randomized clinical trials move the field forward. *Child Abuse and Neglect, 29*, 103–105.

Black, M., Dubowitz, H., & Harrington, D. (1994). Sexual abuse: Developmental differences in children's behavior and self-perception. *Child Abuse and Neglect, 18*, 85–95.

Bolger, K. E., & Patterson, C. J. (2001). Developmental pathways from child maltreatment to peer rejection. *Child Development, 72*, 549–568.

Bonanno, G. A. (2004). Loss, trauma, and human resilience: Have we underestimated the human capacity to thrive after extremely aversive events? *American Psychologist, 59*, 20–28.

Bonner, B. L. (2004). Cognitive-behavioral and dynamic play therapy for children with sexual behavior problems and their caregivers. In B. E. Saunders, L. Berliner, & R. F. Hanson (Eds.), *Child physical and sexual abuse: Guidelines for treatment (Revised Report: April 26, 2004)* (pp. 34–35). Charleston, SC: National Crime Victims Research and Treatment Center.

Bonner, B. L., & Silovsky, J. F. (2004, November). *Working with children with sexual behavior problems*. Workshop presented in Calgary, AB.

Bonner, B. L., Walker, C. E., & Berliner, L. (2000). *Final Report. Children with sexual behavior problems: Assessment and treatment*. (Grant No. 90-CA-1469). Washington, DC: National Clearinghouse on Child Abuse and Neglect.

Boris, N. W., Hinshaw-Fuselier, S., Smyke, A. T., Scheeringa, M. S., Heller, S. S., & Zeanah, C. H. (2004). Comparing criteria for attachment disorders: Establishing reliability and validity in high-risk samples. *Journal of the American Academy of Child and Adolescent Psychiatry, 43*, 568–577.

Bowers, L., Smith, P. K., & Binney, V. (1994). Perceived family relationships of bullies, victims, and bully victims in middle childhood. *Journal of Social and Personal Relationships, 11*, 215–232.

Bowlby, J. (1944). Forty-four juvenile thieves: Their characters and home life. *International Journal of Psycho-Analysis, 25*, 19–52, 107–127.

Bowlby, J. (1958). The nature of the child's tie to his mother. *International Journal of Psycho-Anaylsis, 39*, 350–373.

Bowlby, J. (1969). *Attachment and loss: Vol. 1. Attachment*. New York: Basic Books.

Bowlby, J. (1973). *Attachment and loss: Vol. 2. Separation: Anxiety and anger*. New York: Basic Books.

Bowlby, J. (1980). *Attachment and loss: Vol. 3. Loss*. New York: Basic Books.

Bowlby, J. (1982). *Attachment and loss: Vol. 1. Attachment* (2nd ed.). New York: Basic Books.

Bowlby, J. (1988a). Developmental psychiatry comes of age. *American Journal of Psychiatry, 145*, 1–10.

Bowlby, J. (1988b). *A secure base: Parent–child attachment and healthy human development*. New York: Basic Books.

Bowman, B. (1989). Culturally sensitive inquiry. In J. Garbarino, F. M. Stott, & Faculty of the Erikson Institute, *What children can tell us* (pp. 92–107). San Francisco: Jossey-Bass.

Brady, C. A., & Friedrich, W. N. (1982). Levels of intervention: A model for training in play therapy. *Journal of Clinical Child Psychology, 11*, 39–43.

Braun, B. G. (1986). *Treatment of multiple personality disorder.* Washington, DC: American Psychiatric Press.

Bretherton, I. (1987). New perspectives on attachment relations. In J. Osofsky (Ed.), *Handbook of infant development* (2nd ed., pp. 1061–1100). New York: Wiley.

Bretherton, I., & Beeghly, M. (1982). Talking about internal states: The acquisition of an explicit theory of mind. *Developmental Psychology, 18*, 906–921.

Bretherton, I., Oppenheim, D., Buchsbaum, H., Emde, R. N., & the MacArthur Narrative Group (1990). *MacArthur Story Stem Battery.* Unpublished manuscript.

Bretherton, I., Ridgeway, D., & Cassidy, J. (1990). Assessing internal working models of the attachment relationship. In M. Greenberg, D. Cicchetti, & E. M. Cummings (Eds.), *Attachment in the preschool years* (pp. 273–308). Chicago: University of Chicago Press.

Brewin, C. R. (1989). Cognitive change processes in psychotherapy. *Psychological Review, 96*, 379–394.

Briere, J. N. (1989). *Therapy for adults molested as children: Beyond survival.* New York: Springer.

Briere, J. N. (1992). *Child abuse trauma.* Newbury Park, CA: Sage.

Briere, J. N. (1996). *Professional manual for the Trauma Symptom Checklist for Children (TSCC).* Odessa, FL: Psychological Assessment Resources.

Brisch, K. H. (2002). *Treating attachment disorders: From theory to therapy* (K. Kronenberg, Trans.). New York: Guilford Press.

Broder, E. A., & Hood, E. (1983). A guide to the assessment of child and family. In P. D. Steinhauer & Q. Rae-Grant (Eds.), *Psychological problems of the child in the family* (pp. 130–149). New York: Basic Books.

Bronfman, E., Parsons, E., & Lyons-Ruth, K. (n. d.). *Atypical Maternal Behavior Instrument for Assessment and Classification (AMBIANCE): Manual for coding disrupted affective communication.* Unpublished manuscript, Harvard Medical School, Boston.

Brown, E., & Kolko, D. (1999). Child victims' attributions about being physically abused: An examination of factors associated with symptom severity. *Journal of Abnormal Child Psychology, 27*, 311–322.

Buchsbaum, H. K., Toth, S. L., Clyman, R. B., Cicchetti, D., & Emde, K. B. (1992). The use of a narrative story stem technique with maltreated children: Implications for theory and practice. *Development and Psychopathology, 4*, 603–625.

Budd, K. S., Felix, E. D., Poindexter, L. M., Naik-Polan, A. T., & Sloss, C. F. (2002). Clinical assessment of children in child protection cases: An empirical analysis. *Professional Psychology: Research and Practice, 33*, 3–12.

Budin, L., & Johnson, D. (1989). Sex abuse prevention programs: Offenders' attitudes about their efficacy. *Child Abuse and Neglect, 13*, 77–87.

Bullard, J. B., Glaser, H. H., Hagarty, M. C., & Pivchik, E. C. (1967). Failure to thrive in the "neglected" child. *American Journal of Orthopsychiatry, 37*, 680–690.

Burgess, A. W., Hartman, C. R., Kelley, S. J., Grant, C. A., & Gray, E. B. (1990). Parental response to child sexual abuse trials involving day care settings. *Journal of Traumatic Stress, 3*, 395–405.

Burke, A. E., Crenshaw, D. A., Greene, J., Schlosser, M. A., & Strocchia-Rivera, L.

(1989). Influence of verbal ability on the expression of aggression in physically abused children. *Journal of the American Academy of Child and Adolescent Psychiatry, 28*, 215–218.

Caffaro-Rouget, A., Lang, R, A., & van Santen, V. (1989). The impact of child sexual abuse. *Annals of Sex Research, 2*, 29–47.

Canino, I. (1988). The transcultural child. In C. J. Kestenbaum & D. T. Williams (Eds.), *Handbook of clinical assessment of children and adolescents* (Vol. II, pp. 1024–1042). New York and London: New York University Press.

Carek, D. J. (1979). Individual psychodynamically oriented therapy. In J. D. Nospitz (Ed.), *Handbook of child psychiatry* (Vol. 3, pp. 35–57). New York: Basic Books.

Carlson, V., Barnett, D., Braunwald, K. G., & Cicchetti, D. (1989). Finding order in disorganizations. In D. Cicchetti & V. Carlson (Eds.), *Child maltreatment: Theory and research on the causes and consequences of child abuse and neglect* (pp. 494–528). New York: Cambridge University Press.

Caruso, K. (1987). *Protective storytelling cards*. Redding, CA: Northwest Psychological.

Cassidy, J., & Berlin, L. J. (1994). The insecure/ambivalent pattern of attachment: Theory and research. *Child Development, 65*, 121–134.

Cassidy, J., & Kobak, R. (1988). Avoidance and its relation to other defensive processes. In J. Belsky & T. Nezworski (Eds.), *Clinical implications of attachment* (pp. 300–326). Hillsdale, NJ: Erlbaum.

Cassidy, J., & Mohr, J. J. (2001). Unresolvable fear, trauma, and psychopathology: Theory, research, and clinical considerations related to disorganized attachment across the life span. *Clinical Psychology: Science and Practice, 8*, 275–298.

Celano, M., Hazzard, A., Campbell, S. K., & Lang, C. B. (2002). Attribution retraining with sexually abused children: Review of techniques. *Child Maltreatment, 7*, 65–76.

Chadwick Center for Children and Families. (2004). *Closing the quality chasm in child abuse treatment: Identifying and disseminating best practices*. San Diego, CA: Author.

Chaffin, M., & Bonner, B. (1998). "Don't shoot, we're your children": Have we gone too far in our response to adolescent sexual offenders and children with sexual behavior problems? *Child Maltreatment, 3*, 314–316.

Chaffin, M., Hanson, R., Saunders, B. E., Nicols, T., Barnett, D., Zeanah, C., et al. (2006). Report of the APSAC Task Force on attachment therapy, reactive attachment disorder, and attachment problems. *Child Maltreatment, 11*, 76–89.

Chaffin, M., Silovsky, J. F., Funderburk, F., Valle, L. A., Brestan, E. V., Babchova, T., et al. (2004). Parent–child interaction therapy with physically abusive parents: Efficacy for reducing future abuse reports. *Journal of Consulting and Clinical Psychology, 72*, 500–510.

Chaffin, M., Wherry, J. N., & Dykman, R. (1997). School age children's coping with sexual abuse: Abuse stresses and symptoms associated with four coping strategies. *Child Abuse and Neglect, 21*, 227–240.

Chambless, D. L., Baker, M. J., Baucom, D. H., Beutler, L. E., Calhoun, K. S., Daiuto, A., et al. (1998). Update on empirically validated therapies. II. *Clinical Psychologist, 51*, 3–16.

Chisholm, K. (1998). A three year follow-up of attachment and indiscriminate friendliness in children adopted from Romanian orphanages. *Child Development, 69*, 1092–1106.

Cicchetti, D. (1989). How research on child maltreatment has informed the study of child development: Perspectives from developmental psychopathology. In D. Cicchetti & V. Carlson (Eds.), *Child maltreatment: Theory and research on the causes and consequences of child abuse and neglect* (pp. 377–431). New York: Cambridge University Press.

Cicchetti, D. (2004). An odyssey of discovery: Lessons learned through three decades of research on child maltreatment. *American Psychologist, 59*, 731–741.

Cicchetti, D., & Barnett, D. (1991). Attachment organization in maltreated preschoolers. *Development and Psychopathology, 3*, 397–411.

Cicchetti, D., & Beeghly, M. (1987). Symbolic development in maltreated youngsters: An organizational perspective. In D. Cicchetti & M. Beeghly (Eds.), *Atypical symbolic development* (pp. 47–68). San Francisco: Jossey-Bass.

Cicchetti, D., Lynch, M., Shonk, S., & Manley, J. (1992). An organizational perspective on peer relations in maltreated children. In R. D. Parke & G. W. Ladd (Eds.), *Family–peer relationships: Modes of linkage* (pp. 345–383). Hillsdale, NJ: Erlbaum.

Cicchetti, D., & Olsen, K. (1990). The developmental psychopathology of child maltreatment. In M. Lewis & S. M. Miller (Eds.), *Handbook of developmental psychopathology* (pp. 261–279). New York: Plenum Press.

Cicchetti, D., & Rizley, R. (1981). Developmental perspectives on the etiology, intergenerational transmission, and sequelae of child maltreatment. *New Directions for Child Development, 11*, 31–55.

Cicchetti, D., & Rogosch, F. A. (1994). The toll of child maltreatment on the developing child. *Child and Adolescent Psychiatric Clinics of North America, 3*, 759–776.

Cicchetti, D., Rogosch, F., Maughan, A., Toth, S. L., & Bruce, J. (2003). False belief understanding in maltreated children. *Development and Psychopathology, 15*, 1067–1091.

Cicchetti, D., & Toth, S. L. (1995). A developmental psychopathology perspective on child abuse and neglect. *Journal of the American Academy of Child and Adolescent Psychiatry, 34*, 541–565.

Cohen, H., & Weil, G. R. (1971). *Tasks of Emotional Development test manual.* Brookline, MA: T. E. D. Associates.

Cohen, J. A., & Deblinger, E. (2004). Trauma-focused cognitive-behavioral therapy (CBT). In B. E. Saunders, L. Berliner, & R. F. Hanson (Eds.), *Child physical and sexual abuse: Guidelines for treatment (Revised Report: April 26, 2004)* (pp. 49–51). Charleston, SC: National Crime Victims Research and Treatment Center.

Cohen, J. A., Deblinger, E., Mannarino, A. P., & de Arellano, M. A. (2001). The importance of culture in treating abused and neglected children: An empirical review. *Child Maltreatment, 6*, 148–157.

Cohen, J. A., Deblinger, E., Mannarino, A. P., & Steer, R. A. (2004). A multisite, randomized controlled trial for children with sexual-abuse-related PTSD symptoms. *Journal of the American Academy of Child and Adolescent Psychiatry, 43*, 393–402.

Cohen, J. A., & Mannarino, A. P. (1988). Psychological symptoms in sexually abused girls. *Child Abuse and Neglect, 12*, 571–577.

Cohen, J. A., & Mannarino, A. P. (1996a). Factors that mediate treatment outcome of sexually abused preschool children. *Journal of the American Academy of Child and Adolescent Psychiatry, 34*, 1402–1410.

Cohen, J. A., & Mannarino, A. P. (1996b). A treatment outcome study for sexually abused preschool children: Initial findings. *Journal of the American Academy of Child and Adolescent Psychiatry, 35*, 42–50.

Cohen, J. A., & Mannarino, A. P. (1997). A treatment study for sexually abused preschool children: Outcome during a one-year follow-up. *Journal of the American Academy of Child and Adolescent Psychiatry, 36*, 1228–1235.

Cohen, J. A., & Mannarino, A. P. (1998a). Factors that mediate treatment outcome of sexually abused preschool children: Six- and 12-month follow-up. *Journal of the American Academy of Child and Adolescent Psychiatry, 37*, 44–51.

Cohen, J. A., & Mannarino, A. P. (1998b). Interventions for sexually abused children: Initial treatment outcome studies. *Child Maltreatment, 3*, 17–26.

Cohen, J. A., & Mannarino, A. P. (2000). Predictors of treatment outcome in sexually abused children. *Child Abuse and Neglect, 24*, 983–994.

Cohen, J. A., & Mannarino, A. P. (2002). Addressing attributions in treating abused children. *Child Maltreatment, 7*, 82–86.

Cohen, J. A., Mannarino, A. P., & Knudsen, K. (2005). Treating sexually abused children: One-year follow-up of a randomized controlled trial. *Child Abuse and Neglect, 29*, 135–145.

Cole, P. M., Woolger, C., Power, T. G., & Smith, K. D. (1992). Parenting difficulties among adult survivors of father–daughter incest. *Child Abuse and Neglect, 16*, 239–249.

Conduct Problems Prevention Research Group. (1992). A developmental and clinical model for the prevention of conduct disorder: The FAST Track Program. *Development and Psychopathology, 4*, 509–527.

Conte, J. R., & Schuerman, J. R. (1987). Factors associated with an increased impact of child sexual abuse. *Child Abuse and Neglect, 11*, 201–211.

Conte, J. R., Wolf, S., & Smith, T. (1989). What sexual offenders tell us about prevention strategies. *Child Abuse and Neglect, 13*, 293–301.

Coster, W., Gersten, M., Beeghly, M., & Cicchetti, D. (1989). Communicative functioning in maltreated toddlers. *Developmental Psychology, 25*, 1020–1029.

Crittenden, P. M. (1988). Relationships at risk. In J. Belsky & T. Nezworski (Eds.), *Clinical applications of attachment* (pp. 136–174). New York: Plenum Press.

Crittenden, P. M. (1992a). Children's strategies for coping with adverse home environments: An interpretation using attachment theory. *Child Abuse and Neglect, 16*, 329–343.

Crittenden, P. M. (1992b). Treatment of anxious attachment in infancy and early childhood. *Development and Psychopathology, 4*, 575–602.

Crittenden, P. M., & DiLalla, D. (1988). Compulsive compliance: The development of an inhibitory coping strategy in infancy. *Journal of Abnormal Child Psychology, 16*, 585–599.

Cummings, N. A. (1986). The dismantling of our health system. *American Psychologist, 41*, 426–431.

Cunningham, C., & MacFarlane, K. (1991). *When children molest other children: Group treatment strategies for young sexual abusers*. Orwell, VT: Safer Society Press.

Dahlenberg, D. J., & Jacobs, D. A. (1994). Attributional analyses of child sexual abuse episodes: Empirical and clinical issues. *Journal of Child Sexual Abuse, 3*, 37–50.

Dalgleish, T. (2004). Cognitive approaches to posttraumatic stress disorder: The evolution of multi-representational theorizing. *Psychological Bulletin, 130*, 228–260.

Damon, W. (1980). Patterns of change in children's social reasoning: A two year longitudinal study. *Child Development, 51*, 1011.

Daro, D. (1991). Child sexual abuse prevention: Separating fact from fiction. *Child Abuse and Neglect, 15*, 1–4.

Davis, N. (1990). *Once upon a time: Therapeutic stories to heal abused children*. New York: Institute for Rational Living.

De Bellis, M. D. (2001). Developmental traumatology: The psychobiological development of maltreated children and its implications for research, treatment, and policy. *Development and Psychopathology, 13*, 539–564.

De Bellis, M. D. (2005). The psychobiology of neglect. *Child Maltreatment, 10*, 150–172.

De Bellis, M. D., Keshavan, M. S., & Harenski, K. A. (2001). Anterior cingulate N-acetylaspartate/creatine ratios during clonidine treatment in a maltreated child with posttraumatic stress disorder. *Journal of Child and Adolescent Psychopharmacology, 11*, 311–316.

Deblinger, E., Lippmann, J., & Steer, R. (1996). Sexually abused children suffering posttraumatic stress symptoms: Initial treatment outcome findings. *Child Maltreatment, 1*, 310–321.

Deblinger, E., McLeer, S. W., & Henry, D. (1990). Cognitive behavioral treatment for sexually abused children suffering post-traumatic stress: Preliminary findings. *Journal of the American Academy of Child and Adolescent Psychiatry, 29*, 747–752.

Deblinger, E., Stauffer, L., & Landsberg, C. (1994). The impact of a history of child sexual abuse on maternal response to allegations of sexual abuse concerning her child. *Journal of Child Sexual Abuse, 3*, 67–75.

Deblinger, E., Stauffer, L. B., & Steer, R. A. (2001). Comparative efficacies of supportive and cognitive behavioral group therapies for young children who have been sexually abused and their nonoffending mothers. *Child Maltreatment, 6*, 332–343.

Deblinger, E., Steer, R. A., & Lippmann, J. (1999). Two-year follow-up study of cognitive behavioral therapy for sexually abused children suffering post-traumatic stress disorder. *Child Abuse and Neglect, 23*, 1371–1378.

Demb, J. M. (1991). Reported hyperphagia in foster children. *Child Abuse and Neglect, 15*, 77–88.

Denham, S. A., McKinley, M., Couchoud, E. A., & Holt, R. (1990). Emotional and behavioral predictors of preschool ratings. *Child Development, 61*, 1145–1152.

Dodds, J. B. (1985). *A child psychotherapy primer*. New York: Human Services Press.

Dodge, K. A., Bates, J. E., & Pettit, G. S. (1990). Mechanisms in the cycle of violence. *Science, 250*, 1678–1683.

Dodge, K. A., Pettit, G. S., & Bates, J. E. (1994). Effects of physical maltreatment on the development of peer relations. *Development and Psychopathology, 6*, 43–55.

Dodge, K. A., Pettit, G. S., & Bates, J. E. (1997). How the experience of early physical abuse leads children to become chronically aggressive. In D. Cicchetti & S. L. Toth (Eds.), *Developmental perspectives on trauma: Theory, research, and intervention* (pp. 263–288). Rochester, NY: University of Rochester Press.

Downey, G., Feldman, S., Khuri, J., & Friedman, S. (1994). Maltreatment and childhood depression. In W. M. Reynolds & H. F. Johnston (Eds.), *Handbook of depression in children and adolescents: Issues in clinical psychology* (pp. 481–508). New York: Plenum Press.

Downing, J., Jenkins, S. J., & Fisher, G. L. (1988). A comparison of psychodynamic and reinforcement treatment with sexually abused children. *Elementary School Guidance Counseling, 22*, 291–298.

Dubowitz, H., Black, M., Harrington, D., & Verschoore, A. (1993). A follow-up study of behavior problems associated with child sexual abuse. *Child Abuse and Neglect, 17*, 743–754.

Duncan, G. J., Brooks-Gunn, J., & Klebanov, P. K. (1994). Economic deprivation and early childhood development. *Child Development, 65*, 296–318.

Dunn, J. (1995). Children as psychologists: The later correlates of individual differences in understanding of emotions and other minds. *Cognition and Emotion, 9*, 187–201.

Egeland, B., Jacobvitz, D., & Sroufe, L. A. (1988). Breaking the cycle of abuse. *Child Development, 59*, 1080–1088.

Elliott, A. N., & Carnes, C. N. (2001). Reactions of nonoffending parents to the sexual abuse of their child: A review of the literature. *Child Maltreatment, 6*, 314–331.

Elliott, D. M., & Briere, J. (1994). Forensic sexual abuse evaluations of older children: Disclosures and symptomatology. *Behavioral Sciences and the Law, 12*, 261–277.

Eltz, M. J., Shirk, S. R., & Sarlin, N. (1995). Alliance formation and treatment outcome among maltreated adolescents. *Child Abuse and Neglect, 19*, 419–431.

Emery, R. E., & Laumann-Billings, L. (1998). An overview of the nature, causes, and consequences of abusive family relationships: Toward differentiating maltreatment and violence. *American Psychologist, 53*, 121–135.

Ethier, L. S., Lemelin, J. P., & Lacharité, C. (2004). A longitudinal study of the effects of chronic maltreatment on children's behavioral and emotional problems. *Child Abuse and Neglect, 28*, 1265–1278.

Evans, E., Hawton, K., & Rodham, K. (2005). Suicidal phenomena and abuse in adolescents: A review of epidemiological studies. *Child Abuse and Neglect, 29*, 45–58.

Everson, M. D., Hunter, W. M., Runyon, D. K., Edelsohn, G. A., & Coulter, M. L. (1989). Maternal support following disclosure of incest. *American Journal of Orthopsychiatry, 59*, 197–207.

Fago, D. P. (2003) Evaluation and treatment of neurodevelopmental deficits in sexually aggressive children and adolescents. *Professional Psychology: Research and Practice, 34*, 248–257.

Famularo, R., Fenton, T., Kinscherff, R., Ayoub, C., & Barnum, R. (1994). Maternal and child posttraumatic stress disorder among child victims of sexual abuse. *Child Abuse and Neglect, 18*, 27–36.

Farrell, S. P., Hains, A. A., & Davies, W. H. (1998). Cognitive behavioral interventions for sexually abused children exhibiting PTSD symptomatology. *Behavior Therapy, 29*, 241–255.

Feeny, N. C., Foa, E. B., Treadwell, K. R. H., & March, J. (2004). Posttraumatic stress disorder in youth: A critical review of the cognitive and behavioral treatment outcome literature. *Professional Psychology: Research and Practice, 35*, 466–476.

Feiring, C., Taska, L., & Chen, K. (2002). Trying to understand why horrible things happen: Attribution, shame, and symptom development following sexual abuse. *Child Maltreatment, 7*, 26–41.

Feiring, C., Taska, L., & Lewis, M. (1998). The role of shame and attributional style in children's and adolescent's adaptation to sexual abuse. *Child Maltreatment, 3*, 129–142.

Feshbach, N. D., Feshbach, S., Fauvre, M., & Ballard-Campbell, M. (1983). *Learning to care*. Glenview, IL: Scott, Foresman.

Finkelhor, D. (1995). The victimization of children: A developmental perspective. *American Journal of Orthopsychiatry, 65*, 177–193.

Finkelhor, D., & Browne, A. (1985). The traumatic impact of child sexual abuse: A conceptualization. *American Journal of Orthopsychiatry, 55*, 530–541.

Finkelhor, D., Ormrod, R., Turner, H., & Hamby, S. L. (2005). The victimization of children and youth: A comprehensive, national survey. *Child Maltreatment, 10*, 5–25.

Flaherty, J. A., & Richman, J. A. (1986). Effects of childhood relationships on the adult's capacity to form social supports. *American Journal of Psychiatry, 143*, 851–855.

Foa, E. B., Cashman, L., Jaycox, L., & Perry, K. (1997). The validation of a self-report measure of posttraumatic stress disorder: The Posttraumatic Diagnostic Scale. *Psychological Assessment, 9*, 445–451.

Foa, E. B., Johnson, K. M., Feeny, N. C., & Treadwell, K. R. H. (2001). The Child PTSD Symptom Scale: A preliminary examination of its psychometric properties. *Journal of Clinical Child Psychology, 30*, 376–384.

Foa, E. B., Steketee, G., & Rothbaum, B. (1989). Behavioral/cognitive conceptualizations of post-traumatic stress disorder. *Behavior Therapy, 20*, 155–176.

Fonagy, P. (1991). Thinking about thinking: Some clinical and theoretical considerations in the treatment of the borderline patient. *International Journal of Psycho-Analysis, 72*, 639–656.

Fonagy, P., Gergely, G., Jurist, E., & Target, M. (2002). *Affect regulation, mentalization, and the development of the self*. New York: Other Press.

Fonagy, P., Redfern, S., & Charman, T. (1997). The relationship between belief–desire reasoning and a projective measure of attachment security (SAT). *British Journal of Developmental Psychology, 15*, 51–61.

Fonagy, P., & Target, M. (1997). Attachment and reflective function: Their role in self-organization. *Development and Psychopathology, 9*, 679–700.

Frazier, D., & Levine, E. (1983). Reattachment therapy: Intervention with the very young physically abused child. *Psychotherapy: Theory, Research and Practice, 20*, 90–100.

Freedenfeld, R. N., Ornduff, S. R., & Kelsey, R. M. (1995). Object relations and physical abuse: A TAT analysis. *Journal of Personality Assessment, 64*, 552–568.

Friedrich, W. N. (1990). *Psychotherapy of sexually abused children and their families*. New York: Norton.

Friedrich, W. N., Fisher, J. L., Dittner, C. A., Acton, R., Berliner, L., Butler, J., et al. (2001). Child Sexual Behavior Inventory: Normative, psychiatric, and sexual abuse comparisons. *Child Maltreatment, 6*, 37–49.

Friedrich, W. N., Grambsch, P., Broughton, D., Kuiper, J., & Beilke, R. L. (1991). Normative sexual behavior in children. *Pediatrics, 88*, 456–646.

Friedrich, W. N., Grambsch, P., Damon, L., Hewitt, S., Koverola, C., Lang, R., et al. (1992). The Child Sexual Behavior Inventory: Normative and clinical findings. *Psychological Assessment, 4*, 303–311.

Garb, H. N., Wood, J. M., & Nezworkski, M. T. (2000). Projective techniques and the detection of child sexual abuse. *Child Maltreatment, 5*, 161–168.

Garbarino, J., Guttman, E., & Seeley, J. (1986). *The psychologically battered child: Strategies for identification, assessment and intervention*. San Francisco: Jossey-Bass.

Garbarino, J., Stott, F. M., & Faculty of the Erikson Institute. (1989). *What children can tell us*. San Francisco: Jossey-Bass.

Gardner, L. I. (1972). Deprivation dwarfism. *Scientific American, 227*, 76–82.

Gardner, R. A. (1971). *Therapeutic communication with children: The mutual storytelling technique*. New York: Jason Aronson.

Garmezy, N., & Streitman, S. (1974). Children at risk: The search for antecedents to schizophrenia. Part I: Conceptual models and research methods. *Schizophrenia Bulletin, 8*, 14–90.

Garralda, M. E. (1996). Somatization in children. *Journal of Child Psychology and Psychiatry and Allied Disciplines, 37*, 13–33.

Gauthier, Y., Fortin, G., & Jéliu, G. (2004). Clinical application of attachment theory in permanency planning for children in foster care: The importance of continuity of care. *Infant Mental Health Journal, 25*, 39–396.

Gil, E. (1991). *The healing power of play: Working with abused children*. New York: Guilford Press.

Gil, E., & Johnson, T. C. (1993). *Sexualized children: Assessment and treatment of sexualized children and children who molest*. Rockville, MD: Launch Press.

Ginott, H. G. (1965). *Between parent and child*. New York: Avon Books.

Gladwell, M. (2005). *Blink: The power of thinking without thinking*. New York: Little, Brown.

Goldberg, S. (1991). Recent developments in attachment theory and research. *Canadian Journal of Psychiatry, 36*, 393–400.

Goldenson, R. M. (Ed.). (1984). *Longman dictionary of psychology and psychiatry*. New York: Longman.

Goldfarb, W. (1955). Emotional and intellectual consequences of psychosocial deprivation in infancy: A reevaluation. In P. Hoch & D. Zubin (Eds.), *Psychopathology in childhood* (pp. 105–119). New York: Grune & Stratton.

Goldfried, M. R., & Eubanks-Carter, C. (2004). On the need for a new psychotherapy research paradigm: Comment on Westen, Novotny, and Thompson-Brenner (2004). *Psychological Bulletin, 130*, 669–673.

Gomes-Schwartz, B., Horowitz, J. M., Cardarelli, A. P., & Sauzier, M. (1990). The aftermath of child sexual abuse: 18 months later. In B. Gomes-Schwartz, J. M.

Horowitz, & A. P. Cardarelli (Eds.), *Child sexual abuse: The initial effects* (pp. 132–152). Newbury Park, CA: Sage.

Grave, J., & Blissett, J. (2004). Is cognitive behavior therapy developmentally appropriate for young children? A critical review of the evidence. *Clinical Psychology Review, 24*, 399–420.

Gray, A., Pithers, W. D., Busconi, A., & Houchens, P. (1999). Developmental and etiological characteristics of children with sexual behavior problems: Treatment implications. *Child Abuse and Neglect, 23*, 601–621.

Graziano, A. M., & Wells, J. R. (1992). Treatment for abused children: When is a partial solution acceptable? *Child Abuse and Neglect, 16*, 217–228.

Greenberg, M. T. (1999). Attachment and psychopathology in childhood. In J. Cassidy & P. R. Shaver (Eds.), *Handbook of attachment: Theory, research, and clinical applications* (pp. 469–496). New York: Guilford Press.

Grizenko, N., & Pawliuk, N. (1994). Risk and protective factors for disruptive behavior disorders in children. *American Journal of Orthopsychiatry, 64*, 534–544.

Gullone, E., & King, N. J. (1992). Psychometric evaluation of a fear survey schedule for children and adolescents. *Journal of Child Psychology and Psychiatry, 33*, 987–998.

Gutierrez, J. (1989). Using tests and other instruments. In J. Garbarino, F. M. Stott, & Faculty of the Erikson Institute, *What children can tell us* (pp. 203–225). San Francisco: Jossey-Bass.

Hagans, K. B., & Case, J. (1988). *When your child has been molested: A parent's guide to healing and recovery. Putting the pieces back together.* New York: Lexington Books.

Hall, D. K. (1993). *Assessing child trauma.* Toronto: Institute for the Prevention of Child Abuse.

Hall, D. K., Mathews, F., & Pearce, J. (1998). Factors associated with sexual behavior problems in young sexually abused children. *Child Abuse and Neglect, 22*, 1045–1063.

Hall, D. K., Mathews, F., & Pearce, J. (2002). Sexual behavior problems in sexually abused children: A preliminary typology. *Child Abuse and Neglect, 26*, 289–312.

Hall, D. K., Mathews, F., Pearce, J., Sarlo-McGarvey, N., & Gavin, D. (1996). *The development of sexual behavior problems in children and youth.* Toronto: Central Toronto Youth Services.

Hansburg, H. G. (1972). *Adolescent separation anxiety: A method far the study of adolescent separation problems.* Springfield, IL: Charles C. Thomas.

Hanson, R. F., & Spratt, E. G. (2000). Reactive attachment disorder: What we know about the disorder and implications for treatment. *Child Maltreatment, 5*, 137–145.

Harter, S. (1977). A cognitive-developmental approach to children's expression of conflicting feelings and a technique to facilitate such expression in play therapy. *Journal of Consulting and Clinical Psychology, 45*, 417–432.

Harter, S. (1982). The Perceived Competence Scale for Children. *Child Development, 53*, 87–97.

Harter, S. (1983). Cognitive-developmental considerations in the conduct of play therapy. In C. E. Schaeffer & K. J. O'Connor (Eds.), *Handbook of play therapy* (pp. 95–127). New York: Wiley.

Haugaard, J. J. (2004a). Recognizing and treating uncommon behavioral and emotional disorders in children and adolescents who have been severely maltreated: Dissociative disorders. *Child Maltreatment, 9*, 146–153.

Haugaard, J. J. (2004b). Recognizing and treating uncommon behavioral and emotional disorders in children and adolescents who have been severely maltreated: Introduction. *Child Maltreatment, 9*, 123–130.

Haugaard, J. J. (2004c). Recognizing and treating uncommon behavioral and emotional disorders in children and adolescents who have been severely maltreated: Somatization and other somatoform disorders. *Child Maltreatment, 9*, 169–176.

Hazzard, A. (1995). Structured treatment and prevention activities for sexually abused children. *Directions in Clinical Psychology, 5*, 1–10.

Hembree-Kigin, T. L., & McNeil, C. B. (1995). *Parent–child interaction therapy.* New York: Plenum Press.

Heriot, J (1996). Maternal protectiveness following the disclosure of intrafamilial child sexual abuse. *Journal of Interpersonal Violence, 11*, 181–194.

Herrenkohl, E. C., Herrenkohl, R. C., & Egolf, B. P. (2003). The psychosocial consequences of living environment instability on maltreated children. *American Journal of Orthopsychiatry, 73*, 367–380.

Hewitt, S. K., & Friedrich, W. N. (1991, January). *Preschool children's responses to alleged sexual abuse at intake and one-year follow up*. Paper presented at the annual meeting of the American Professional Society on the Abuse of Children, San Diego, CA.

Hibbard, R. A., & Hartman, G. L. (1992). Behavioral problems of alleged sexual abuse victims. *Child Abuse and Neglect, 16*, 755–762.

Hoffman-Plotkin, D., & Twentyman, C. T. (1984). A multi-modal assessment of behavioral and cognitive deficits in abused and neglected preschoolers. *Child Development, 55*, 794–802.

Howes, C. (1984). Social interactions and patterns of friendships in normal and emotionally disturbed children. In T. Field, J. Roopnarine, & M. Segal (Eds.), *Friendships in normal and handicapped children* (pp. 163–185). Norwood, NJ: Ablex.

Howes, C., & Eldredge, R. (1985). Responses of abused, neglected, and non-maltreated children to the behaviors of their peers. *Journal of Applied Developmental Psychology, 6*, 261–270.

Howes, C., & Espinosa, M. P. (1985). The consequences of child abuse for the formation of relationships with peers. *Child Abuse and Neglect, 9*, 397–404.

Hufton, I. W., & Gates, R, K. (1977). Nonorganic failure to thrive: A long term follow-up. *Pediatrics, 59*, 73–77.

Hughes, D. (2004). An attachment-based treatment of maltreated children and young people. *Attachment and Human Development, 6*, 263–278.

Jaffee, S. R., Caspi, A., Moffitt, T. E., Dodge, K. A., Rutter, M., Taylor, A., et al. (2005). Nature × nurture: Genetic vulnerabilities interact with physical maltreatment to promote conduct problems. *Development and Psychopathology, 17*, 67–84.

Jaffee, S. R., Caspi, A., Moffitt, T. E., & Taylor, A. (2004). Physical maltreatment victim to antisocial child: Evidence of an environmentally mediated process. *Journal of Abnormal Psychology, 113*, 44–55.

James, B. (1989). *Treating traumatized children: New insights and creative interventions*. Lexington, MA: Lexington Books.

James, B. (1994). *Handbook for treatment of attachment-trauma problems in children*. Lexington, MA: Lexington Books.

Johnson, R. M., Kotch, J. B., Catellier, D. J., Winsor, J. R, Dufort, V., Hunter, W., et al. (2002). Adverse behavioral and emotional outcomes from child abuse and witnessed violence. *Child Maltreatment, 7*, 179–186.

Johnson, T. C. (1988). Child perpetrators—children who molest other children: Preliminary findings. *Child Abuse and Neglect, 12*, 219–229.

Johnson, T. C. (1989). Female child perpetrators: Children who molest other children. *Child Abuse and Neglect, 13*, 571–585.

Jouriles, E. N., McDonald, R., Spiller, L., Norwood, W. D., Swank, P. R., Stephens, N., et al. (2001). Reducing conduct problems among children of battered women. *Journal of Consulting and Clinical Psychology, 69*, 774–785.

Kagan, R. M. (1986). Game therapy for children in placement. In C. E. Schaefer & S. Reid (Eds.), *Game play: Therapeutic use of childhood games* (pp. 73–94). New York: Wiley.

Karen, R. (1994). *Becoming attached*. New York: Warner Books.

Karp, C. L., & Butler, T. L. (1996). *Treatment strategies for abused children: From victim to survivor.* Thousand Oaks, CA: Sage.

Katz, K. (1992). Communication problems in maltreated children: A tutorial. *Journal of Childhood Communication Disorders, 14*, 147–163.

Kaufman, J., & Cicchetti, D. (1989). Effects of maltreatment on school-age children's socio-emotional development: Assessments in a day camp setting. *Developmental Psychology, 25*, 516–524.

Kelley, S. J. (1990). Parental stress response to sexual abuse and ritualistic abuse of children in day-care centers. *Nursing Research, 39*, 25–29.

Kendall, P. C. (Ed.). (1991). *Child and adolescent therapy: Cognitive-behavioral procedures*. New York: Guilford Press.

Kendall, P. C., & Braswell, L. (1993). *Cognitive-behavioral therapy for impulsive children* (2nd ed.). New York: Guilford Press.

Kendall-Tackett, K. A., & Eckenrode, J. (1996). The effects of neglect on academic achievement and disciplinary problems: A developmental perspective. *Child Abuse and Neglect, 20*, 161–169.

Kendall-Tackett, K. A., Williams, L. M., & Finkelhor, D. (1993). Impact of sexual abuse on children: A review and synthesis of recent empirical studies. *Psychological Bulletin, 113*, 164–180.

King, N. J., Tonge, B. J., Mullen, P., Myerson, N., Heyne, D., Rollings, S., et al. (2000). Treating sexually abused children with posttraumatic stress symptoms: A randomized clinical trial. *Journal of the American Academy of Child and Adolescent Psychiatry, 39*, 1347–1355.

Kinzl, J. F., Traweger, C., & Biebl, W. (1995). Family background and sexual abuse associated with somatization. *Psychotherapy and Psychosomatic Medicine, 64*, 82–87.

Kirby, K. M., & Hardesty, P. H. (1998). Evaluating older pre-adoptive foster children. *Professional Psychology: Research and Practice, 29*, 428–436.

Kiser, L. J., Heston, J., Millsap, P. A., & Pruitt, D. B. (1991). Physical and sexual abuse in childhood: Relationship with posttraumatic stress disorder. *Journal of the American Academy of Child and Adolescent Psychiatry, 30*, 776–783.

Kitzman, K. M., Gaylord, N. K., Holt, A. R., & Kenny, E. D. (2003). Child witnesses to domestic violence: A meta-analytic review. *Journal of Consulting and Clinical Psychology, 71*, 339–352.

Klagsbrun, M., & Bowlby, J. (1976). Responses to separation from parents: A clinical test for young children. *British Journal of Protective Psychology, 21*, 7–21.

Kluft, R. P. (1984). Multiple personality disorder in children. *Psychiatric Clinics of North America, 7*, 121–134.

Kluft, R. P. (1996). Outpatient treatment of dissociative identity disorder and allied forms of dissociative disorder not otherwise specified in children and adolescents. *Child and Adolescent Psychiatric Clinics of North America, 5*, 471–494.

Koenen, K. C., Moffit, T. E., Caspi, A., Taylor, A., & Purcell, S. (2003). Domestic violence is associated with environmental suppression of IQ in young children. *Development and Psychopathology, 15*, 297–311.

Kolko, D. J. (1996). Individual cognitive behavioral treatment and family therapy for physically abused children and their offending parents: A comparison of clinical outcomes. *Child Maltreatment, 1*, 322–342.

Kolko, D. J., Brown, E. J., & Berliner, L. (2002). Children's perceptions of their abusive experience: Measurement and preliminary findings. *Child Maltreatment, 7*, 42–55.

Kolko, D. J., & Feiring, C. (2002). "Explaining why": A closer look at attributions in child abuse victims. *Child Maltreatment, 7*, 5–8.

Kot, S., & Tyndall-Lind, A. (2005). Intensive play therapy with child witnesses of domestic violence. In L. A. Reddy, T. M. Files-Hall, & C. E. Schaefer (Eds.), *Empirically based play interventions for children* (pp. 31–49). Washington, DC: American Psychological Association.

Kovacs, M. (2003). *The Children's Depression Inventory: Technical manual.* Tonawanda, NY: Multi-Health Systems.

Kretchmar, M. D., Worsham, N. L., & Swenson, N. (2005). Anna's story: A qualitative analysis of an at-risk mother's experience in an attachment-based foster care program. *Attachment and Human Development, 7*, 31–49.

Kurtz, K. J., Gaudin, J. M., Wodarski, J. S., & Rowing, P. T. (1993). Maltreatment and the school-aged child: School performance consequences. *Child Abuse and Neglect, 17*, 581–590.

Lamb, S. (1986). Treating sexually abused children: Issues of blame and responsibility. *American Journal of Orthopsychiatry, 56*, 303–307.

Landreth, G. L. (2002). Therapeutic limit setting in the play therapy relationship. *Professional Psychology: Research and Practice, 33*, 529–535.

Lansford, J. E., Dodge, K. A., Pettit, G. S., Bates, J. E., Crozier, J., & Kaplow, J. (2002). Long-term effects of early child physical maltreatment on psychological, behavioral, and academic problems in adolescence: A 12-year prospective study. *Archives of Pediatric and Adolescent Medicine, 156*, 824–830.

Leifer, M., Shapiro, J. P., & Kassem, L. (1993). The impact of maternal history and behavior upon foster placement and adjustment in sexually abused children. *Child Abuse and Neglect, 17*, 755–766.

Levine, M. D. (1996). *The ANSER System*. Cambridge, MA: Educators Publishing Service.

Levy, D. (1939). Release therapy. *American Journal of Orthopsychiatry, 9*, 713–736.

Lewandowdski, L. A., & Baranoski, M. V. (1994). Psychological aspects of acute trauma: Intervening with children and families in the inpatient setting. *Child and Adolescent Psychiatric Clinics of North America, 3*, 513–592.

Lewis, D. O. (1992). From abuse to violence: Psychophysiological consequences of maltreatment. *Journal of the American Academy of Child and Adolescent Psychiatry, 31*, 383–391.

Lewis, D. O. (1996). Diagnostic evaluation of the child with dissociative identity disorder/multiple personality disorder. *Child and Adolescent Psychiatric Clinics of North America, 5*, 303–331.

Lewis, D. O., Lovely, E., Yeager, C., & Delia Femina, D. (1989). Toward a theory of the genesis of violence: A follow-up study of delinquents. *Journal of the American Academy of Child and Adolescent Psychiatry, 28*, 431–436.

Lewis, D. O., Lovely, E., Yeager, C., Ferguson, G., Friedman, M., Sloane, G., et al. (1988). Intrinsic and environmental characteristics of juvenile murderers. *Journal of the American Academy of Child and Adolescent Psychiatry, 27*, 582–587.

Lewis, D. O., & Yeager, C. A. (1994). Abuse, dissociative phenomena, and childhood multiple personality disorder. *Child and Adolescent Psychiatric Clinics of North America, 3*, 729–743.

Lewis, D. O., Yeager, C. A., Cobham-Portorreal, C. S., Klein, N., Showalter, C., & Anthony, A. (1991). A follow-up of female delinquents: Maternal contributions to the perpetuation of deviance. *Journal of the American Academy of Child and Adolescent Psychiatry, 30*, 197–201.

Lieberman, A. F., Van Horn, P., & Ozer, E. J. (2005). Preschooler witnesses of marital violence: Predictors and mediators of child behavior problems. *Development and Psychopathology, 17*, 385–396.

Lieberman, A. F., & Zeanah, C. H. (1995). Disorders of attachment in infancy. *Child and Adolescent Psychiatric Clinics of North America, 4*, 571–587.

Liotti, G. (1999). Understanding the dissociative processes: The contribution of attachment. *Psychoanalytic Inquiry, 19*, 757–783.

Lipman, E. L., Offord, D. R., & Boyle, M. H. (1994). Relation between economic disadvantage and psychosocial morbidity in children. *Canadian Medical Association Journal, 151*, 431–437.

Littner, N. (1960). The child's need to repeat his past: Some implications for placement. *Social Services Review, 34*, 128–148.

Lochman, J. E., White, K. J., & Wayland, K. K. (1991). Cognitive-behavioral assessment and treatment with aggressive children. In P. C. Kendall (Ed.), *Child and adolescent therapy: Cognitive-behavioral procedures* (pp. 25–65). New York: Guilford Press.

Looney, J. G. (1984). Treatment planning in child psychiatry. *Journal of the American Academy of Child Psychiatry, 23*, 529–536.

Lyon, E. (1993). Hospital staff reactions to accounts by survivors of childhood abuse. *American Journal of Orthopsychiatry, 63*, 410–416.

Lyons-Ruth, K., Alpern, L., & Repacholi, B. (1993). Disorganized infant attachment classification and maternal psychosocial problems as predictors of hostile–aggressive behavior in the preschool classroom. *Child Development, 64*, 572–585.

Lyons-Ruth, K., Easterbrooks, A., & Cibelli, C. (1997). Infant attachment strategies, infant mental lag, and maternal depressive symptoms: Predictors of internalizing and externalizing problems at age 7. *Developmental Psychology, 33*, 681–692.

Lyons-Ruth, K., & Jacobvitz, D. (1999). Attachment disorganization: Unresolved loss, relational violence, and lapses in behavioral and attentional strategies. In J. Cassidy & P. R. Shaver (Eds.), *Handbook of attachment: Theory, research, and clinical applications* (pp. 520–554). New York: Guilford Press.

Lyons-Ruth, K., Repacholi, B., McLeod, S., & Silva, E. (1991). Disorganized attachment behavior in infancy: Short-term stability, maternal and infant correlates, risk-related subtypes. *Development and Psychopathology, 3*, 377–396.

MacDonald, R. (1985). The Hutterites in Alberta. In H. Palmer & T. Palmer (Eds.), *Peoples of Alberta: Portraits of cultural diversity* (pp. 348–364). Saskatoon, SK: Western Producer Prairie Books.

MacFarlane, K., & Cunningham, C. (1988). *Steps to healthy touching*. Mt. Dora, FL: Kidsrights.

MacFie, J., Cicchetti, D., & Toth, S. L. (2001). The development of dissociation in maltreated preschool-aged children. *Development and Psychopathology, 13*, 233–254.

MacLean, K. (2003). The impact of institutionalization on child development. *Development and Psychopathology, 15*, 853–884.

Main, M. (1981). Avoidance in the service of attachment: A working paper. In K. Immelman, G. Barlow, L. Petrinovich, & M. Main (Eds.), *Behavioral development* (pp. 651–693). Cambridge, UK: Cambridge University Press.

Main, M. (1990). Cross-cultural studies of attachment organization: Recent studies, changing methodologies, and the concept of conditional strategies. *Human Development, 33*, 48–61.

Main, M., & Cassidy, J. (1988). Categories of response to reunion with the parent at age 6: Predictable from infant classifications and stable over a 1-month period. *Developmental Psychology, 24*, 425–426.

Main, M., & George, C. (1985). Response of abused and disadvantaged toddlers to distress in agemates: A study in the day care setting. *Developmental Psychology, 21*, 407–412.

Main, M., & Goldwyn, R. (1984). Predicting rejection of her infant from other's representation of her own experience: Implications for the abused–abusing intergenerational cycle. *Child Abuse and Neglect, 8*, 203–217.

Main, M., & Hesse, E. (1990). Parents' unresolved traumatic experiences are related to infant disorganized attachment status: Is frightened and/or frightening parental behavior the linking mechanism? In M. Greenberg, D. Cicchetti, & E. M. Cummings (Eds.), *Attachment in the preschool years: Theory, research and intervention* (pp. 161–184). Chicago: University of Chicago Press.

Main, M., Kaplan, N., & Cassidy, J. (1985). Security in infancy, childhood, and adulthood: A move to the level of representation. In I. Bretherton & E. Waters (Eds.), Growing points of attachment theory and research. *Monographs of the Society for Research in Child Development*, 50(1–2, Serial No. 209), 66–104.

Main, M., & Solomon, J. (1986). Discovery of an insecure disorganized/disoriented attachment pattern. In T. B. Brazelton & M. W. Yogman (Eds.), *Affective development in infancy* (pp. 95–124). Norwood, NJ: Ablex.

Main, M., & Solomon, J. (1990). Procedures for identifying infants as disorganized/disoriented during the Ainsworth strange situation. In M. Greenberg, D. Cicchetti, & M. Cummings (Eds.), *Attachment in the preschool years* (pp. 121–160). Chicago: University of Chicago Press.

Main, M., & Weston, D. (1982). Avoidance of the attachment figure in infancy: Descriptions and interpretations. In C. M. Parkes & J. Stevenson-Hinde (Eds.), *The place of attachment in human behavior* (Vol. 8, pp. 203–217). London: Tavistock.

Malinosky-Rummell, R., & Hansen, D. J. (1993). Long-term consequences of childhood physical abuse. *Psychological Bulletin, 114*, 68–79.

Malinosky-Rummell, R., & Hoeir, T. S. (1991). Validating measures of dissociation in sexually abused and nonabused children. *Behavioral Assessment, 13*, 341–357.

Mandell, J. G., & Damon, L. (1989). *Group treatment for sexually abused children.* New York: Guilford Press.

Manly, J. T., Cicchetti, D., & Barnett, D. (1994). The impact of maltreatment on child outcome: An exploration of dimensions within maltreatment. *Development and Psychopathology, 6*, 121–143.

Mannarino, A. P., & Cohen, J. A. (1986). A clinical–demographic study of sexually abused children. *Child Abuse and Neglect, 10*, 17–23.

Mannarino, A. P., & Cohen, J. A. (1996a). Abuse-related attributions and perceptions, general attributions, and locus of control in sexually abused girls. *Journal of Interpersonal Violence, 11*, 162–180.

Mannarino, A. P., & Cohen, J. A. (1996b). A follow-up study of factors that mediate the development of psychological symptomatology in sexually abused girls. *Child Maltreatment, 1*, 246–260.

Mannarino, A. P., Cohen, J. A., & Berman, S. R, (1994). The Children's Attributions and Perceptions Scale: A new measure of sexual abuse-related factors. *Journal of Clinical Child Psychology, 23*, 204–211.

Mantzicopoulos, P. Y., & Morrison, D. (1994). A comparison of boys and girls with attention problems: Kindergarten through second grade. *American Journal of Orthopsychiatry, 64*, 522–533.

Martin, H. P., Beezley, P., Conway, E. F., & Kempe, C. H. (1974). The development of the abused child. *Advances in Pediatrics, 21*, 25–73.

Mash, E. J. , & Terdal, L. G. (Eds.). (1997). *Assessment of childhood disorders* (3rd ed.). New York: Guilford Press.

Massat, C. R., & Lundy, M. (1998). "Reporting costs" to nonoffending parents in cases of intrafamilial child sexual abuse. *Child Welfare, 11*, 371–388.

Masten, A. S., Best, K. M., & Garmezy, N. (1990). Resilience and development: Contributions from the study of children who overcome adversity. *Development and Psychopathology, 2*, 425–444.

McArthur, D. S., & Roberts, G. E. (1982). *Roberts Apperception Test for Children manual.* Los Angeles: Western Psychological Services.

McCabe, O. L. (2004). Crossing the quality chasm in behavioral health care: The role of evidence-based practice. *Professional Psychology: Research and Practice, 35*, 571–579.

McCrone, E. R, Egeland, B., Kalkoske, M., & Carlson, E. A. (1994). Relations between early maltreatment and mental representations of relationships assessed with projective storytelling in middle childhood. *Development and Psychopathology, 6*, 99–120.

McKibbon, A., Eady, A., & Marks, S. (1999). *PDQ: Evidence-based principles and practice*. Lewiston, NY: Decker.

McLeer, S. V., Deblinger, E., Henry, D., & Orvaschel, H. (1992). Sexually abused children at high risk for posttraumatic stress disorder. *Journal of the American Academy of Child and Adolescent Psychiatry, 31*, 875–879.

Messer, S. B. (2004). Evidence-based practice: Beyond empirically supported treatments. *Professional Psychology: Research and Practice, 35*, 580–588.

Messer, S. B., & Wampold, B. E. (2002). Let's face facts: Common factors are more potent than specific therapy ingredients. *Clinical Psychology: Science and Practice, 9*, 21–25.

Miller-Perrin, C. L., Wurtele, S. K., & Kondrick, P. A. (1990). Sexually abused and nonabused children's conceptions of personal body safety. *Child Abuse and Neglect, 14*, 99–112.

Mills, B., & Allan, J. (1992). Play therapy with the maltreated child: Impact upon aggressive and withdrawn patterns of interaction. *International Journal of Play Therapy, 1*, 1–20.

Mills, J. C., & Crowley, R, J. (1986). *Therapeutic metaphors for children and the child within*. New York: Brunner/Mazel.

Money, J. (1977). The syndrome of abuse dwarfism (psychosocial dwarfism or reversible hyposomatotropism). *American Journal of Diseases in Childhood, 131*, 508–513.

Money, J., & Annecillo, C. (1976). IQ change following change of domicile in the syndrome of reversible hyposomatotropism: Pilot investigation. *Psychoneuroendocrinology, 1*, 427–239.

Money, J., Annecillo, C., & Kelly, J. F. (1983). Abuse-dwarfism syndrome: After rescue, statural and intellectual catchup growth correlate. *Journal of Clinical Child Psychology, 12*, 279–283.

Mowrer, O. H. (1960). *Learning theory and behavior.* New York: Wiley.

Mueller, E., & Silverman, N. (1989). Peer relations in maltreated children. In D. Cicchetti & V. Carlson (Eds.), *Child maltreatment: Theory and research on the causes and consequences of child abuse and neglect* (pp. 529–578). New York: Cambridge University Press.

Murray, H. (1938). *Explorations in personality.* New York: Oxford University Press.

Murray, H. (1943). *Thematic Apperception Test—manual*. Cambridge, MA: Harvard University Press.

Nelson, C. A., & Bloom, F. E. (1997). Child development and neuroscience. *Child Development, 68*, 970–987.

Nelson, C. A., Bloom, F. E., Cameron, J. L., Amaral, D., Dahl, R. E., & Pine, D. (2002). An integrative, multidisciplinary approach to the study of brain–behavior relations in the context of typical and atypical development. *Development and Psychopathology, 14*, 499–520.

Newton, R. R., Litrownik, A. J., & Landsverk, J. A. (2000). Children and youth in foster care: Disentangling the relationship between problem behaviors and number of placements. *Child Abuse and Neglect, 24*, 1363–1374.

Norcross, J. C. (2002). *Psychotherapy relationships that work.* New York: Oxford University Press.

Oates, R. K., Peacock, A., & Forrest, D. (1985). Long-term effects of nonorganic failure to thrive. *Pediatrics, 75*, 36–40.

O'Connor, T. G., Bredenkamp, D., Rutter, M., & The English and Romanian Adoptees (ERA) Study Team. (1999). Attachment disturbances and disorders in children exposed to early severe deprivation. *Infant Mental Health Journal, 20*, 10–29.

O'Connor, T. G., Marvin, R. S., Rutter, M., Olrick, J. T., Britner, P. A., & the English and Romanian Adoptees Study Team. (2003). Parent–child attachment following early institutional deprivation. *Development and Psychopathology, 15*, 19–38.

O'Connor, T. G., Rutter, M., & the ERA Study Team. (2000). Attachment disorder behavior following early severe deprivation: Extension and longitudinal follow-up. *Journal of the American Academy of Child and Adolescent Psychiatry, 39*, 703–712.

Ogawa, J. R., Sroufe, L. A., Weinfeld, N. S., Carlson, E. A., & Egeland, B. (1997). Development and the fragmented self: A longitudinal study of dissociative symptomatology in a normative sample. *Development and Psychopathology, 9*, 855–879.

Owen, M. T., & Cox, M. J. (1997). Marital conflict and the development of infant–parent attachment relationships. *Journal of Family Psychology, 11*, 152–164.

Palmer, L., Farrar, A. R., Valle, M., Ghahary, N., Panella, M., & DeGraw, D. (2000). An investigation of the clinical use of the House-Tree-Person projective drawings in the psychological evaluation of child sexual abuse. *Child Maltreatment, 5*, 169–175.

Parker, G. B., Barrett, B. A., & Hickie, I. B. (1992). From nurture to network: Examining links between perceptions of parenting received in childhood and social bonds in adulthood. *American Journal of Psychiatry, 149*, 877–885.

Patterson, G. R. (1980). *Living with children: New methods for parents and teachers.* Champaign, IL: Research Press.

Patterson, G. R., Redi, J. B., Jones, R. R., & Conger, R. E. (1975). *A social learning approach to family intervention: Vol. 1. Families with aggressive children.* Eugene, OR: Castalia.

Pearce, J. (2001). Sexual behavior problems in preadolescent children. *Journal of Child and Youth Care, 14*, 65–82.

Pearce, J. W., & Pezzot-Pearce, T. D. (1994). Attachment theory and its implications for psychotherapy with maltreated children. *Child Abuse and Neglect, 18*, 425–438.

Pearce, J. W., & Pezzot-Pearce, T. D. (1997). *Psychotherapy of abused and neglected children.* New York: Guilford Press.

Pears, K. C., & Fisher, P. A. (2005). Emotion understanding and theory of mind among maltreated children in foster care: Evidence of deficits. *Development and Psychopathology, 17*, 47–65.

Persons, J. (1991). Psychotherapy outcome studies do not accurately represent current models of psychotherapy. *American Psychologist, 46*, 99–106.

Pezzot, T. D. (1978). *Battered and neglected children: Developmental characteristics and the familial–environmental factors involved in abuse*. Unpublished master's thesis, University of Manitoba, Winnipeg, Manitoba, Canada.

Pezzot-Pearce, T. D., & Pearce, J. (2004). *Parenting assessments in child welfare cases: A practical guide*. Toronto: University of Toronto Press.

Piaget, J. (1952). *The origins of intelligence*. New York: Norton.

Piaget, J. (1967). *Six psychological studies*. New York: Random House.

Piers, E. V., Harris, D. B., & Herzberg, D. S. (2002). *The Piers–Harris Children's Self-Concept Scale: Second edition manual*. Los Angeles: Western Psychological Services.

Pithers, W. D., Gray, A., Busconi, A., & Houchens, P. (1998a). Caregivers of children with sexual behavior problems: Psychological and familial functioning. *Child Abuse and Neglect, 22*, 129–141.

Pithers, W. D., Gray, A., Busconi, A., & Houchens, P. (1998b). Children with sexual behavior problems: Identification of five distinct child types and related treatment considerations. *Child Maltreatment, 3*, 384–406.

Pollak, S. D., Cicchetti, D., Hornung, K., & Reed, A. (2000). Recognizing emotion in faces: Developmental effects of child abuse and neglect. *Developmental Psychology, 36*, 679–688.

Pollak, S. D., & Sinha, P. (2002). Effects of early experience on children's recognition of facial displays of emotion. *Developmental Psychology, 38*, 784–791.

Pollak, S. D., & Tolley-Schell, S. A. (2003). Selective attention to facial emotion in physically abused children. *Journal of Abnormal Psychology, 112*, 323–338.

Polansky, N. A., Chalmers, M. A., Buttenwieser, E., & Williams, D. P. (1981). *Damaged parents: An anatomy of child neglect*. Chicago: University of Chicago Press.

Post, R. M., & Weiss, S. R. B. (2002). Psychological complexity: Barriers to its integration into the neurobiology of major psychiatric disorders. *Development and Psychopathology, 14*, 635–651.

Powell, G. F., Brasel, J. A., & Blizzard, R. M. (1967). Emotional deprivation and growth retardation simulating idiopathic hypopituitarism: I. Clinical evaluation of the syndrome. *New England Journal of Medicine, 276*, 1271–1278.

Powell, G. F., Brasel, J. A., Raiti, S., & Blizzard, R. M. (1967). Emotional deprivation and growth retardation simulating idiopathic hypopituitarism: II. Endocrinologic evaluation of the syndrome. *New England Journal of Medicine, 276*, 1279–1283.

Psychological Corporation. (2002). *Wechsler Individual Achievement Test–II manual*. San Antonio, TX: Author.

Putnam, F. W. (1989). *Diagnosis and treatment of multiple personality disorder*. New York: Guilford Press.

Putnam, F. W. (1993). Dissociative disorders in children: Behavioral profiles and problems. *Child Abuse and Neglect, 17*, 39–45.

Putnam, F. W., Helmers, K., & Trickett, P. K. (1993). Development, reliability, and validity of a child dissociation scale. *Child Abuse and Neglect, 17*, 731–741.

Pynoos, R. S., & Eth, S. (1986). Witness to violence: The child interview. *Journal of the American Academy of Child Psychiatry, 25*, 306–319.

Pynoos, R. S., Frederick, C., Nader, K., Arroyo, W., Steinburg, A., Eth, S., et al.

(1987). Life threat and posttraumatic stress in school-age children. *Archives of General Psychiatry, 44*, 1057–1063.

Realmuto, G. M., Masten, A., Carole, L. F., Hubbard, J., Groteluschen, A., & Chhun, B. (1992). Adolescent survivors of massive childhood trauma in Cambodia: Life events and current symptoms. *Journal of Traumatic Stress, 5*, 589–599.

Regehr, C. (1990). Parental responses to extrafamilial child sexual assault. *Child Abuse and Neglect, 14*, 113–120.

Resick, P. A, & Schnicke, M. K. (1992). Cognitive processing therapy for sexual assault victims. *Journal of Consulting and Clinical Psychology, 60*, 748–756.

Resick, P. A, & Schnicke, M. K. (1993). *Cognitive processing therapy for rape victims: A treatment manual.* Newbury Park, CA: Sage.

Reynolds, C. R., & Kamphaus, R. W. (2004). *Manual for Behavior Assessment System for Children: Second edition.* Circle Pines, MN: American Guidance Service.

Reynolds, C. R, & Richmond, B. O. (1978). What I think and feel: A revised measure of children's anxiety. *Journal of Abnormal Child Psychology, 6*, 271–280.

Rieder, C., & Cicchetti, D. (1989). An organizational perspective on cognitive control functioning and cognitive–affective balance in maltreated children. *Developmental Psychology, 25*, 382–393.

Roid, G. H. (2003). *Stanford-Binet Intelligence Scale—Fifth Edition: Examiner's manual.* Itasca, IL: Riverside.

Ronen, T. (1997). *Cognitive developmental therapy with children.* Chichester, UK: Wiley.

Ross, A. O. (1964). Interruptions and termination of treatment. In M. R. Haworth (Ed.), *Child psychotherapy: Practice and theory* (pp. 292–297). New York: Basic Books.

Runyan, D. K., Everson, M. D., Edelsohn, G. A., Hunter, W. M., & Coulter, M. L. (1988). Impact of legal intervention on sexually abused children. *Journal of Pediatrics, 113*, 647–653.

Runyan, M. K., & Kenny, M. C. (2002). Relationship of attributional style, depression, and posttrauma distress among children who suffered physical or sexual abuse. *Child Maltreatment, 7*, 254–264.

Rutter, M. (1985). Resilience in the face of adversity: Protective factors and resistance to psychiatric disorder. *British Journal of Psychiatry, 147*, 598–611.

Rutter, M. (1993). Resilience: Some conceptual considerations. *Journal of Adolescent Health, 14*, 626–631.

Ryan, G. (1989). Victim to victimizer: Rethinking victim treatment. *Journal of Interpersonal Violence, 4*, 325–341.

Ryan, G. (2000). Childhood sexuality: A decade of study. Part I: Research and curriculum development. *Child Abuse and Neglect, 24*, 33–48.

Saigh, P. A. (1986). In vitro flooding in the treatment of a 6-year-old boy's posttraumatic stress disorder. *Behavior Research and Therapy, 24*, 685–688.

Saigh, P. A. (1987a). In vitro flooding of an adolescent's posttramatic stress disorder. *Journal of Clinical Child Psychology, 16*, 147–150.

Saigh, P. A. (1987b). In vitro flooding of a childhood posttraumatic disorder. *School Psychology Review, 16*, 203–211.

Saigh, P. A. (1987c). In vitro flooding of childhood posttraumatic stress disorders: A systematic replication. *Professional School Psychology, 2*, 133–145.

Saigh, P. A. (1989). The use of in vitro flooding in the treatment of traumatized adolescents. *Developmental and Behavioral Pediatrics, 10*, 17–21.

Salt, P., Myer, M., Coleman, L., & Sauzier, M. (1990). The myth of the mother as "accomplice" to sexual abuse. In B. Gomes-Schwartz, J. M. Horowitz, & A. P. Cardarelli (Eds.), *Child sexual abuse: The initial effects* (pp. 109–131). Newbury Park, CA: Sage.

Salzinger, S., Feldman, R. S., Hammer, M., & Rosario, M. (1993). The effects of physical abuse on children's social relationships. *Child Development, 64*, 169–187.

Salzinger, S., Feldman, R. S., Ng-Mak, D. S., Mojica, E., & Stockhammer, T. F. (2001). The effect of physical abuse on children's social and affective status: A model of cognitive and behavioral processes explaining the association. *Development and Psychopathology, 13*, 805–825.

Sandler, J., Kennedy, H., & Tyson, R L. (1980). *The technique of child psychoanalysis—Discussions with Anna Freud*. Cambridge, MA: Harvard University Press.

Saunders, B. E., Berliner, L., & Hanson, R. F. (Eds.). (2004). *Child physical and sexual abuse: Guidelines for treatment (Revised Report: April 26, 2004)*. Charleston, SC: National Crime Victims Research and Treatment Center.

Sauzier, M., Salt, P., & Calhoun, R. (1990). The effects of child sexual abuse. In B. Gomes-Schwartz, J. M. Horowits, & A. P. Cardarelli (Eds.), *Child sexual abuse: The initial effects* (pp. 75–108), Newbury Park, CA: Sage.

Schofield, G., & Beek, M. (2005). Providing a secure base: Parenting children in long-term foster family care. *Attachment and Human Development, 7*, 3–25.

Schowalter, J. E. (1985). Counter-transference in work with children: Review of a neglected concept. *Journal of the American Academy of Child Psychiatry, 25*, 40–45.

Schutz, B. M., Dixon, E. B., Lindenberger, N. J., & Ruther, N. J. (1989). *Solomon's sword*. San Francisco: Jossey-Bass.

Schwartz, J. M., Stoessel, P. W., Baxter, L. R., Jr., Martin, K. M., & Phelps, M. E. (1996). Systematic changes in cerebral glucose metabolic rate after successful behavior modification treatment of obsessive–compulsive disorder. *Archives of General Psychiatry, 53*, 109–113.

Scully, L. (Writer/Director). (1992). *Good things can still happen* [Video]. Montreal: National Film Board of Canada.

Shelby, J. S., & Felix, E. (2005). Posttraumatic play therapy: The need for an integrated model of directive and nondirective approaches. In L. A. Reddy, T. M. Files-Hall, & C. E. Schaefer (Eds.), *Empirically based play intervention for children* (pp. 79–103). Washington, DC: American Psychological Association.

Shields, A. M., Cicchetti, D., & Ryan, R M. (1994). The development of emotional and behavioral self-regulation and social competence among maltreated school-age children. *Development and Psychopathology, 6*, 57–76.

Shirk, S. R. (1998). Interpersonal schemata in child psychotherapy: A cognitive-interpersonal perspective. *Journal of Clinical Child Psychology, 27* 4–16.

Shirk, S. R., & Karver, M. (2003). Prediction of treatment outcome from relationship variables in child and adolescent therapy: A meta-analytic review. *Journal of Consulting and Clinical Psychology, 71*, 452–464.

Shirk, S. R., & Russell, R. L. (1996). *Change processes in child psychotherapy: Revitalizing treatment and research*. New York: Guilford Press.

Shirk, S. R., & Saiz, C. C. (1992). Clinical, empirical, and developmental perspectives on the therapeutic relationship in child psychotherapy. *Development and Psychopathology, 4*, 713–728.

Shouldice, A., & Stevenson-Hinde, J. (1992). Coping with security distress: The Separation Anxiety Test and attachment classification at 4.5 years. *Journal of Child Psychology and Psychiatry, 33*, 331–348.

Silberg, J. (1996). *The dissociative child: Diagnosis, treatment, and management.* Baltimore: Sidran.

Silberg, J. (2000). Fifteen years of dissociation in maltreated children: Where do we go from here? *Child Maltreatment, 5*, 119–136.

Silovsky, J. F., & Niec, L. (2002). Characteristics of young children with sexual behavior problems: A pilot study. *Child Maltreatment, 7*, 187–197.

Silverman, W. K., & Nelles, W. B. (1988). The Anxiety Disorders Interview Schedule for Children. *Journal of the American Academy of Child and Adolescent Psychiatry, 27*, 772–778.

Slade, A. (2004). The move from categories to process: Attachment phenomena and clinical evaluation. *Infant Mental Health Journal, 25*, 269–283.

Smith, J. D., Walsh, R T., & Richardson, M. A. (1985). The Clown Club: A structured fantasy approach to group therapy with the latency-age child. *International Journal of Group Psychotherapy, 35*, 49–64.

Smyke, A. T., Dumitrescu, A., & Zeanah, C. H. (2002). Attachment disturbances in young children. I: The continuum of caretaking casualty. *Journal of the American Academy of Child and Adolescent Psychiatry, 41*, 972–982.

Solomon, J., & George, C. (1999). The measurement of attachment security in infancy and childhood. In J. Cassidy & P. R. Shaver (Eds.), *Handbook of attachment: Theory, research, and clinical applications* (pp. 287–316). New York: Guilford Press.

Solomon, J., George, C., & De Jong, A. (1995). Children classified as controlling at age six: Evidence of disorganized representational strategies and aggression at home and at school. *Development and Psychopathology, 7*, 447–463.

Southam-Gerow, M., & Kendall, P. C. (1996). Long-term follow-up of cognitive behavioral therapy for anxiety disordered youth. *Journal of Consulting and Clinical Psychology, 64*, 724–730.

Spaccarelli, S., & Kim, S. (1995). Resilience criteria and factors associated with resilience in sexually abused girls. *Child Abuse and Neglect, 19*, 1171–1182.

Sparrow, S., Balla, D., & Cicchetti, D. (2005). *Vineland Adaptive Behavior Scales–2.* Circle Pines, MN: American Guidance Service.

Spielberger, C. D. (1973). *State–Trait Anxiety Inventory for Children.* Palo Alto, CA: Consulting Psychologists Press.

Spitz, R. (1945). Hospitalism: An inquiry into the genesis of psychiatric conditions in early childhood. *Psychoanalytic Study of the Child, 1*, 53–74.

Spitz, R. (1946). Anaclitic depression. *Psychoanalytic Study of the Child, 2*, 313–342.

Spivak, G., Platt, J. J., & Shure, M. B. (1976). *The problem-solving approach to adjustment.* San Francisco: Jossey-Bass.

Sroufe, L. A. (1979). The coherence of individual development: Early care, attachment, and subsequent developmental issues. *American Psychologist, 34*, 834–841.

Sroufe, L. A. (1983). Infant–caregiver attachment and patterns of adaptation in preschool: The roots of maladaptation and competence. In *Minnesota Symposium in Child Psychology* (Vol. 16, pp. 41–83). Hillsdale, NJ: Erlbaum.

Sroufe, L. A. (1988). The role of infant–caregiver attachment in development. In J. Belsky & T. Nezworski (Eds.), *Clinical implications of attachment* (pp. 18–38). Hillsdale, NJ: Erlbaum.

Sroufe, L. A., Carlson, E. A., Levy, A. K., & Egeland, B. (1999). Implications of attachment theory for developmental psychopathology. *Development and Psychopathology, 11*, 1–13.

Sroufe, L. A., & Fleeson, J. (1986). Attachment and the construction of relationships. In W. Hartup & Z. Rubin (Eds.), *Relationships and development* (pp. 51–71). Hillsdale, NJ: Erlbaum.

Sroufe, L. A., & Rutter, M. (1984). The domain of developmental psychopathology. *Child Development, 55*, 17–29.

Stauffer, L. B., & Deblinger, E. (1996). Cognitive behavioral groups for nonoffending mothers and their young sexually abused children: A preliminary treatment outcome study. *Child Maltreatment, 1*, 65–76.

Steele, B. F., & Pollock, C. B. (1968). A psychiatric study of parents who abuse infants and small children. In C. H. Kempe & R. E. Heifer (Eds.), *The battered child* (pp. 103–147). Chicago: University of Chicago Press.

Stern, J. B., & Fodor, I. G. (1989). Anger control in children: A review of social skills and cognitive behavioral approaches to dealing with aggressive children. *Child and Family Behavior Therapy, 11*, 1–20.

Steward, M. S., Bussey, K., Goodman, G. S., & Saywitz, K. J. (1993). Implications of developmental research for interviewing children. *Child Abuse and Neglect, 17*, 25–38.

Stovall, G., & Craig, R. J. (1990). Mental representations of physically and sexually abused latency-aged females. *Child Abuse and Neglect, 14*, 233–242.

Streissguth, A. P. (1997). *Fetal alcohol syndrome: A guide for families and communities*. Baltimore: Paul H. Brookes.

Suess, G. J., Grossmann, K. E., & Sroufe, L. A. (1992). Effects of infant attachment to mother and father on quality of adaptation in preschool: From dyadic to individual organization of self. *International Journal of Behavioral Development, 15*, 43–66.

Swenson, C. C., Brown, E. J., & Sheidow, A. J. (2003). Medical, legal, and mental health service utilization by physically abused children and their caregivers. *Child Maltreatment, 8*, 138–144.

Target, M., Shmueli-Goetz, Y, & Fonagy, P. (2002). Attachment representations in school-age children: The early development of the Child Attachment Interview (CAI). *Journal of Child and Adolescent Psychotherapy, 2*, 91–105.

Task Force on Promotion and Dissemination of Psychological Procedures. (1995). Training in and dissemination of empirically-validated psychological treatments. *The Clinical Psychologist, 48*, 3–23.

Terr, L. C. (1990). *Too scared to cry.* New York: Harper & Row.

Terr, L. C. (1991). Childhood traumas: An outline and overview. *American Journal of Psychiatry, 148*, 10–20.

Thompson, R. A. (1999). Early attachment and later development. In J. Cassidy & P.

R. Shaver (Eds.), *Handbook of attachment: Theory, research, and clinical applications* (pp. 265–286). New York: Guilford Press.

Thompson, R. A., Briggs, E., English, D. J., Dubowitz, H., Lee, L. C., Brody, K., et al. (2005). Suicidal ideation among 8-year-olds who are maltreated and at risk: Findings from the LONGSCAN studies. *Child Maltreatment, 10*, 26–36.

Thompson, R. A., & Nelson, C. A. (2001). Developmental science and the media: Early brain development. *American Psychologist, 56*, 5–15.

Thorsteinsson, E. B., James, J. E., & Gregg, M. E. (1998). Effects of video-relayed social support on hemodynamic reactivity and salivary cortisol during laboratory-based behavioral challenge. *Health Psychology, 17*, 436–444.

Timmer, S. G., Urquiza, A. J., Zebell, N. M., & McGrath, J. M. (2005). Parent–child interaction therapy: Application to maltreating parent–child dyads. *Child Abuse and Neglect, 29*, 825–842.

Timmons-Mitchell, J., Chandler-Holtz, D., & Semple, W. E. (1996). Post-traumatic stress symptoms in mothers following children's reports of sexual abuse. *American Journal of Orthopsychiatry, 66*, 463–467.

Timmons-Mitchell, J., Chandler-Holtz, D., & Semple, W. E. (1997). Post-traumatic stress disorder symptoms in child sexual abuse victims and their mothers. *Journal of Child Sexual Abuse, 6*, 1–14.

Tong, L., Gates, K., & McDowell, M. (1987). Personality development following sexual abuse. *Child Abuse and Neglect, 11*, 371–383.

Toth, S. L., Cicchetti, D., MacFie, J., & Emde, R. N. (1997). Representations of self and other in the narratives of neglected, physically abused, and sexually abused preschoolers. *Development and Psychopathology, 9*, 781–796.

Tremblay, C., Hebert, M., & Piché, C. (1999). Coping strategies and social support as mediators of consequences in child sexual abuse victims. *Child Abuse and Neglect, 23*, 929–945.

Trickett, P. K., McBride-Chang, C., & Putnam, F. W. (1994). The classroom performance and behavior of sexually abused females. *Development and Psychopathology, 6*, 183–194.

Troy, M., & Sroufe, L. A. (1987). Victimization among preschoolers: The role of attachment relationship history. *Journal of the American Academy of Child and Adolescent Psychiatry, 26*, 166–172.

Trupin, E., Tarico, V., Low, B., Jemelka, R., & McClellan, J. (1993). Children on child protective service caseloads: Prevalence and nature of serious emotional disturbance. *Child Abuse and Neglect, 17*, 345–355.

Tuft's New England Medical Center, Division of Psychiatry. (1984). *Sexually exploited children: Service and research project: Final report for the Office of Juvenile Justice and Delinquency Prevention*. Washington, DC: U. S. Department of Justice.

Tutty, L. (1994). Developmental issues in young children's learning of sexual abuse prevention concepts. *Child Abuse and Neglect, 18*, 179–192.

Urquiza, A. J., & Winn, C. (1994). *Treatment far abused and neglected children: Infancy to age 18*. Washington, DC: U. S. Department of Health and Human Services Administration for Children and Families.

Valle, L. A., & Silovsky, J. F. (2002). Attributions and adjustment following child sexual and physical abuse. *Child Maltreatment, 7*, 9–25.

Van de Putte, S. J. (1995). A paradigm for working with child survivors of sexual abuse who exhibit sexualized behaviors during play therapy. *International Journal of Play Therapy, 4*, 27–49.

van IJzendoorn, M. H., Schuengel, C., & Bakermans-Kranenburg, M. J. (1999). Disorganized attachment in early childhood: Meta-analysis of precursors, concomitants, and sequelae. *Development and Psychopathology, 11*, 225–249.

Vissing, Y. M., Straus, M. A., Gelles, R. J., & Harrop, J. W. (1991). Verbal aggression by parents and psychosocial problems of children. *Child Abuse and Neglect, 15*, 223–238.

Vondra, J., Barnett, D., & Cicchetti, D. (1990). Self-concept, motivation, and competence among preschoolers from maltreating and comparison families. *Child Abuse and Neglect, 14*, 525–540.

Wachtel, P. L. (1973). *Psychoanalysis and behavior therapy: Toward an integration.* New York: Basic Books.

Wallach, H., & Dollinger, S. (1999). Dissociative disorders in childhood and adolescence. In S. Netherton, D. Holmes, & C. Walker (Eds.), *Child and adolescent psychological disorders* (pp. 344–366). New York: Oxford University Press.

Wampold, B. E. (2001). *The great psychotherapy debate: Model, methods, and findings*. Mahwah, NJ: Erlbaum.

Wampold, B. E., & Bhati, K. S. (2004). Attending to omissions: A historical examination of evidence-based practice movements. *Professional Psychology: Research and Practice, 35*, 563–570.

Weaver, T. L., & Clum, G. A. (1995). Psychological distress associated with interpersonal violence: A meta-analysis. *Clinical Psychology Review, 15*, 115–140.

Wechsler, D. (2003). *WISC-IV manual.* San Antonio, TX: Psychological Corporation.

Werner, E. E. (1989). High risk children in young adulthood: A longitudinal study from birth to 32 years. *American Journal of Orthopsychiatry, 59*, 72–81.

Werner, E. E. (1993). Risk, resilience, and recovery: Perspectives from the Kauai Longitudinal Study. *Development and Psychopathology, 5*, 503–515.

Westen, D., Novotny, C. M., & Thompson-Brenner, H. (2004). The empirical status of empirically supported psychotherapies: Assumptions, findings, and reporting in controlled clinical trials. *Psychological Bulletin, 130*, 631–663.

Widom, C. S. (1999). Posttraumatic stress disorder in abused and neglected children grown up. *American Journal of Psychiatry, 156*, 1223–1229.

Widom, C. S., & Maxfield, M. G. (2001). *An update on the "cycle of violence"* (NCJ 184894). Washington, DC: National Institute of Justice.

Wieckowski, E., Hartsoe, P., Mayer, A., & Shortz, J. (1998). Deviant sexual behavior in children and young adolescents: Frequency and patterns. *Sexual Abuse: A Journal of Research and Treatment, 10*, 293–303.

Wieland, S. (1997). *Hearing the internal trauma: Working with children and adolescents who have been sexually abused.* Thousand Oaks, CA: Sage.

Wilkinson, G. S. (1993). *The Wide Range Achievement Test–3: Administration manual.* Wilmington, DE: Wide Range.

Wilson, T. (2002). *Strangers to ourselves: Discovering the adaptive unconscious.* Cambridge, MA: Harvard University Press.

Winnicott, D. (1965). *The family and individual development.* London: Tavistock.

Wolfe, D. A. (1988). Child abuse and neglect. In E. J. Mash & L. G. Terdal (Eds.), *Be-*

havioral assessment of childhood disorders (2nd ed., pp. 627–669). New York: Guilford Press.

Wolfe, D. A., Sas, L., & Wekerle, C. (1994). Factors associated with the development of posttraumatic stress disorder among child victims of sexual abuse. *Child Abuse and Neglect, 18*, 37–50.

Wolfe, V. V., Gentile, C., Michienzi, T., Sas, L., & Wolfe, D. A. (1991). The Children's Impact of Traumatic Events Scale: A measure of post-sexual-abuse PTSD symptoms. *Behavioral Assessment, 13*, 359–383.

Wolfe, V. V., Gentile, C., & Wolfe, D. A. (1989). The impact of sexual abuse on children: A PTSD formulation. *Behavior Therapy, 20*, 215–228.

Wolfe, V. V., & Wolfe, D. A. (1988). The sexually abused child. In E. J. Mash & L. G. Terdal (Eds.), *Behavioral assessment of childhood disorders* (2nd ed., pp. 670–714). New York: Guilford Press.

Wright, J. D., Binney, V., & Smith, P. K. (1995). Security of attachment in 8–12 year-olds: A revised version of the Separation Anxiety Test, its psychometric properties and clinical interpretation. *Journal of Child Psychology and Psychiatry, 36*, 757–774.

Yates, T. M., Dodds, M. F., Sroufe, L. A., & Egeland, B. (2003). Exposure to partner violence and child behavior problems: A prospective study controlling for child physical abuse and neglect, child cognitive ability, socioeconomic status, and life stress. *Development and Psychopathology, 15*, 199–218.

Yeager, C. A., & Lewis, D. O. (1996). The intergenerational transmission of violence and dissociation. *Child and Adolescent Psychiatric Clinics of North America, 5*, 393–430.

Zeanah, C. H., Nelson, C. A., Fox, N. A., Smyke, A. T., Marshall, P., Parker, S. W., et al. (2003). Designing research to study the effects of institutionalization on brain and behavioral development: The Bucharest Early Intervention Project. *Development and Psychopathology, 15*, 885–907.

Zeanah, C. H., Scheeringa, M., Boris, N. W., Heller, S. S., Smyke, A. T., & Trapani, J. (2004). Reactive attachment disorder in maltreated toddlers. *Child Abuse and Neglect, 28*, 877–888.

Zeanah, C. H., Smyke, A. T., & Dumitrescu, A. (2002). Attachment disturbances in young children. II. Indiscriminate behavior and institutional care. *Journal of the American Academy of Child and Adolescent Psychiatry, 41*, 983–989.

Index

Page numbers followed by *f* indicate figure; *t* indicate table

B

C

V

W